Myelomeningocele

Grune & Stratton Rapid Manuscript Reproduction

Proceedings of a Multidisciplinary Symposium
University of Cincinnati, Cincinnati, Ohio
March 11–13, 1976

MYELOMENINGOCELE

Edited by

Robert L. McLaurin, M.D.

Section Editors

Sonya Oppenheimer, M.D.
Robert L. McLaurin, M.D.
Richard A. Jolson, M.D.
Pramod R. Rege, M.D.

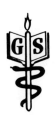

Grune & Stratton
A Subsidiary of Harcourt Brace Jovanovich, Publishers
New York   San Francisco   London

Grune & Stratton, Inc.
111 Fifth Avenue
New York, New York 10003

Distributed in the United Kingdom by
Academic Press, Inc. (London) Ltd.
24/28 Oval Road, London NW 1

Library of Congress Catalog Number 77-80637
International Standard Book Number 0-8089-1001-9

Printed in the United States of America

CONTENTS

FOREWORD

A multidisciplinary symposium dealing with spinal dysraphism and related problems was held at the University of Cincinnati, March 11–13, 1976. The symposium was conceived and organized by the Cincinnati Myelomeningocele Team which functions as a unit of the University-affiliated Cincinnati Center for Developmental Disorders. The team was organized in 1964 to give centralized and consistent care to children with spinal dysraphism and related disorders. The multidisciplinary team approach has been involved in each stage of the child's development. Team members have included a pediatrician, neurosurgeon, urologist, orthopedist, orthotist, occupational and physical therapist, nutritionist, clinical nursing specialist, social worker, psychologist, and special educator.

The symposium was designed to stimulate communication and discussion within specialty groups concerned with myelodysplasia as well as between the specialties. In addition the symposium was held concurrently with the annual meeting of the Spina Bifida Association of America, permitting interchange between this parents' organization and the professional participants.

The members of the Cincinnati myelomeningocele team have edited the following proceedings in the hope that they will document the present "state of the art" and stimulate further interest and progress in the care of myelodysplastic children.

Robert L. McLaurin, M.D.

Part I
GENERAL CONSIDERATIONS

Participants

Mary Anne Barry, A.C.S.W.
Northwestern University, Chicago, Illinois

Abby S. Cutright, R.N., M.S.N.
University of Cincinnati, Cincinnati, Ohio

W. James Gardner, M.D.
Cleveland Clinic Foundation, Cleveland, Ohio

Leonard Harris, M.D.
University of Cincinnati, Cincinnati, Ohio

Linda Custis Land, M.S.
Columbus, Ohio

Eva Nakos, L.P.T.
Children's Hospital Medical Center, Cincinnati, Ohio

Sonya Oppenheimer, M.D.
University of Cincinnati, Cincinnati, Ohio

Susan Taylor, O.T.R.
Children's Hospital Medical Center, Cincinnati, Ohio

Josef Warkany, M.D.
University of Cincinnati, Cincinnati, Ohio

ETIOLOGY AND PATHOGENESIS OF THE
DEVELOPMENT OF MYELOMENINGOCELE

W. James Gardner, M.D.

In medicine it is an accepted principle that a theory
which attributes a single cause to a disease process is more
likely to prove correct than one which implicates several.
Further, that there is no more effective way to stifle
thinking concerning a disease process than to apply to it
some misleading title such as "dysraphia". Whereas
"araphia", meaning nonclosure of the neural tube, may
constitute an anatomic entity, "dysraphia" implying faulty
closure is purely hypothetical. The theory has been
advanced that all dysraphic states with their accompanying
distortions and adhesions to surrounding non-neural
structures may be explained on the basis of a single factor-,
over-distention of the neural tube resulting from inadequate
passage of cerebrospinal fluid at varying stages of embryonal
and fetal development; that myelomeningocele, subsequently
referred to as myelocele, results from rupture of the neural
tube (myeloschisis) not from its failure to close. The
physiological expansion of the cerebrospinal fluid spaces,
beautifully described by Weed,[27] cannot be seen through the
microscope.

MYELOSCHISIS

The combination of hydrocephalus with myelocele indicates a causal relationship between these two abnormal collections of fluid. Two centuries ago Morgagni,[14] unencumbered with the knowledge that the sac of the myelocele consists of an open neural tube, naively concluded that these "watery tumors of the vertebrae" resulted from the pressure of fluid descending from the hydrocephalic head through the tube of the spine and pressing the bones asunder. More than a century later this hydrodynamic theory of Morgagni was discredited by von Recklinghausen.[17] (See footnote.) Because his microscope revealed an open portion of the neural tube in the wall of the sac, he stated that it was the result of failure of the neural tube to close. Since then his belief has been confirmed repeatedly, albeit by investigators who based their studies upon this idea. This theory may be correct in some instances. However, it does not explain how a neural tube that fails to close can become overdistended, as is the case in most of the dysraphic states. For this reason alone, Morgagni's disruption hypothesis surely merits reconsideration. Furthermore, his theory will explain every single feature of the distorted anatomy; not only in the case of the myelocele and its associated hindbrain hernia, but also of related malformations ranging from syringomyelia of adulthood, to diastematomyelia of adolescence, to congenital hydrocephalus, to meningocele, to encephalocele, and finally to anencephalus of the stillborn.[7] One cannot understand these instances of abnormal development of the cerebrospinal fluid (CSF) spaces without a knowledge of their normal

"...in every...art fundamental matters are perennially being discovered, discredited, forgotten, rediscovered and reaffirmed." (A Textbook of Surgery, John Homans, C.C. Thomas, Springfield, Illinois, 1936).

development which was so beautifully described by Weed[27] in
1917.   Aside from its embryonal outpouchings, the eye and
the internal ear, the CNS is the only organ with such a
third circulation.   These outpouchings also are subject to
disturbances of their third circulations.   The hydrodynamic
stresses, imparted by the cerebrospinal fluid on the
developing CNS, cannot be seen through the microscope.

THE HYDRODYNAMIC MECHANISM

     The central nervous system originates as an elongated,
multilayered area of ectodermal cells which form a groove
that progressively deepens and finally closes to constitute
a tube which has no outlets.   Fluid is then secreted into
this tube causing it to distend throughout its length
(hydrocephalomyelia).   This intraluminal fluid must establish
its own means of returning to the circulation.   This it
accomplishes by dissecting a false (i.e. unlined by its
epithelium) passage way through the surrounding mesenchyme.
With this dissection the internal hydromyelia becomes
external (Fig. 1).   It is not surprising that this factitious
method of fluid escape sometimes proves inadequate.

     In 1958 Warkany et al[19] produced myelocele in rat
embryos by treating the maternal rat with trypan blue.   They
found that occult spina bifida, meningocele, syringomyelia
and myelocele may be present at different levels in the same
animal.   Their embryos of less than 18 days with an open
neural tube (myeloschisis), had no Arnold Chiari malformation,
whereas all of more than 21 days had the malformation.   This
finding supports Chiari's belief that the hindbrain hernia
develops as the cerebellum grows.   None of the rats with
myeloschisis had hydrocephalus while many litter mates
without myeloschisis did have hydrocephalus.   The authors

failed to consider the possibility that these litter mates
may have started out with the same defect and that hydrocephalus developed only in those in which excess fluid could
not escape because the neural tube had not ruptured.

Dorcas Padget[15] became converted to the rupture theory[6]
by her fortuitous discovery of a monkey embryo which had an
extensive reopening of the previously closed roof plate of
the neural tube. This rupture was covered by a fluid filled
subcutaneous bleb extending from head to tail (Fig. 2).
Only in one small area between the leg buds had the single
cell layer of cutaneous ectoderm ruptured into the amniotic
sac. Since closure of cutaneous ectoderm can occur *only* as
a result of closure of neuroectoderm, this neural tube had
certainly closed with subsequent overdistention and rupture
of its roof plate allowing CSF to infiltrate mesenchyme and
to be extruded beneath the largely intact layer of overlying
cutaneous ectoderm to form a bleb. It is obvious that this
thin covering of skin ectoderm, deprived of its supporting
mesoderm, would soon have parted throughout its entire
length to produce the so-called craniorachischisis totalis.
The duration of such a bleb stage may be only a matter of
seconds which would explain the extreme rarity of its
discovery. The underlying mesenchymal changes have been
referred to as somite necrosis.[12]

In her continuing studies of the marvelous collection
of human embryos at the Carnegie Institution in Washington,
Padget,[15] found that encephaloschisis, the forerunner of
exencephalus and anencephalus, occurs posterior to a closed
anterior neuropore and, therefore, could not be the result
of its failure to close. Her studies also established that
opening of the caudal end of the neural tube, resulted from

rupture (myeloschisis) not from failure of closure.
Browne,[1] through a window in the skull of a fertilized
chicken egg that had been treated by a teratogen, watched
the closed neural tube overdistend with consequent rupture
of the bulging mesencephalon (i.e. posterior to the closed
anterior neuropore). The mammalian teratologist is handicapped by his inability to actually see these events take
place. Browne explained the overdistention, which occurred
prior to the appearance of the choroid plexus, on the
progressive basis of an abnormal increase of the osmotic
tension of the neural tube fluid.

In each of the dysraphic states, except anencephalus,
not only is the central canal usually overdistended but the
same may be said of the bony canal. The bony distention in
these cases, beautifully illustrated by Feller and Sternberg[5]
(Fig. 3), has a form that can be explained only by overdistention of the neural tube during the precartilagenous
somite stage.[7]

It is an axiom in medicine that to obtain a proper
perspective of a disease process, one should begin with the
study of its early or mild stages and then progress to the
later and more severe. In congenital malformations as
compared with acquired diseases this sequence is reversed.
Here the severe forms, such as a swollen head, meningocele,
myelocele, and anencephaly are obvious at birth, whereas
the milder forms become symptomatic either in adolescence, as
in diastematomyelia, or in adult life as in syringomyelia.
By serendipity, it was established that the cause of syringomyelia is not in the spinal cord but in the malformed
hindbrain;[7] that fluid from the 4th ventricle enters and
distends the patent central canal to form a syrinx because

of a partial obstruction of the outlets of the 4th ventricle.
On account of this obstruction, the ventricular fluid pulse
wave is augmented and continues to be funneled into the
patent central canal with each arterial systole. Further
study has disclosed that the adult with syringomyelia may
have all of the anatomical abnormalities present in the
infant with myelocele except an open neural tube (Table 1).
Further, that most of these are probably present in the
adolescent with diastematomyelia, although there are few
opportunities to expose them. Naturally in these milder
forms of the dysraphic states, these abnormalities are less
severe, less frequent and more difficult to demonstrate.

THE FOUR STAGES OF HYDROMYELIA

     The results of overdistention of the spinal portion of
the neural tube may be arbitrarily divided into four progressive stages (Fig. 4). In stage I (Fig. 5A) the central
canal is only moderately overdistended but sufficiently so
that the surrounding mesenchyme is stretched, and the
bordering somites containing the precartilagenous sclerotomes
are mildly distorted and displaced laterally. Such overdistention may permit tethering of neuroepithelium to
cutaneous epithelium which may eventuate in a connecting
dermal sinus. If such a sinus becomes pinched off by
invading mesoderm, it may result in an isolated epidermoid
attached to the posterior surface of the cord. If the
rhombic roof then becomes adequately permeable, the subarachnoid space will be dissected open although the prior spread-
ing of the bordering sclerotomes may result in a dilated and
perhaps bifid spinal canal. If the dissection of the
subarachnoid space is delayed, some degree of internal
hydromyelia may persist to constitute the forerunner of

syringomyelia. If the delayed dissection of the subarachnoid
space becomes adequate, the internal hydromyelia may be
completely replaced by an overlarge subarachnoid space
enclosed within a bony canal which is also enlarged, because
it had been overdistended during its precartilagenous stage.
During the stage of internal hydromyelia, the tip of the
conus pressing caudally may become tethered to mesoderm
resulting in an intraspinal lipoma (Fig. 5B). The sclerotomes, displaced laterally during this stage, may fail to
close posteriorly resulting either in occult spina bifida or
in a posteriorly bulging meningocele. The latter constitutes
an extraspinal diverticulum of the external hydromyelia.
Since the subarachnoid fluid is still confined by mesodermal
tissue reinforced by overlying skin, the hydrodynamic
dissection of the subarachnoid space continues, and the
arachnoid villi become adequately permeable. This stage of
hydrocephalomyelia usually becomes completely compensated,
though at a later stage than in the normal. This compensation explains why the surgical removal of the sac of a
meningocele is seldom followed by recurrence of hydrocephalus.

If the obstructive phase becomes compensated sufficiently
early, the newborn may appear normal with perhaps an
enlargement of the head so slight that it is overlooked.
However, a sphere 12 cm in diameter weighs 73% more than one
of 10 cm. The human spine was not designed to be carried
vertically, but since fond mothers like to brag about how
early Johnny sat up, the base of the large thin skull may be
pushed in. The resulting basilar impression, unrecognizable
until adulthood, therefore is not congenital but acquired.[8]
Because of distorted sclerotomes, scoliosis may become
obvious in adolescence and symptoms of syringomyelia may
appear in adulthood. Pneumoencephalography will disclose

the congenital hindbrain hernia.

Even the smallest degree of overdistention of the
embryonic central canal will cause it to push caudally. In
some adult patients with syringomyelia, the conus is not
only located abnormally low, indicating some degree of
tethering, but the central canal, which normally terminates
at the tip of the conus, has been found to protrude into the
filum terminale for its entire length.[10] Some patients whose
symptoms of syringomyelia develop in adulthood, will have a
history of operation for sacral meningocele in infancy that
disclosed tethering of the conus or cauda equina to a lipoma
within the dilated and bifid sacral canal.[7]

Stage 2. During the obstructive phase, if the overdistention is somewhat more severe (Fig. 6A), the thick
lateral neural plates may be pressed so far laterally that
separation of the thin roof and floor plates (A,B) of the
hydromyelic cord occurs (combined anterior and posterior
internal myeloschisis). The disconnnected lateral plates
then will close independently to form two separate hemicords.
Such closure results from the tendency for epithelium to
grow until it meets epithelium. As the internal hydromyelia
becomes external, the two hemicords may be contained in an
enlarged subarachnoid space within a dilated spinal canal
(C) or each may develop its own dural sac (D). During the
phase of external hydromyelia, the fetus may or may not
develop a meningocele, which constitutes an extra spinal
protrusion of the external hydromyelia (E). In adolescence
he may or may not develop symptoms of diastematomyelia. One
hemicord may become so overdistended that it protrudes
externally as a syringomyelocele; an extraspinal protrusion
of an internal hydromyelia (F). The spine is usually
scoliotic, the bony canal will be locally widened, shortened

and the bodies may be fused to constitute a Klippel-Feil
syndrome at the involved level. A midline bony spur usually
develops because of the tendency for precartilagenous
sclerotomes to surround neural tissue.[11] If the stretched
sclerotomes fail to come together both anteriorly and
posteriorly the result will be combined anterior and posterior spinal bifida occulta (bilateral hemivertebrae). The
anterior gap may have permitted adhesion between the floor
plate of the neural tube and the primitive gut. With the
subsequent interposition of mesoderm, this previous tethering
of gut to spinal cord may result in an elongated stalk
connecting gut to cord. This stalk may or may not contain
gut elements but entodermal cells adhering to the anterior
aspect of the spinal cord may persist to form an enterogenous
cyst. Similarly, a prior posterior tethering to cutaneous
ectoderm may result in a dermal sinus or a dermoid attached
to the posterior surface of the cord which may be diastema-
tomyelic (Fig. 6C,D). If the split in the roof plate includes
the as yet undivided midline wedge of cells that constitute
the earliest evidence of the neural crest,[13] one or possibly
both hemicords, in addition to their set of normal nerve
roots, may present the rudiments of a second set. This has
been responsible for the suggestion that the spinal cord has
doubled, thus the term diplomyelia.

Though seldom sought, Doran and Guthkelch[4] demonstrated
8 instances of diastematomyelia at operation in a series of
197 cases of meningocele. In diastematomyelia as in
meningocele, pneumoencephalography has shown a picture
similar to that of syringomyelia, namely, a lack of ventricular filling and the shadow of a congenital hindbrain
hernia in the cisterna magna.[7] The spinal cord at and above
the two hemicords may remain hydromyelic although, because

of postmortem shrinkage, the pathologist may consider the
central canal to be of normal size. Rarely, the degree of
internal hydromyelia is so severe that it protrudes externally
 in the form of a syringomyelocele, which constitutes the
extra spinal protrusion of an internal hydromyelia. In one
such case there were two extra spinal protrusions, a meningocele and below it a diastematomyelia of which the enormously
distended right hemicord protruded in the form of syringomyelocele[7] (Fig. 6E). This patient therefore had both an
extra spinal protrusion of an external hydromyelia as well
as an extra spinal protrusion of an internal hydromyelia
that involved one hemicord. In diastematomyelia, one hemicord is always larger, suggesting that its central canal is
more distended.

Stage 3. If the obstructive phase of hydromyelia is
still more severe (Fig. 7A) the roof plate of the neural tube
will rupture through cutaneous ectoderm into the amniotic sac
to constitute external myeloschisis, the forerunner of myelocele. As the rhombic roof becomes permeable a belated and
inadequate dissection of the subarachnoid space begins. When
this hydrodissection reaches the site of the myeloschisis,
the ruptured neural tube is turned inside out by the pressure
of the subarachnoid fluid and is extruded to form a myelocele.
The latter in turn may rupture permitting the escape of CSF,
in which case the infant may be born microcephalic, although
roentgenography will disclose craniolacunia, the result of
embryonal hydrocephalus.[9] The spinal cord above the
myeloschisis remains hydromyelic and below this there
frequently is diastematomyelia, and the lateral plates in
their unclosed state, may continue into the myelocele[2] to
constitute diastematomyelia aperta (Fig. 7B). The occult
diastematomyelia and hydromyelia which are present cephalad

to the myelocele cannot be explained by failure of closure
of the neural tube. In myelocele the bony canal is short,
wide, bifid and the bodies may be fused to constitute a
Klippel-Feil syndrome at this level (Fig. 7C). There is a
severe hindbrain hernia and the hydrocephalus seldom becomes
compensated because, on account of the rupture, there was
inadequate dissecting pressure in the subarachnoid space at
the time when its complete dissection should have occurred.
Since the central canal is kinked off by the severe caudal
displacement and subsequent telescoping at the cervicomedullary junction, the existing internal hydromyelia[2] does
not progress.

If rupture of the neural tube occurs at the level of the
bulging mesencephalon, the result is encephaloschisis, the
forerunner of anencephalus. In this case the intraluminal
pressure is immediately and permanently lost, the dissection
of the subarachnoid space, if started prior to rupture,
cannot continue and the normal cellular reproduction in the
spinal cord may close the central canal. In encephaloschisis
the exposed choroid plexus pumps its product directly into
the amniotic sac causing severe hydramnios. The anencephalic
cannot survive spontaneous delivery because the part of the
brain that remains is exposed to an amniotic pressure of
100 mmHg during labor contractions. If rupture of the roof
plate affects the entire length of the neural tube, the
result is craniorachischisis totalis.

Stage 4. During the obstructive phase, a localized
area of overdistention may be so severe as to result in
simultaneous rupture of the roof plate into the amniotic sac
and also rupture of the floor plate down to or even through
the wall of the primitive gut (Fig. 8A). This constitutes

anterior and posterior diastematomyelia aperta. In rare
instances, this lesion may heal to form a posterior enteric
fistula presenting between a divided spine containing a
divided hydromyelic cord[16] (Fig. 8B,C). In one such case[3]
in which there was an imperforate anus, the unruptured
enteric canal was herniated onto the back through the split
spine. In this case, the enlarged skull showed severe
craniolacunia, evidence of embryonal hydrocephalus[9] (Fig. 8D).

CONCLUSIONS

These four progressive stages of hydromyelia are
proposed because they offer a reasonable explanation for each
and all of the so-called dysraphic states. Furthermore, they
represent a morphologic continuum since stage 1 is present in
stage 2, both are present in stage 3 and the preceding three
stages in all probability are present in the rare stage 4.
The evidence indicates that they all result from a pathologic
degree of the physiologic hydrocephalomyelia that plays a
major part in the shaping of the embryo.

REFERENCES

1. Browne, J.M.: Normal and abnormal changes in cerebro-
    spinal fluid and their relation to morphogenesis of the
    chick brain (abstract). *Teratology, 3*:199, 1970.
2. Cameron, A.H.: Arnold-Chiari and other neuroanatomical
    malformations associated with spina bifida. *J. Path.
    Bact., 73*:195, 1957.
3. Denes, J., Honti, J., Leb, J.: Dorsal herniation of a
    gut: a rare manifestation of the split notochord syn-
    drome. *J. Pediat. Surg., 2*:359, 1967.

4. Doran, P.A. and Guthkelch, A.N.: Studies in spina bifida cystica. I. General survey and reassessment of problem. *J. Neurol. Neurosurg. Psychiat.*, *24*:331, 1961.

5. Feller, A. and Sternberg, H.: Zur Kenntnis der Fehlbildungen der Wirbelsaule; die anatomischen Grundlagen des Kurzhalses (Klippel-Feilschen Syndroms). *Virchows Arch. path. Anat.*, *285*:112, 1932.

6. Gardner, W.J.: Rupture of the neural tube. *Arch. Neurol.*, *4*:1, 1960.

7. Gardner, W.J.: The dysraphic states; from syringomyelia to anencephaly. IN Excerpta Medica, Amsterdam, 1973, pp. 201.

8. Gardner, W.J.: Anomalies of the craniovertebral junction. IN Neurological Surgery, Vol. I, J.R. Youmans, (ed.), Philadelphia, W.B. Saunders Co., 1973, pp. 628.

9. Gardner, W.J., Poolos, P.N., Jr.: Craniolacunia - The result of embryonal hydrocephalus? *Teratology*, *13*:189, 1976.

10. Gardner, W.J., Bell, H.S., Poolos, P.N., Jr., Dohn,D.F., and Steinberg, M.: Terminal ventriculostomy for syringomyelia. In preparation.

11. Holtzer, H.: Experimental analysis of development of spinal column. I. Response of precartilage cells to size variations of spinal cord. *J. Exp. Zool.*, *121*: 121, 1952.

12. Marin-Padilla, M., and Ferm, V.: Somite necrosis and developmental malformation induced by vitamin A in the golden hamster. *J. Embryol. Exper. Morph.*, *13*:1, 1965.

13. Marin-Padilla, M.: The closure of the neural tube in the golden hamster. *Teratology*, *3*:39, 1970.

14. Morgagni, J.B.: The seats and causes of diseases investigated by anatomy, 3 volumes, translated by

Benjamin Alexander, London, A. Millar and T. Cadell, Publishers, 1769.

15. Padget, D.H.: Development of so-called dysraphism: with embryologic evidence of clinical Arnold-Chiari and Dandy-Walker malformations. *Johns Hopkins Med. J., 130*: 127, 1972. Reproduced by permission of author and publisher.

16. Saunders, R.L. de C.H.: Combined anterior and posterior spina bifida in living neonatal human female. *Anat. Rec., 87*:255, 1943.

17. von Recklinghausen, E.: Untersuchungen uber die Spina bifida. *Arch. path. Anat., 105*:243, 1886.

18. Walker, W.E.: Dilatation of vertebral canal associated with congenital anomalies of spinal cord. *Amer. J. Roentgenol., 52*:571, 1944.

19. Warkany, J., Wilson, J.G. and Geiger, J.I.: Myeloschisis and myelomeningocele produced experimentally in the rat. *J. comp. Neurol., 109*:35, 1958.

TABLE 1.

Features Common to Myelomeningocele and Syringomyelia

Hindbrain hernia

Upward coursing nerve roots

Hydrocephalus

Hydromyelia

Failure perforation median foramen

Tethered conus

Glial cell rests in arachnoid

Dilated spinal canal

Scoliosis

Klippel-Feil fusion

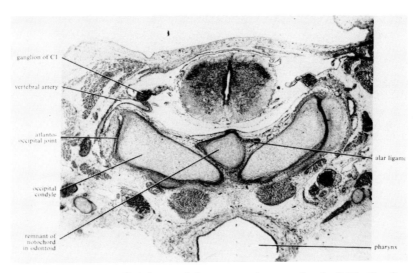

Fig. 1. Cross section of eight week human embryo at level of C1. The former internal hydromyelia has become external. (Reproduced from "Cervical Spondylosis" (1976) by Brain and Wilkinson by permission of authors and publisher, W.B. Saunders).

17

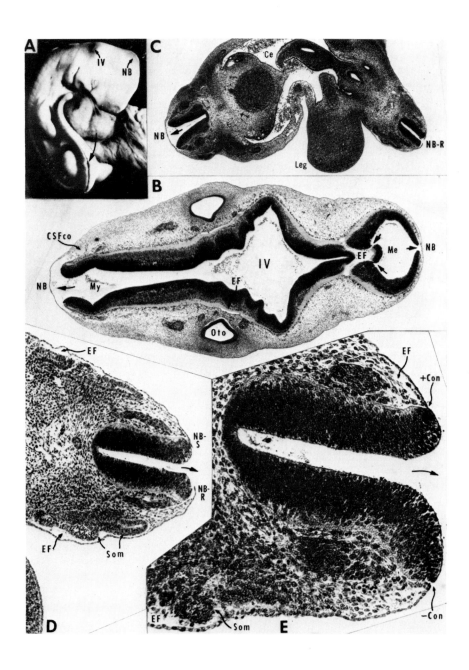

Fig. 2. (facing page). Padget's monkey embryo of 6.7 mm: A is oblique lateral view; B to E are progressively caudal transverse sections of 7.5μ, right side below in all. Abnormal body twist in A may be related to extravasated blood cells in coelom (CE). In A an elongated external opening (arrow) of neural tube between leg buds is surely abnormal, but not an unclosed neuropore. Just visible in front and behind rhombic cavity (IV) are neuroschistic blebs (NB). The findings in this embryo suggest that there is a common origin for spina bifida aperta, cystica and occulta, and their cranial counterparts.

Section B traverses normal rhombic neuromeres and 4 abnormal neural clefts (neuroschisis: large arrows). The two ventral clefts split open caudal end of the primitive midbrain (Me). The dorsal clefts produce neuroschistic blebs (NB), voluminous over the wide open medullary cleft (My). Bleb fluid invades mesenchyme on left side as marked by blood cells in ventricular coagulum (CSFco). This extraneous fluid (EF) courses lateroventrally around neural tube (arrow), is traversed by unbroken capillaries and borders right otocyst (Oto). The bleb continues over the normally closed neural tube in upper thorax, and then over the tube where it is again split open throughout lower trunk (to left in C).

Sections C to E, through the external opening in A, show its cause to be a rupture of the long bleb wall. Its bilateral remnants (NB-R) shown in C and D get progressively shorter before being secondarily attached (NB-S) either to the left neural margins, or to nearby mesenchyme as in E. Here the rounded edges of divided neural wall are slightly and asymmetrically everted. Within a few sections, remnants of ruptured bleb wall reappear, get progressively longer (to right in C) and reconstitute the bleb, which ends together with the dorsal neural cleft in the proximal portion of the tail. Note in D and E the separated cell nuclei in the neural cleft margins which are less everted on left; the secondary development of neural and cutaneous ectodermal continuity (+Con), also a lack of such true continuity (−Con); and the somite (Som) damage by extended bleb fluid (EF). (Reproduced by permission of author's literary executor and the publisher[15].)

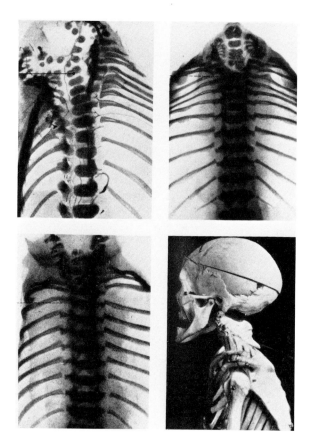

Fig. 3. The three radiographs are from stillborn infants with severe Klippel-Feil syndrome. The skeleton is from an adult with the same syndrome. This extreme enlargement of the bony canal can only result from overdistention of the neural tube in the precartilagenous somite stage. This skeletal syndrome may be present in the adult with syringomyelia and in the lumbar spine of the infant with myelocele. (Reproduced from Feller and Sternberg[5].)

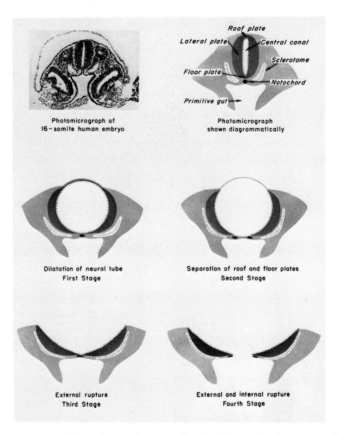

Photomicrograph of
16-somite human embryo

Photomicrograph
shown diagrammatically

Roof plate
Lateral plate
Central canal
Sclerotome
Floor plate
Notochord
Primitive gut

Dilatation of neural tube
First Stage

Separation of roof and floor plates
Second Stage

External rupture
Third Stage

External and internal rupture
Fourth Stage

Fig. 4. The photomicrograph of a 16 somite human embryo is reproduced diagrammatically. The central canal remains a sagittal slit prior to closure of the neuropores. Note that the roof and floor plates are much thinner than the lateral plates and therefore less able to tolerate overdistension. The onset of each of four stages that occur shortly after closure are represented. In stage one the overdistension becomes compensated prior to rupture. In stage two the roof and floor plates have ruptured internally. In stage three the roof plate has ruptured externally. In stage four both roof and floor plates have ruptured.

Fig. 5A. Stage 1.

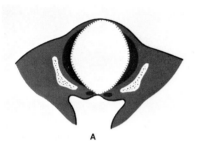

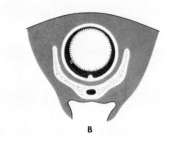

A. As the formerly slit-like neural tube begins to expand, mesoderm inserts itself between cutaneous ectoderm and neuroectoderm.

B. The central canal has overdistended, but the subarachnoid space is beginning to be dissected open despite the pathologic degree of internal hydromyelia.

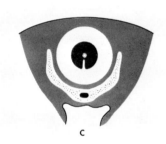

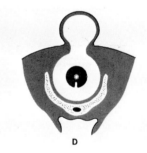

C. The internal hydromyelia has become compensated leaving an abnormally large subarachnoid space (external hydromyelia).

D. The meningocele is an extraspinal protrusion of an external hydromyelia.

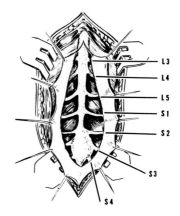

Fig. 5B. The conus is tethered to a lipoma within a dilated subarachnoid space contained within a dilated spinal canal. (Reproduced from Walker[15]).

Fig. 6A. Stage 2.

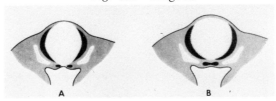

A, B. Splitting of roof and floor plates prior to dissection of the subarachnoid space. The split may or may not include notochord.

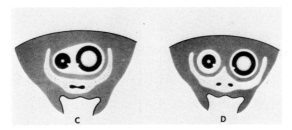

C, D. Each hemicord has closed and the subarachnoid space has been dissected open.

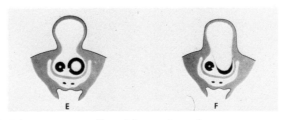

E. Diastematomyelia with menigocele.
F. Diastematomyelia with syringomyelocele of one hemicord.

Fig. 6B. Diastematomyelia within
a dilated subarachnoid space.
(Reproduced from Walker[15]). This
cord was tethered at the sacral level.
During the phase of internal
hydromyelia that caused the
splitting, the sclerotomes had been
spread producing a wide bony canal.

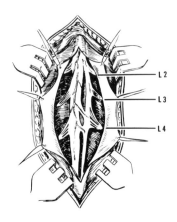

L 2

L 3

L 4

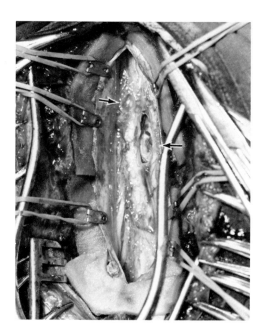

Fig. 6C. Diastematomyelia. The larger size of the left
hemicord is probably the result of a dilated central
canal. The upper arrow indicates an epidermoid, the
lower the midline bony spur.

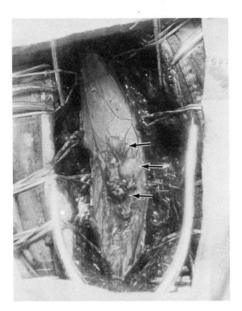

Fig. 6D. Diastematomyelia. The very severe hydromyelia above the split also involved the right hemicord. The upper arrow indicates a dermoid, the middle a lipoma, the lower the bony spur.

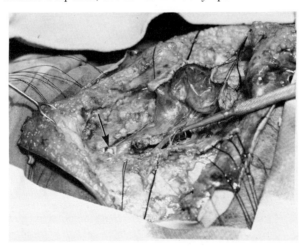

Fig. 6E. This surgical exposure shows a combination of E and F as shown in Fig. 6A. The small left hemicord is elevated on a spatula whose tip is in contact with the bony spur. Arrow indicates location of the severed stalk of the removed meningocele. The enormously distended right hemicord has been extruded extraspinally to form a syringomyelocele. Its thin covering of skin is being retracted by sutures.

25

Fig. 7A. Stage 3.

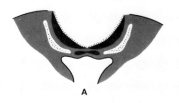

A. The roof plate of the overdistended neural tube has ruptured through cutaneous ectoderm into the amniotic sac.

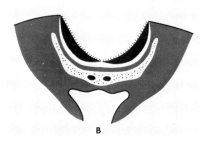

B. A belated dissection of the subarachnoid space then begins.

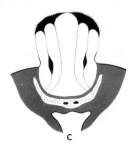

C. The open, everted neural tube becomes extruded to form a myelocele.

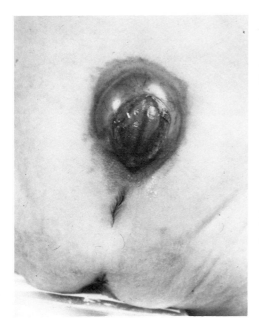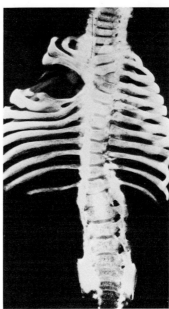

Fig. 7B (left). In this myelocele the two separated lateral plates may be seen. This constitutes diastematomyelia aperta. Cameron[2] has found the hemicords above the myelocele are closed as shown in Fig. 6A. This constitutes diastematomyelia occulta at this level.

Fig. 7C (right). This roentgenogram of the skeleton of a newborn with Arnold-Chiari malformation and myelocele reveals distorted fused ribs with associated hemivertebrae resulting from the distortion of sclerotomes during the stage of overdistention of the central canal. The lumbosacral canal is wide. The bodies of L1 and 2 are fused (Klippel-Feil syndrome) by the midline bony spur of a diastematomyelia located cephalad to the myelocele. (Reproduced from Cameron[2] with permission of author and publisher.)

27

Fig. 8A. Stage 4.

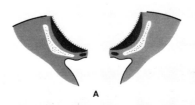

A

A. Rupture of both roof plate externally into the amniotic sac and the floor plate into the primitive gut.

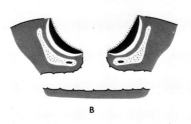

B

B. The subarachnoid space is developing.

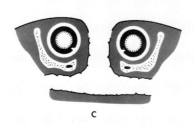

C

C. If healing occurs, the fetus may survive with a posterior enteric fistula.

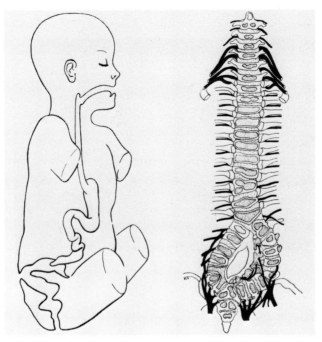

Fig. 8B. This infant survived for 7 months with a fistula of the colon discharging through the split spine. (Reproduced from Saunders[16].)

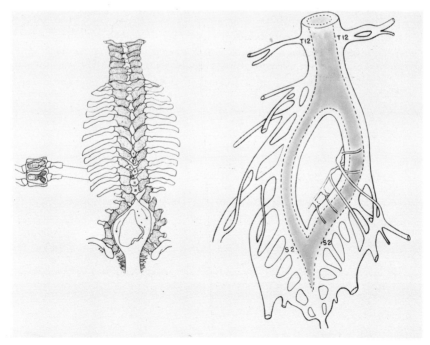

Fig. 8C. There was hydromyelia of the cord and of both hemicords. One hemicord possessed a rudimentary second set of nerve roots.

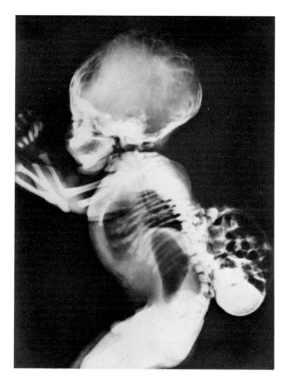

Fig. 8D. In this case, due to an imperforate anus, the abdominal contents had herniated onto the back through the split spinal column. Note the large head and craniolacunia, evidence of hydrocephalus in embryonal life. (Reproduced from Denes, et al.[3] with permission of authors and publisher.)

MORPHOGENESIS OF SPINA BIFIDA

Josef Warkany, M.D.

In this discussion I shall emphasize the morphogenesis
of the common spina bifida cystica or myelomeningocele as
seen in newborn children and describe its development in
experimental animals.

At birth a tumor of a rather puzzling appearance is seen
in the lumbosacral area of the child (Fig. 1). There is a
central area of red, raw and often bleeding tissue on top of
the sac which is sometimes mistaken for an ulcer. Around
this central area one observes a paper-thin wrinkled zone
that in turn is surrounded by an area consisting of skin.
What is the origin of such a lesion?

Ninety years ago an astute pathologist, Friedrich von
Recklinghausen,[5] developed the concept, still acknowledged
today by most investigators, which implies that this lesion
begins with a failure of the embryonic neural plate to close
in its caudal part and that from this initial error the
changes of surrounding tissues follow. In rat embryos of 10
days, the open neural plate lies on the dorsal surface, not
covered by skin, connective tissue and bone; but on the 12th
day the neural plate of the normal rat embryo has been
converted into a tube, covered by epithelium (Fig. 2) which
later is transformed into skin. If closure of the neural
plate is prevented by adverse factors, the nervous tissue

31

lies on the dorsal surface unprotected by skin, connective
tissue and bone (Fig. 3). At first the neural plate
differentiates further, forming anterior horns in their
proper place while the normally posterior areas develop in
the lateral aspects of the plate. As seen in Fig. 4 the
neural plate lies "like an open book" on the body surface
where it is exposed to amniotic fluid and stretched beyond
its normal confines. Consequently it degenerates and undergoes progressive destruction. The resulting wound may become
epithelialized and partly covered up by skin. Regeneration
of new tissues gives the lesion a certain protection but
repair of destroyed nervous tissues does not take place.
Recklinghausen named the central area "zona medullovasculosa":
it consists of neural remnants and blood vessels. Outside
of it there is a "zona epitheliosa" surrounded by a "zona
cutanea" (Fig. 1).

An old diagram of a myelomeningocele by Bockenheimer[1]
(Fig. 5) nicely shows how the remnants of nervous tissue are
pushed to the surface of the body and how nerves originating
from the anterior horn cells course ventrad to their muscles.
Fig. 6 is a corresponding diagram of a meningocele which
contains an intact spinal cord, the nerves taking a more
natural course through the vertebral foramina.

Sixty years after Recklinghausen, Gillman and coworkers[2]
found a method to produce spina bifidas and other congenital
malformations in rats by injecting trypan blue solutions into
pregnant animals. There are now many other methods available
which have similar effects and curiously aspirin can be used
to the same purpose in rats[6] (Fig. 7). Like trypan blue,
salicylates produce various kinds of spina bifida which can
be used as models of their human counterparts. Such animal
models have advantages and disadvantages. They permit us to

follow the development of a malformation, from its earliest
recognizable stages to birth; and we can obtain fresh and
well-preserved specimens that can be sectioned serially
which is difficult in human embryos obtained by chance. Such
sections can serve us better than diagrams in our explanations. On the other hand, we all know that there are sometimes great differences between animal models and human
specimens so that caution is needed in interpretations from
one species to another.

With this in mind we can follow the development of the
common spina bifida in rats treated with trypan blue or other
teratogens. As you know, the spinal cord is formed by
folding of the neural plate, with the rostral and caudal ends
closing last. In the rat the neural tube should be closed
by the 12th day of gestation (Fig. 2). But Fig. 3 shows a
rat embryo on the 14th day which still has a wide-open neural
tube that represents one of the earliest stages of spina
bifida.

A few days later (Fig. 8) the neural plate is already
in a state of degeneration; it is also undermined by epithelium that creeps in from the adjacent skin separating the
nervous tissue from its base and causing its sloughing off.
And finally there are hardly any structures left of the
neural plate, but some remnants can be recognized because
they are still connected with the nerves which course ventrad
through the fluid-filled cystic space. This is a perfect
confirmation of the diagram of 1902 (Fig. 9)[1].

Are there any signs of rupture of the neural tube in
these experimental animals? Are there blebs in early embryos
like those emphasized by Padget[4]? Recently Lendon[3] has
described blebs in rat embryos treated by trypan blue. But
these blood filled blebs are beneath previously formed

myeloceles; they are not the cause but the result of the anomalies. They, according to Lendon, do not support the concept of secondary opening of previously closed neural tubes.

Of course, there are other forms of cystic spina bifidas such as the myelocystoceles or hydromyelias. They are very rare forms seen in association with exstrophy of the cloaca. Myelocystoceles are covered by skin and when opened one can show that they represent huge expansions of the central canal.

Spina bifidas have been interpreted by pathologists, neurosurgeons and relatively recently by experimental teratologists. Some developed their opinions through observations in children, others through observations in rats or mice. Some looked at gross specimens weeks after birth; others at microscopic sections of embryos or fetuses. It is not surprising that differences of opinion exist as to the earliest minute deviations from the normal which nobody has actually seen. We all interpret and extrapolate our limited findings and there is no room for expressions of certainty or heated debate.

Does it make any difference whether spina bifida is due to <u>lack of closure</u> of the neural plate or due to <u>rupture</u> of a previously formed neural tube? Is this just an argument of scholars who want their opinion imposed on others? There could be practical and even legal consequences. If spina bifida begins with nonclosure of the posterior neuropore, it begins (in human embryos) <u>at the latest</u> by the end of the first month (28th day of gestation). Events after that time cannot initiate a spina bifida. But if this anomaly is due to rupture of an established neural tube, events in the second or third month of pregnancy or even later could be the cause of spina bifida. There are scientific and even legal

implications associated with these differing concepts, the
most important question being: How late in pregnancy can
spina bifida be caused by an environmental event?

REFERENCES

1. Bockenheimer, P.:   Zur Kenntniss der Spina bifida.   *Arch.*
    fur klinsche Chirurgie, 65:697, 1902.

2. Gillman, J., Gilbert, C. and Gillman, T.:   A preliminary
    report on hydrocephalus, spina bifida and other
    congenital anomalies in the rat produced by trypan blue.
    S. Afr. J. Med. Sci., 13:47, 1948.

3. Lendon, R.G.:   The embryogenesis of trypan-blue induced
    spina bifida aperta and short tail in the rat.   *Devel.*
    Med. Child Neurol., 17:3, 1975.

4. Padget, D.H.:   Neuroschisis and human embryonic malde-
    velopment.   *J. Neuropathol. Exp. Neurol., 29*:192, 1970.

5. Recklinghausen, F., von: Untersuchungen uber die Spina
    bifida.   *Virchow. Arch. Path. Anat., 105*:243, 1886.

6. Warkany, J. and Takacs, E.:   Experimental production of
    congenital malformations in rats by salicylate poisoning.
    J. Path., 35:315, 1959.

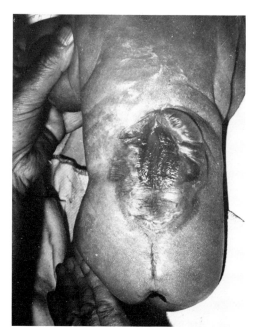

Fig. 1. Myelomeningocele in an infant. In the center there is a zona medullovasculosa surrounded by zona epitheliosa and zona cutanea.

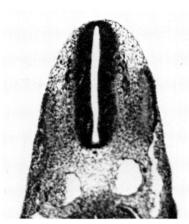

Fig. 2. Neural tube of a rat embryo on the 12th day.

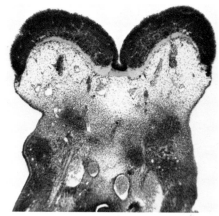

Fig. 3. Neural plate of a rat embryo on the 14th day. At that age the neural plate should have been converted into a tube. This was prevented by injections of the mother with trypan blue (8th to 10th day) of pregnancy.

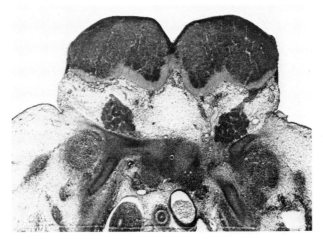

Fig. 4. Open neural plate in a rat embryo (16th day). "Open book stage" produced by injection of the mother with methysalicylate on the 10th day of pregnancy.

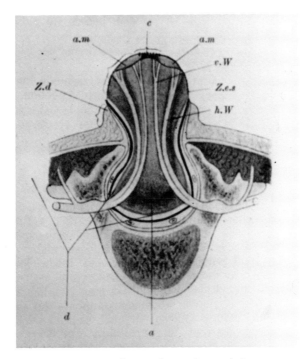

Fig. 5. Diagram of a myelomeningocele[2]. am: area medullaris. Z.e.s.: Zona epithelio-serosa. Z.d.: Zona dermatica. d: dura. v.W.: anterior root. h.W.: posterior root. a: fluid in arachnoid space.

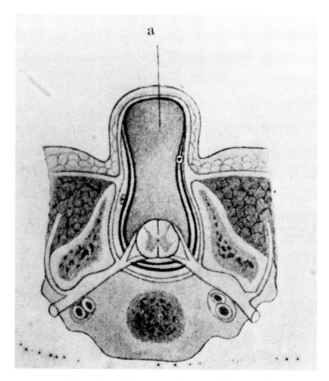

Fig. 6. Diagram of a meningocele.[2]

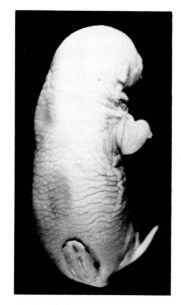

Fig. 7. Spina bifida (in a 21-day rat fetus) produced by aspirin given orally to mother on 10th day of pregnancy

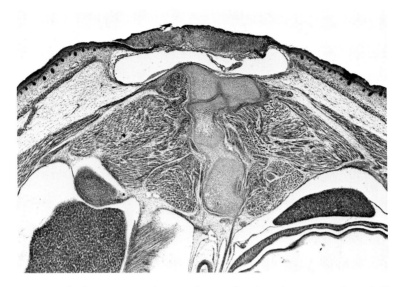

Fig. 8. Neural plate in a 21-day rat fetus, showing degenerated medullary plate, undermined by epithelium continuous with skin. Abnormal vertebrae are seen under arachnoid.

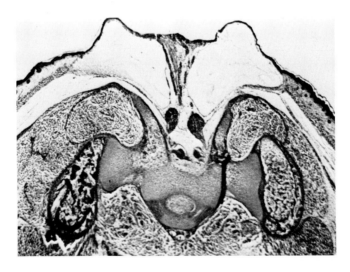

Fig. 9. Further degeneration of the neural plate. Its former existence is demonstrated by nerve roots which course ventrad through arachnoid space. Compare this section through spina bifida of a 21-day rat fetus with the diagram of Fig. 5 derived from observation of human myelomeningoceles.

COMPARATIVE STATISTICS - TREATMENT
VERSUS NON-TREATMENT

Sonya Oppenheimer, M.D.

The major purpose of Dr. Lorber's article,[2] "Results of
Treatment of Myelomeningocele, puslished in 1971, is to raise
the question of selective treatment for infants with myelomeningocele. He established criteria of selection based on
data obtained from 524 unselected cases treated in Sheffield
over a twelve year period. The article states that "It may
now be wiser to abandon immediate back repair for all such
children as initially advocated in 1963 by Zachary, leaving
the most severely affected children unrepaired and allowing
for further energetic treatment of the less severely affected
children."

Currently, centers dealing with the treatment of the
child with myelomeningocele are searching for additional
criteria which would be more predictive of poor prognosis for
quality of life. Thus the pendulum has swung from non-
treatment because it was not surgically feasible to Zachary's[3]
plea to treat all, to the current plea for selective
treatment.

I would like to present the results of treatment of 139
children followed over a 10 year period by Cincinnati
Myelomeningocele Team and compare this data with similar
data from other larger centers. The purpose, however, is not

to confirm that a certain group of children should not be
treated but instead, to encourage collection of data from
other centers to identify weak areas of treatment and to
encourage strengthening and improvement of treatment of all
children with myelomeningocele.

A total of 139 children with myelomeningocele have been
seen from 1964 through September of 1974. These children
are followed in the Myelomeningocele Program which offers a
multidisciplinary team approach. The team includes a neurosurgeon, orthopedist, urologist, pediatrician, psychiatrist,
orthotist, physical therapist, occupational therapist,
nutritionist, social worker, psychologist, special educator
and clinical specialist nurse. A newborn infant is referred
by the private pediatrician or obstetrician to the team
neurosurgeon and then comes under the auspices of the Myelomeningocele Team. The back lesion if open is repaired as an
emergency procedure within the first 24 hours of life. Those
children who have signs of developing hydrocephalus are
shunted as soon as possible. The appropriate team members
see the child in the intensive care nursery. At that time,
the child is totally evaluated including general physical,
neurological examinations, and level of lesion is determined.

Prior to discharge, renal functioning is determined by
intravenous pyelograms, cinecystogram and urine culture, BUN
and creatinine.

The team pediatrician, nurse and/or social worker
contacts the family and assists the family with understanding
the multiplicity of problems that this child will have. One
month following discharge, the child is seen in the clinic
by all team members and the plan of treatment is continued.
Initially, the child is seen monthly and eventually every
three months. Responsibility for general pediatric care

remains with the private physician.

The team pediatrician serves as coordinator and is responsible for keeping the private physician informed of the child's progress plus coordinating other services involved.

Ambulation is a primary goal regardless of the level of lesion. Surgery is undertaken when indicated to help the child achieve a functional position for bracing. Physical therapist, occupational therapist, orthotist work jointly with the orthopedic surgeon toward early ambulation.

Urinalysis and/or cultures are obtained at regular intervals and treatment instituted where indicated. Yearly evaluations of kidney function are obtained. Bowel training is begun as early as possible. A variety of methods are used to assist with urinary incontinence as the child gets older. Management of the urinary tract problem is under the direction of the team urologist.

Developmental data is obtained yearly. A variety of programs ranging from an infant stimulation problem to an adolescent group are offered to the children. As the children reach schoolage, a special educator helps with appropriate school planning and where possible, regular school placement is encouraged.

Nutritionist involvement begins with the first clinic visit both to help prevent obesity and to establish early good dietary habits.

Complete genetic histories are obtained on each family and genetic counselling is provided.

The following statistics are a comparative analysis of the Cincinnati results versus those of five other major articles published within the past several years that describe treatment results in both selective and non-selective populations. Lorber's study is based on unselective

treatment of 270 children. Ames and Schut's[1] study in
Philadelphia describes treatment results on 171 children.
Smith's[5] series from Australia describes the results of
selective treatment on a total of 295 children, 88 of whom
survived. Stark and Drummond[6] from Edinburough also described treatment results based on 78 children treated
selectively. Shurtleff's[4] results are based on 98 children
who had unselective treatment.

Lorber's selective criteria for non-treatment is as
follows:

1. Severe paraplegia, level L2 and above.

2. Gross hydrocephalus, head circumference 2 cms above
the 90th percentile.

3. Kyphosis.

4. Associated gross congenital anomalies.

Fig. 1 indicates overall mortality figures. Because one
of the major criteria used for non-selection is level of
lesion, I have emphasized this in all of the figures. The
dark lines would indicate mortality figures for those
children who theoretically would fit the criteria for non-
treatment. The blank space is the total overall results.

Lorber's overall mortality figures are 50% including
a small second series he reported where he tried to do more
active selection. Therefore, even in his selective series,
there was an overall mortality rate of 60%.

Cincinnati mortality for a 10 year period for levels of
L2 is 29%; total mortality 22% (Table I). Philadelphia's
study for children with L2 lesion is 35%; overall mortality
is 20%. Smith's series overall mortality was 40%; mortality
for children with levels of L2 and above were 60%. Those
children who were selected for treatment had a mortality rate

of 22%. Stark's series shows an 80% mortality for those
children who were not treated; for those children who fit the
selective criteria, there was a mortality figure of 40%,
which leads the authors to conclude that even stricter
criteria for selection is needed. Shurtleff's series would
show an overall mortality in both the L2 lesion and total
mortality of 40%.

Fig. 2 shows statistical results of IQ testing. Again
one of the standards for quality of life is that the child
function in the normal range intellectually. Using the AAMD
standard (American Association Mental Deficiency) normal IQ is
classified as above 68, mildly retarded is 52 to 67, moderate
36 to 51. However, statistics for what is considered normal
IQ varies in the different articles. Forty-four percent of
the children with lesions above L2 in Cincinnati have an IQ
of greater than 84. A total of 67% of the children in Cincinnati with lesions above L2 have an IQ above 68 which falls
into the category of normal. Eighty-one percent of all
children followed by the Cincinnati team have an IQ in the
normal range. Twenty-one percent have IQ's below 50 with
lesions above L2. In comparison,in Lorber's series 41% have
IQ's above 84 with lesions above L2, 28% have IQ's below 50.
In Ames series, 42% have IQs in the normal range. In Smith's
selective series, 63% have IQ's in the normal range with
lesions of L2. The confusion here is that even though some
of his children were selected, some did end up having lesions
above L2 and these would be "the best survivors". His total
figure for children with selective treatment would indicate
that 77% have a normal IQ and only less than 3% have an IQ
below 50. In Stark's selective series, a total of only 15%
have IQ's below 50, 64% of his L2's have an IQ of above
normal for a total of 85% functioning in the normal range

intellectually. Shurtleff's series would indicate that 33%
of children with lesions above L2 have IQ's of above 84, 15%
have IQ's between 68 and 83 or a total of 48%, and 33% have
IQ's below 50.

Another criteria for quality of life is ambulation.
Fig. 3 illustrates the Cincinnati results. All series were
consistent in that children with lesions above L2 were unable
to ambulate without appliances. In Lorber's series, no
children with lesions above L2 were considered community
ambulators. Twenty-three percent with lesions above L2 in
Cincinnati were community ambulators. In Lorber's series,
those children with lesions above L2, 96% were confined to
wheelchairs completely. In Cincinnati, 21% were confined to
wheelchairs while another 36% were considered household
ambulators.

Urinary statistics will be presented in detail in a
subsequent paper. Sixty-three percent of children with
lesions above L2 have had a urinary diversion compared to
34% in Lorber's series and 44% in Ames and 25% in Smith's
series. The type of urinary procedures followed is dependent
on the team urologist. Thirty percent of the children in
Cincinnati are on intermittent catheterization.

Table I summarizes the results of treatment of the
children followed in Cincinnati. Perhaps most significant is
the comparison of children with lesions at L3-L4 where
treatment is advocated and children with a higher level of
paralysis above L2. Eighty-two percent with lower level of
paralysis have shunts compared to 95% in the higher level of
paralysis. Seventy-five percent have IQ's in the normal
range compared to 67% normal intellect and 63% are able to
ambulate with appliances compared to 23% who can ambulate
with appliances in the higher level of paralysis.

These statistics would indeed indicate that children with high lesions who fit some of the criteria that Dr. Lorber advocates for non-treatment, do not do as well as children without these criteria as predicted by Dr. Lorber.

The children followed in Cincinnati overall regardless of level of lesion seem to have "better quality of survival". The multi-disciplinary approach is time-consuming, requires effort by all team members including availability of all the medical team, and a great deal of participation by both parents and children. Funding is a never ending problem. Frequent hospitalizations are difficult for the child, family and house staff, who have strong feelings concerning caring for these handicapped children.

The ethical questions involved in selection have become a prime concern at all meetings. Physicians continue to refine criteria of predictability of poor prognosis. Perhaps, however, the question should be, "how can we improve care for these children so that the children who do have adverse factors, do not suffer from a self-fulfilling prophecy?" The handicap of the child with myelomeningocele is not that different from the handicap of children with other developmental defects. What is different is that the child with myelomeningocele can be diagnosed at birth and the physicians have available surgical treatment which can prevent death. Therefore, such a child becomes a prime target for selective treatment.

This project was supported by Grant No. MCT-000912-11-0, awarded the Bureau of Community Health Services, Health Services Administration, Public Health Service, DHEW & Grant No. 59-P-25297/5.05, awarded by Region V, Social & Rehabilitation Service, DHEW.

REFERENCES

1. Ames, M.D. and Schut, L.: Results of treatment of myelomeningocele. *Pediat., 50*:466, 1972.

2. Lorber, J.: Results of treatment of myelomeningocele. An analysis of 524 unselected cases with special reference to possible selection for treatment. *Develop. Med. Child Neurol., 13*:279, 1971.

3. Sharrard, W.J.W., Zachary, R.B., Lorber, J. and Bruce, A.M.: A controlled trial of immediate and delayed closure of spina bifida cystica. *Arch. Dis. Child., 38*:18, 1963.

4. Shurtleff, D.B., Hayden, P.W. Chapman, W.H., et al: Myelodysplasia - Problems of long term survival and social function. *West. J. Med., 122*:199, 1975.

5. Smith, G.K. and Smith, E.D.: Selection for treatment in spina bifida cystica. *Brit. Med. J., 2*:189, 1973.

6. Stark, G.P. and Drummond, M.: Results of selected early operation on myelomeningocele. *Arch. Dis Child., 48*: 676, 1973.

TABLE 1.

Cincinnati Statistics

	SHUNT		INTELLIGENCE					
	C	S	84–100	68–83	52–67	36–51	20–35	>20
Grade I 10 S_3	40%	60%	90% (100%)	10%	0	0	0	0
Grade II 32 S_1–S_3	69%	31%	84% (93%)	9%	3%	0	0	0
Grade III 33 L_3–L_4	82%	18%	45% (75%)	30%	21%	0	0	4%
Grades IV & V 34 >L_2	95%	5%	44% (67%)	23%	12%	6%	3%	12%
TOTAL	77%	23%	61%	20%	11%	2%	1%	5%

49

TABLE 1. (cont)

	AMBULATION				SCHOOL		GENITO-URINARY		
	W/O	C	H	W	REG	OR	CONT	IN	COND
Grade I 10 S_3	100%	0	0	0	100%		60%	30%	10%
Grade II 32 S_1-S_3	25%	75%	0	0	46%	54%	6%		18%
Grade III 33 L_3-L_4	0	63%	28%	9%	55%	40%	0		48%
Grades IV & V 34 > L_2	0	23%	56%	21%	28%	54%	0	63%	
TOTAL	17%	51%	20%	12%	54%	40%	18%		43%

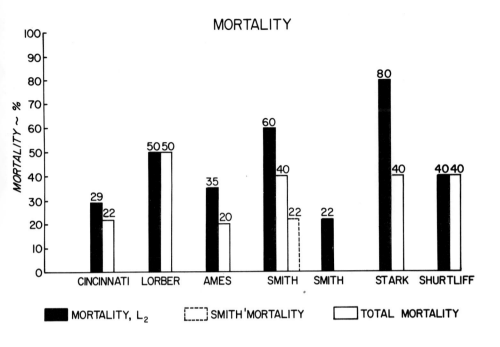

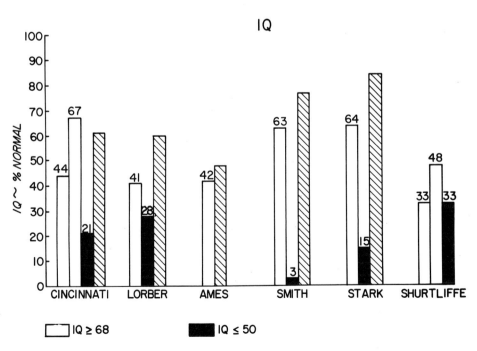

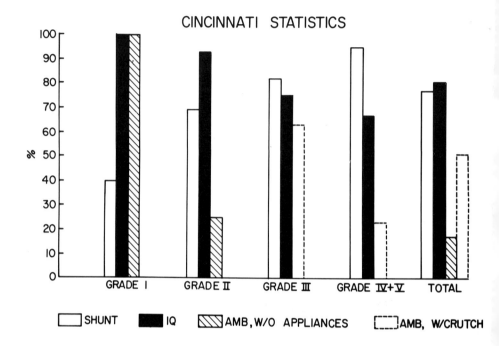

CINCINNATI STATISTICS

FOUNDATIONS OF PARENTAL ADJUSTMENT: EARLY INTERVENTION, CRISIS INTERVENTION*

Abby S. Cutright, R.N., M.S.N.

When an infant is born with an extensive physical defect such as myelomeningocele, the impact on the total family is great and there are a multitude of immediate and long-term needs to be met. In this Center a treatment team for total care of the child with myelomeningocele has existed since 1964. Services to these children and their families have gradually been expanded. A recently identified priority has been that of early intensive intervention with parents of the newly-born infant with myelomeningocele. This need was identified as a result of two related assumptions: 1) that for the infant born with myelomeningocele, the first months of life are a time of great stress and crisis for the family and 2) that difficulties in adjustment in later childhood or adolescence may be minimized by early intensive intervention that helps the parents cope with negative feelings about having a child who is handicapped and assists them to have positive interactions with their infants.

*This project was supported by Grant No. MCT-000912-10-0, awarded the Bureau of Community Health Services, Health Services Administration, Public Health Service, DHEW & Grant No. 59-P-25297/03, awarded by Region V, Social & Rehabilitation Service, DHEW.

From a theoretical viewpoint we know that coping with
the birth of a child with a handicap involves relinquishing
the "whole" or "perfect" child anticipated before birth.[9]
In every healthy mother-infant relationship there is a
gradual working-through of discrepancies between the
idealized perfect infant and the actual infant with all its
urgent needs and lovable and unlovable characteristics. With
the infant born with myelomeningocele, the discrepancy
between idealized, anticipated infant and actual infant is
great, and the result is interruption or alteration of the
mother's developing capacity to accept and "mother" her
infant. She may need to alter previous patterns of mothering
(if this is not her firstborn) or she may need to alter
anticipated patterns of mothering. At a time when she may
be eager to get on with the process of mothering, the
infant's critical needs hinder this. These alterations and
delays affect not just the mother but hinder the whole
family's incorporation of this new member. Thus, it is
important to direct our efforts toward helping parents and
other significant family members to work through the grief
they experience in "losing" the anticipated perfect child,
so they will be free to assist their child in maximizing his
potential. It has been our experience that many of our
families with children who have reached adolescence and who
have myelomeningocele experience increased stress related to
the limitations imposed by the handicap. Many of the
adolescents experienced extremely stormy first years of life
and the parents' expectations were that their child's life
would be short. Solnit and Stark have stated that "the ghost
of the desired, expected healthy child continues to interfere
with the family's adaptation to the child with a developmental disability if the mourning process becomes fixed as a

sustained atmosphere of the family."[8] E. Waechter has said
that "the importance of supportive, informative and therapeutic assistance to parents during this time cannot be
over-estimated, for patterns of parent-child interaction are
formed during the first few months and are later very
resistive to change."[10] The interventions described below
were based on the belief that intensive intervention during
infancy can facilitate optimum adjustment of the family and
thus, of the person with myelomeningocele.

One of the goals of the treatment team is the earliest
possible referral of the infant with myelomeningocele to the
team. This enables the team to begin working with the
family, helping them begin to cope with this crisis as early
as the first few days of life. As the nursing clinical
specialist for the team, my role with the family of a newly-
born infant with myelomeningocele has been 1) to reinforce
and, as necessary, further clarify information regarding the
physical defect itself, 2) to encourage verbalization of
feelings about what has been happening to them, how they
perceive their child's handicap and what immediate and long-
range fears and expectations they have and 3) to help them
plan for and assist them following their baby's initial
homecoming. My initial contact with the family is ideally
made as soon after birth as possible in the form of a home
visit with both parents and/or other significant family
members, and focuses on the above mentioned goals. Depending
on the circumstances surrounding the child's birth and early
treatment and the needs of the parents, one or more home
visits may be scheduled. The infant's initial hospitalization constitutes a separation that is often difficult for
the mother, as well as other family members, but the delay
can be used constructively to assist parents to identify

feelings and mobilize resources to cope with situations ahead
of them. When possible, a time is arranged when the nurse
can accompany the mother as she visits her baby in the newborn intensive care unit. The purpose of this visit is to
assess mother's reaction to her infant (first as an infant
and second as an infant with special needs); to support her
if necessary in relating to hospital staff; and to give her
another opportunity to verbalize her questions, fears and
expectations. A subsequent home visit is arranged as soon as
possible following the baby's discharge from the hospital.
This visit usually involves only the mother or other principle mother-figure and focuses on physical care of the
infant related to the defect, important observations she must
be aware of, infant stimulation techniques (in general and
in specific as they relate to her child's handicap) and
preparation for the initial clinic visit. In all of these
contacts with the family the nurse must be sensitive to how
the family members are coping with their feelings and the
degree to which they are ready to assimilate new information.
Depending on assessment of how the parents are coping with
the crisis of birth, additional home visits may be needed to
accompany them throughout their first clinic visit as their
child is seen by various members of the myelomeningocele
team. Goals at this time include reducing anxiety, providing
clarification as necessary, supporting them in asking
questions of other team members and further orienting them to
what they can expect from the team. At this time the child
is usually two to three months old and the family has,
hopefully, regained equilibrium as a result of having
verbalized feelings, assimilated some helpful factual information and begun to care effectively for and have positive
interactions with their infant. They would then be

encouraged to begin their infant in the infant stimulation program.   If resolution of the crisis is progressing more slowly, this step would be delayed and individual assistance would be continued.

The infant stimulation program was a group program initiated in 1972 for the purpose of 1) stimulating children under age two years primarily in areas of motor, visual-perceptual and social growth and development and 2) increasing parents' ability to meet their child's special needs by relating normal early child development to special needs/adaptations for the child with myelomeningocele, by facilitating positive interaction between parent and child, by providing a discussion group where parents can explore mutual concerns and share successes.

The program was organized as follows: an infant group with an age range of three to twelve months (actual range at start of program was three to ten months), and a toddler group between one and two years of age. (This older group was later discontinued. A major factor seemed to be that by the time the child reached a year of age, many of the parents were coping quite well and were drawing on the Parents' Organization as a major source of support.) This discussion will be confined to the infant group. The therapists were a physical therapist, an occupational therapist and a nursing clinical specialist for multihandicapped children. The general format was that the first hour emphasized gross motor, fine motor, language and social interaction activities with therapists, parents and children all actively involved. The second hour was used for a discussion group, conducted by the nursing clinical specialist as group leader and the occupational therapist as observer-recorder. This discussion group took place in a separate room apart from the children,

this separation being considered essential to the development
and success of the group. At the request of the parents,
some of the discussion hours were used for guest speakers.
Assessment of each infant and family prior to the first
session included evaluation of motor abilities, especially of
the lower extremities and an assessment of developmental
level by the occupational therapist using the Denver Developmental Screening Test. A nursing assessment, within the
home, evaluated the child's level of functioning within the
home environment, resources available within the home,
parent's level of coping physically and emotionally with
their child and the child's impact on the total family.

This group met twice-monthly for a total of twelve two-
hour sessions. During the first session the parents
completed a questionnaire designed to be non-threatening and
to tap understanding of normal growth and development and of
basic aspects of their child's handicap. Understanding of
normal growth and development was adequate in all group
members except one. There were some gaps in most of the
mothers' understanding of basic medical aspects of the handicap and these were reviewed as the sessions progressed. The
first hour of each session occurred in a large room supplied
with mats and other appropriate equipment and toys. The
second hour of each session took place in a smaller room
where members could sit in a circle and where coffee was
available. The group composition was diverse in terms of age,
cultural background, financial resources and severity of the
child's defect. Only one family represented had another
child with a significant birth defect, in this case being
cleft lip. Two of the children in the group came from
families where they were the youngest of four children, two
were the youngest of two children, and two were firstborn and

only children. In each of these groups of two, one child
with myelomeningocele was minimally involved and one was more
extensively involved. The seventh child in the group was the
youngest of seven children and was extensively involved. The
sessions were primarily attended by infants and mothers.
Occasionally an older sibling would accompany them; one
father attended several sessions but was not comfortable to
participate in the discussion group.

The format for the first hour of each session was
primarily the responsibility of the physical and occupational
therapists. They along with the nurse assisted the parents
in carrying out activities or techniques demonstrated at the
beginning of each session and in using equipment available
in the room. (For example, the occupational therapist and
the physical therapist might focus on head and trunk control
and balance and the session would be devoted to activities
that encourage development of this control.) Informal conversation with each parent during this time allowed the
therapists to evaluate what activities were being attempted
at home and whether any problems were encountered. Spontaneous conversation between the mothers increased dramatically as the sessions progressed. Since details of specific
infant stimulation techniques will be covered elsewhere, the
remainder of this paper will detail the mothers' discussion
group.

During the twelve sessions there was a definite
progression of topics discussed and of the way in which the
group handled these topics. During the first two sessions
they directed considerable anger at health professionals
specifically surrounding the birth and initial treatment of
their children with considerable sharing of experiences and
feelings. They felt they had often been given misinformation

or that there was a lack of helpful information; further,
they expressed concern about the pessimism that was conveyed
regarding their child's prognosis (apparently irregardless of
extent of defect). During the second session this ventilation progressed to "what can we do about it?" Other significant themes during the first three sessions were fear of
retardation and meaning of developmental lag, risk of having
a second child with this defect, and feelings related to
brief or prolonged separation from their child. Several
aspects of separation were discussed: the long, initial
separation, separation during subsequent hospitalizations
(frequent for this age group), and separations (brief) which
allow the parents to meet their own individual needs and/or
those of other siblings. Feelings were discussed freely
during the first three sessions. Then during the next three
sessions the group avoided free discussion of feelings and
focused on factual topics. The remaining six sessions dealt
more with feelings again: for example, with family relationships, treating the child as "normal" and again with aspects
of separation. There was also more looking to the future in
terms of situations they and their children would encounter.
Throughout these latter sessions, a number of the children
had major or minor surgery, and the mothers were very
supportive of each other.

Data gathered via a formal questionnaire completed by
the participating parents at the end of sessions indicated
that they saw the sessions as valuable, having met some of
their needs, having contributed significantly to their
understanding of the defect, having value in the care of
their non-handicapped children as well, and having
significant, positive influence on their child's physical and
social development. All the mothers strongly agreed that the

program should be offered to other parents of newly-born
infants with myelomeningocele. The majority felt that the
number and length of sessions were adequate. They felt that
the program helped them feel more comfortable in physically
handling their child. (Three of the seven children were over
six months old at the beginning of the program.) The mothers
felt that their husbands had benefited from the program in
that they had discussed together at home the problems and
solutions discussed in the sessions, the fathers had become
more active in the play and physical stimulation aspect of
their child's care, and that they had become involved in
adapting equipment within the home. The mothers were most
enthusiastic about the guest speaker, herself the mother of
a child with myelomeningocele, who spoke with them about her
fears during a subsequent pregnancy, her experience during
her child's ileo-conduit surgery, and her current experiences
as her child began kindergarten in a regular public school.
During the twelfth session as problems and solutions were
reviewed, the mothers were encouraged to use the Parents'
Organization as a source of support in the same way that they
had used each other as sources of support during the previous
six months.

DISCUSSION

        Much of what has been written regarding development of
a crisis and steps in crisis intervention is applicable to a
stressful situation such as birth of a child with myelomeningocele. Lindemann theorized that during every individual's
life there are events that can be predicted to generate
emotional stress and lead to a series of adaptive mechanisms
directed toward mastery of the stressful situation.[1] Such a
stressful situation becomes a crisis when the individual

cannot, for a time, solve the problem or reduce anxiety by
use of previous coping mechanisms.[5] The outcome of this
crisis will be a new equilibrium that may be better or worse
than the previous equilibrium, depending on what takes place
between the individual and other key figures in his emotional
milieu during the time of crisis.[1] The crisis is by nature,
self-limiting and it is during a crisis that the individual
is most open to alternate modes of coping. Steps in utilizing
the therapeutic technique of crisis intervention may be
summarized as follows: 1) assessment of the person (family)
and the problem (i.e. nature of the defect and how the family
is coping), 2) planning therapeutic intervention, 3) intervention through helping the person (family) intellectually
understand the crisis (facts regarding the physical defect),
through helping them verbalize feelings and thus relieve
immobilizing tension, and through exploration of new ways of
coping with the crisis, and 4) resolution of the crisis and
anticipatory planning.[7] The birth of a child with myelomeningocele unquestionably constitutes a highly stressful
situation for the family with rise of inner strain and
tension. Whether this stressful event becomes a crisis as
defined by Caplan or whether equilibrium is rapidly regained,
depends on the family's perception of the event, their
available coping mechanisms and their use of available
situational supports.[3] When therapeutic intervention can be
begun shortly after birth, the parents can be given factual
information related to their perception of the event, can
begin to verbalize for themselves and with each other their
feelings and concerns, can talk with another parent who has
had a similar experience, and can begin making constructive
plans for their child's homecoming. Without this early
intervention or alternate intensive long-term intervention,

lasting impairment of emotional functioning is likely to
exist within the family. The result, then, is a series of
situational and/or developmental crises throughout childhood
and adolescence, with the likelihood of that person failing
to reach his optimum potential.

In the infant stimulation program described, each of the
parents had reduced anxiety to a level where they could
effectively enter into the group situation. The parents'
discussion group can perhaps best be classified a therapeutic
group as described by Marram.[6] The mothers in the group were
basically healthy individuals experiencing a common crisis or
stress. The stress was developmental in terms of having
given birth to a baby and situational in terms of that baby
having an extensive physical disability. All of the group
members related experiences that indicated a high level of
anxiety following the birth of their child. At the time the
group began, some degree of equilibrium within each family
had been regained by intensive early intervention and/or use
of situational supports (i.e. close supportive marriage
relationship, support of extended family or intervention of
health professionals who assist with problem-solving).[2]
The goal of the group, then, was to further establish the
equilibrium that they had achieved. The fact that the group
was able to readily identify and discuss feelings in the
early sessions may have been due, in part, to continued
experiencing of a significant level of anxiety. The basic
goal of the group as verbalized by various members was to be
better prepared to meet the special needs of their child.
This basic goal was met as they sought factual information
(educational aspect), as they verbalized feelings related to
past and current experiences regarding their child (cathar-
sis), and as they used a problem-solving approach in

considering ways of handling specific problems or situations.
The leader's role in the group was that of a facilitator in
helping the group define problems and explore alternate
solutions. They were encouraged to test out solutions and
evaluate results. As pointed out by Bruce, these mothers
did not want to be told what to do, but rather wanted
guidance and facts, providing a base to enable them to
formulate their own solutions.[4]

The ultimate measure of success in meeting the goals of
the early intervention and infant stimulation programs will
be in relation to how the whole family weathers the developmental states through which the child passes and the degree
to which these children achieve happy and productive lives.

REFERENCES

1. Aquilera, C.C., Messick, J.M. and Farrell, M.S.: Crisis
    Intervention - Theory and Methodology, St. Louis, C.V.
    Mosby Co., 1970, pp. 5.

2. Aquilera, C.C., Messick, J.M. and Farrell, M.S.: Crisis
    Intervention - Theory and Methodology, St. Louis, C.V.
    Mosby Co., 1970, pp. 55.

3. Aquilera, C.C., Messick, J.M. and Farrell, M.S.: Crisis
    Intervention - Theory and Methodology, St. Louis, C.V.
    Mosby Co., 1970, pp. 57.

4. Bruce, S.J.: Group leadership in parent education. IN
    Current Concepts in Clinical Nursing, Vol. 1, St. Louis,
    C.V. Mosby Co., 1967, pp. 414.

5. Caplan, G.: An Approach to Community Mental Health,
    New York, Grune and Stratton, Inc., 1961, pp. 18.

6. Marram, G.D.: The Group Approach in Nursing Practice,
    St. Louis, C.V. Mosby Co., 1973, pp. 24.

7. Morley, W., Messick, J. and Aquilera, D.: Crisis: Paradigms of intervention, *J. Psychiatric Nursing, 5*: 537, 1967.

8. Solnit, A. and Stark, M.H.: Mourning and the birth of a defective child. IN The Psychoanalytic Study of the Child, Vol. XVI, 1961, pp. 532.

9. Solnit, A. and Stark, M.H.: Mourning and the birth of a defective child. IN The Psychoanalytic Study of the Child, Vol. XVI, 1961, pp. 525.

10. Waechter, E.H.: Developmental correlates of physical disability. *Nursing Forum, 9*:90, 1970.

MYELOMENINGOCELE AS A FAMILY PROBLEM: A DEVELOPMENTAL TASK MODEL

Mary Anne Barry, ACSW

This paper will discuss how myelomeningocele is seen, not as a physical, emotional and psychological problem to the patient, but how it affects the systems around the patient, particularly the family, and how helping professionals might intervene in more constructive ways to enable the child and the family to live out their lives with some degree of comfort and independence and zest.

The study of parenthood is a relatively new field of concentration. Until a few decades ago, it was taken for granted that the whole process took place instinctively, that it was all done by the seat of one's pants. Our ancestors had all they could do to survive physically, so that little thought was given to the psychological needs of the child, much less to the needs of the family or the parents.

When we as a society began to be conscious of the needs of the child, it was an important step. Children were no longer chattel, but persons in their own right. We need now to go one step further, to examine in detail what happens to people when they take on the difficult and demanding role of parenthood, and especially parenthood of a handicapped child.

We saw during the age of Spock that Americans are the

most anxious of parents. Sidney Callahan calls it "self-conscious parenthood". Other cultures do not seem to impose this same kind of pressure. And families of Spina Bifida children are part of the total picture, anxious to be good parents, little aware of their own needs. They have gotten the message that the child's needs come first, if they are to be successful parents. And since success in parenting is often seen as success of the child, parents of handicapped children have difficulty in measuring if they are making it or not, if their handicapped child may not be successful in ways that our culture measures success: health, beauty, wealth, independence. My thesis is that we as professionals must shift our attention now to the problems and adjustments of the total family of the child and how it copes with stress.

The professional literature, you will find, is not very helpful. It has only begun to deal with these issues. One can find reams of material on the psychological adjustment of the child to chronic illness, to hospitalization, to separation from parents, to school placement, but almost nothing on what happens to parents when the child is in the hospital, or how they feel when the handicapped child leaves on the school bus for the first time, or what residential placement does to *them*, or what it does to a mother when a cranky and obstinate two year old throws his crutch at her in rage when she has been trying so hard to teach him to walk. How does a dad feel when he is laid off, or when the car won't make it through another winter, when the child must go every week to the clinic 50 miles away? What happens to his self-esteem when he must ask for help from an impersonal hospital system or from a enormous welfare system which is in the public eye only when it is "weeding out the welfare cheaters"?

I am hoping that by working closely with families of

children with spina bifida, and getting feedback from them, by working with the independent parents' organization, and from observation of hundreds of families, to pull out some concept of how families cope, what unique pressures they face, and how helping professionals can best fit in.

When we talk about families with spina bifida, we have to start with certain assumptions. The first is that they experience severe and lasting trauma, and that they need support and encouragement in order to survive and grow as a family. Secondly, we will assume that these families are not the so-called "troubled" families with whom social work has traditionally been linked. Thirdly, we assume that they want and need for themselves what everyone wants and needs for themselves.

Max Lerner, in a column a few years ago, said that in order to grow we need a feeling of growth, selfhood, security, struggle, fulfillment, belonging, and believing. Nathan Ackerman says that families achieve health and well-being insofar as they fulfill the biological potentials of parent-child relations and husband-wife relations. The family must provide survival needs of food and shelter, and be a part of the community, be internally stable but open to change, with realistic and appropriate goals and values, having a climate inducive to the psychological growth and value strivings of its members, with freedom also for individuality. The members of the family need a degree of comfort in their roles, and a method of solving problems and resolving conflicts that works for that family. It must reconcile within its structure the often conflicting needs of the child and parents in ways that promote growth of the total family. That is a heavy assignment for any family. How do we make it apply to the families of children with spina bifida in ways that can make sense to them - and to us professionally?

It seems to me that the first step is to find out what does happen in the family of a child with spina bifida, almost day to day, from the first day, that is *different* from what happens in any family that has a new baby.

To what degree is the family aware of what is happening to them, how do they deal with it, do they see themselves as wanting or needing help, and can they use the help offered to them ? And how can the helping professionals enhance this helping process and pass it on to other families and other professionals? What I am trying to do is to separate out the process, my response to it, and the response of the people around the family, so that the total experience can become a more conscious, planned and refined approach that we can share with the parents, which is open to adaptation and input by parents and members of the team.

Crisis itself is not a pathological experience, and persons in crisis, even disturbed behavior, are not neces-sarily sick and shouldn't be treated as such. The wrong kind of helping can create a large group of very dependent people, or on the other hand, families so defended that they cannot use any kind of help.

And I am beginning to be convinced that social work itself need not, and in some situations, should not, provide all or most of the helping to be done. But my convictions are that early intervention by the social worker into the lives of these families, acting in a planned manner, rather than reacting later to maladaptive coping and family disor-ganization, is most helpful.

This paper will touch upon only one piece of the total picture, the early weeks and months. From that you can see how the approach can be stretched to encompass the

developmental stages of the family throughout its natural
history.

I have constructed a model, which is a way of thinking
about the ordinary family and the special concerns of the
family of the spina bifida child, which has helped me to put
some things in place. It is loosely based on a concept of
family developmental tasks spelled out by Reuben Hill and
Evelyn Millis Duvall in her book, Family Development. Let
me elaborate on the material.

Table 1 shows the relationship between the age of the
child; the medical milestones, or the medical picture typical
to the spina bifida child of that age; the developmental
tasks of any child, and the complications in carrying out
these tasks in light of his unique experience. We are
interested here particularly in the tasks of the ordinary
family of the infant and young child, Table 2; and possible
task complications for a family if the child is born with
spina bifida, Table 3.

In Table 4 we begin to spell out what some of the
supplementary tasks of the family of the infant with spina
bifida might be, and in Table 5 the possible tasks of systems
around the family. For the family of the older child one
could compile a similar schema, breaking down the tasks, the
complications of the tasks, and the supplementary tasks to be
taken on in light of the problems by the family and the
systems around the family.

Now, what precisely are developmental tasks? Generally
the family's (as opposed to the individual spouse's) ongoing
tasks are physical maintenance, allocation of resources,
division of labor and role assignment, reproduction, recruit-
ment, and release of family members, socialization of family

members, maintenance of order (the formation of communication and interaction patterns), placement of the members in the larger society, and the maintenance of motivation and morale.

Duvall says that developmental tasks arise around a certain period in the life of a family, the successful carrying out of which will lead to their happiness and success in later tasks, while failure in carrying them out leads to their unhappiness, disapproval by society and failure in later tasks. It is the response that any family assumes for growing up at any point in its life. Families grow when they see what other families, more mature, are accomplishing; they are forming new conceptions of themselves, they are coping effectively with conflicting demands on themselves, and they are motivated to grow (partly by previous successes) enough to work on it. More specifically, a young couple, engaged and newly married, has gone from the stage of intimacy, which can enrich them and free them up to accept the challenges of the next stage. Erikson calls this the stage of generativity, the stage of the young child-bearing family, concerned in establishing and guiding the next generation. It is one in which a couple have defined for themselves, Erikson says, "what and whom they have come to care for, what they care to do well, and how they plan to take care of what they have started and created."

When we hear what he and other thoughtful persons have to say, and when we look now at Duvall's tasks of the usual child-bearing family, Table 2, we wonder how the parents of children with special problems can be expected to carry out the tasks and grow into further stages. We can see more vividly how the carrying out of these tasks by his family becomes so complicated, frustrating, and exhausting and sets up families for a feeling of failure.

Table 3 lists the possible task complications of the
family of the young child with spina bifida. This list is a
bit overwhelming. It has been changed and added to and
deleted from each time I have presented this material. But
tentative as it might be, it does help to see where the
greatest problems and pressures may occur, and how the usual
developmental tasks may need to be supplemented or modified
or carried out not just by the family itself, but by the
people and the systems around the family. These might
include the visiting nurse, the hospital staff, the social
worker, the relatives, the parents' group. Some of these
supplemental tasks are listed in Table 4 and Table 5. As we
and the parents become aware of the tasks and the problem
areas and the help available, the problems can be less overwhelming, and more manageable. As so many parents have said,
"what we know, we can face. It is the unknown that wipes
us out."

You may be asking at this moment, why the need for a
model? Why spell out what may seem so obvious to families,
or what may never have been a felt need for them? But is all
of this so obvious, to them and to us? I don't think so.

We need a structure to make sense out of it for ourselves (and other professionals) so that our role is clearer
not only to us but to the parents. Back in 1972, when we had
our first multi-disciplinary care clinic at Children's
Memorial Hospital, the team devised a questionnaire to ascertain parent satisfaction with the delivery of service.
Some of the questions related to the role of the social
worker. The responses were disquieting. Fifty percent of
the 131 respondents saw the social worker as very helpful,
and 10% saw her as not helpful at all. The correlations
indicated that the families who saw the social worker as most

helpful wanted the doctors to take more responsibility in planning for their child. The marked passivity in their responses was an area of concern for us. These families tended to become too dependent on social workers as well as on physicians. The families who did not find the social worker helpful at all were those who were inclined to deny problems, and were too highly defended from any helpers to use needed services. But most important, from my point of view, were the correlations which indicated that the role of the social worker was poorly perceived. (And I agree that the social worker's own hazy perception of her role on the team could certainly influence this response.) But in a population which objectively would have great need at some time in their lives for helping professionals, this lack of recognition could be a serious problem.

Could it be, I wondered, that the kind of services traditionally offered by social workers to troubled families are not helpful to these families, and that preventive help is not offered at high-risk times? Do we then need a model which points up more clearly the high-risk periods and the ongoing problems relating to the developmental stages of a family? In this way we can enhance our case work skills, our intuition and empathy, and our wish to be helpful in work with these families, and feel less overwhelmed ourselves. We too may go through some of the same stages the parents go through when faced with this assignment; denial, depression, anger, and a sense of helplessness and failure. We need a structure within which to relate to families. We will see better when and how to reach out and when and why to step back. I feel too that the families, after the early months, and the parent's organization, can profit from knowing this material. It can make them more comfortable in asking for

help. They can know what help is available to them, they can
anticipate and prepare for more difficult times, they may be
less inclined to blame themselves, and less inclined to see
themselves as inadequate.

So we will get some of our real data for the model from
the sociological literature, some from observation, some from
trial and error, and a great deal from the parents.

I think it will be helpful to take you through the first
few days and weeks with a family so that we can see in detail
how it is different for them and what their special needs
might be.

This is probably the single most difficult period in the
life of this family. We see first the father, frightened, at
our hospital, talking to the neurosurgeon, making life and
death decisions about his baby's surgery, with his wife at
another hospital, alone and needing him, in a ward with other
young mothers caring for their healthy babies. This is a
critical time. The literature reports that the manner in
which the parent first hears about his child's problem deeply
influences his subsequent behavior.

He has perhaps only recently become comfortable in his
new role as one who "takes care" of his wife and now his
child. He may have his mother and father with him. He may
have to lean heavily on his parents for emotional support at
a time when he has just won a hard struggle within himself to
be independent of his family of origin. His father and
mother may themselves be experiencing shock and disorganization, and may be unable to be supportive, and may even need
to be protected themselves.

This young man is feeling numb and empty, perhaps
unwilling to allow his wife to know ho upset he is for fear

of upsetting her, and she is doing the same, at a time when
mutual acceptance and support are important. Both may have
uncomfortable ambivalent feelings about the survival of the
child, and both may want to run from this pain, and are
ashamed to verbalize what they see as "unspeakable" thoughts.
He may feel that he must protect her from the realities of
the medical picture, unaware that her fantasies may be worse
than the reality. They are both coping too with the indefiniteness of the medical picture. Doctors find it hard,
understandably, to lay the full weight of it on the parents,
and too, may not be able to say definitely what the future
holds for the child.

The father is worried of course about what all this is
going to cost, and at a time when he is faced with his own
feelings of failure, he may see applying for state funds as
another manifestation of his inadequacy. He may be concerned
about how long he can stay away from his job without jeopar-
dizing it. This young couple may still be working out their
relationship with each other, and now we are asking them to
take on the task of caring for the child with special
problems before they have a chance to grieve over the loss of
the "hoped for" child. Birth itself is a family crisis of
limited duration. The birth of a damaged child is a major
crisis.

This young couple will bring, as we all did, their old
eyes and their prejudices to this event. A crippled child -
that was always "them" - now it is "us". They are certainly
of course, aware of the rejecting and pitying attitude of
our society, and feel defensive about their handicapped,
damaged child. As the weeks go by, the couple's concepts of
themselves as providers and as strong adequate persons are in

question. They are afraid that they will be expected to be
more than they can be. Their friends are having healthy
babies and their anger may not allow them the closeness and
support of these friends. Friends, too, may have pulled
away because they don't know what to say. They are told by
relatives and friends and even sometimes by us "you mustn't
cry", or"you must be brave", or "it could be worse". The
message that they get from us is that their grief makes us
feel uncomfortable, and in order to be accepted and included
by us (and this is one of their greatest needs at this time)
they must keep their feelings to themselves. They are made
to feel guilty about the negative feelings they are having.

This young father is often unable to express what he is
feeling. Our society teaches little boys well the lesson
that "big boys don't cry", very poor mental health advice.
He has no role models to follow and no guidelines. He doesn't
know what is expected of him or whether he is doing it right
or not. Our society has welcoming rituals for the healthy
newborn and his family; flowers, handing out cigars, the
teasing of the new father, the christening parties, snapshot
taking, visiting by relatives. We even have rituals for the
family of the baby who dies. But our families enjoy few such
rituals, and the support and the feeling of being included
and cared for that are built into them.

The young mother cannot "take care" of her baby during
these early days, cannot hold him or feed him, things which
could help her to manage her feelings of helplessness. When
the baby goes home from the hospital, all of the built-in
helps are there, but with the new life-style to be adjusted
to, and the real concerns about the future, it is easy for
the mother and father to feel harassed and exhausted and
resentful. They find it hard to recognize, or have time for,

or even see the legitimacy of their own needs as spouses and
as persons.

This family then is generally experiencing, in the early
days, shock, grief, disorganization and emptiness. As the
realities of the diagnosis become more obvious, they experience a sense of isolation, a wish for flight, feelings of
anger and resentment, and a sense of helplessness and failure.

How does all of this fit into the model? Look now again
at the developmental tasks of the family of the young child,
on Table 2. Some of the tasks listed are "celebrating the
rituals of birth", "learning to care for the child with
competence and assurance" and another few - "maintaining a
satisfactory emotional and sexual relationship with spouse
separate from role as parent", accepting and adjusting to and
enjoying the independence from their family of origin", and
"establishing a new and rewarding relationship with one's own
parents and in-laws". The fulfillment of these tasks for our
families is very difficult. Might there not be other and
better ways of fulfilling these tasks for the family that are
more within their capabilities to carry out? Could a grand-
mother take over some of the roles in the family, can a day-
care center offer some breathing space and help the parents
make the adjustment to a new kind of parenthood, can the
parents seek out other parents to see how they cope with
these unique pressures? Can the visiting nurse help the
parents learn to care for the child with competence? Can the
social worker help the family to understand more fully how
the impact of this can affect them as a couple, emotionally,
sexually, and socially. And probably most importantly, can
the couple themselves, as they grow more aware of their needs
as a family, develop their own unique way to work out these
tasks?

Again, what about the professional helper? Social workers have always offered support and encouragement to families under stress, but the 1972 questionnaire, and the literature, supports the fact that families too often see what we do as something either mysterious and magic and controlling, or, on the other hand, not helpful at all. It is important that the helping process feel more tangible and be more tangible to these families, and it needs to be shared with these families in some creative way. Does the model then, help us to see more clearly what the needs are and how and where the social workers might best intervene?

But before we examine what the social workers do we need to think about what goals we and the family might have that are different from the usual family goals. This can clarify for us what the parent's expectations of themeselves and us, are and should be.

These early goals for the social worker may be:

1) To help the family to acknowledge and work through their grief.

2) To give support, comfort, and acceptance to the family.

3) To help the family to define the problem; medically, socially, financially.

4) To give the family some beginning feeling of mastery over the problem with some success experiences (learning to handle and feed the baby, telling relatives, applying for financial assistance).

5) Helping the family to acknowledge and deal with negative feelings.

6) Helping the family to begin to relate to the hospital system.

7) Helping the family to see the hospital as a helping place.

8) To begin to introduce alternate community, family, and agency support systems (VNA, parent's group, relatives, other parents).

9) To help families to recognize their own needs.

10) To help the family to begin to consider some changes in their life-style.

I see the long range goals for the family as:

1) Their continuing use of the hospital as a helping place.

2) Their recognition of their own legitimate needs and the individual needs of their members.

3) Their feeling of mastery over their own life and problems, with a succession of success experiences (involvement with the parent's group, school planning, helping new parents).

4) Their ability to ask for help when needed.

5) Their ability to use extended family and community resources as supports.

6) Their inclusion of the handicapped child within the family system.

7) Their creation of a new life-style which is satisfying to all family members.

8) Their ability to function independently.

9) Their ability to understand and live with chronic anxiety, rage, and sorrow.

10) Eventual independence of their handicapped child (if that is possible).

My priority, as you can see from these goals, is the family, not the child. My approach is preventive,

anticipating stress and problems, teaching productive ways
of coping and survival, allowing the expression of feelings,
especially "unacceptable" ones, emphasizing family life
education, encouraging families to work with other families,
and teaching ways to get what they want and need from the
hospital system and the community.

My early contacts with a family are almost non-verbal in
content, indicating to them that I and the hospital staff
care about what is happening to them, want to help, and can
help.

My first formal interview with the couple, usually
before the baby is 3 weeks old, is a lengthy one. I may know
the parents slightly by this time, either through phone calls
or bedside visits. I try to help them pinpoint their concerns, medically, financially, whatever. They are encouraged
to express their grief, and their negative feelings. We
discuss their own needs as individuals. We anticipate together what the next few weeks and months might be life.
They are encouraged to talk about themselves, their family,
their parents, as we explore ways they have coped with
pressure in the past. They think about who can be helpful
and supportive to them now, and who will need help. We talk
about how they will be needing support and communication from
each other when it may be very hard to give. I also introduce to them the idea that there are other parents who want
to be helpful to them.

We talk about the hospital system, how it works, and
what their relationship to it will be. During the following
weeks I may see the parents on a regular basis or informally.
When the child goes home, hopefully the family will by now
feel more in control of their lives, less isolated and less
helpless. They usually know their way around the hospital,

call the staff and other parents by name, and are greeted by
name. They know where to get coffee and change, and how to
arrange to sleep overnight in the waiting room. They usually
know by now the extent of the handicap (as far as it is
possible to know) and are hopefully beginning to enter a
period of re-integration with some kind of acknowledgement
(not acceptance - can one ever accept?) of the situation.
They have usually fed and held the baby many times.

They have had conferences with the nurses regarding
special nursing procedures, and with the physical therapist
regarding exercises, which they may already be doing themselves. They are usually impatient to take the baby home but
frightened of the responsibility. They will know that the
visiting nurse is available to them for moral support as well
as for nursing help.

They will have been in touch with the agencies for
financial help. They may have talked with the floor chaplain
and been encouraged to seek out their clergyman for support.
(This is an important step since so many parents and many of
use see the "why" of this as one of the hardest things that
we and they have to struggle with.) They may already be in
touch with the parents' group or have made friends with
another parent in the hospital. They know how they can reach
me. They are encouraged to contact the hospital if medical
problems arise. They have talked many times with the coordinator of the MM/MCD program, know that they have her
support and help and have follow-up clinic visits already
scheduled. So they have a relatively clear picture of what
the pressures of the next months might be, and know how to
get more information and help if they need it. Lydia
Rapoport calls this anticipatory work "emotional immunization".

Another important part of the parents' ability to
survive this difficult time is the independent parents'
organization, a group we work closely with. It can be one of
the most constructive factors in the lives of these families
and offers something very special to them. It meets the
needs of the isolated family, in search of role models; it
offers friendship and practical help; and it gives families
a vehicle through which they can do something about what has
happened to them and their child. One of the major tasks
accomplished by the group is the feeling of mastery the
families have when they can make changes in their communities
and school.s Probably the greatest contribution the organization makes is its outreach to new parents. Routinely now,
we offer new parents a chance to talk with parents of an
older child. All new parents do not use this service, but
those who do report the relief they feel after talking with
thems, and seeing them as ones who have survived. But
another positive thing takes place. The parents who volun-
teer and go to help new parents, feel good, even though old
hurts and memories are activated, because in many ways
reaching out to new parents spells out in a graphic way to
parents of the older child, that they have indeed coped,
they have survived, they do have mastery over their lives
once again.

Specifically, then, what are some of the things that
arise out of our new ways of looking at the family that seem
to be working, so that the family can carry out its developmental tasks and go on to further stages of growth?

We pay serious attention to the parents as individuals
and spouses (as separate from parents) and help them to
recognize and acknowledge the legitimacy of their own needs.
We create some alternate (and maybe temporary) communities

or support groups for the family to deal with the feeling of isolation (the ward, the hospital, the staff, the parents' group). We anticipate with them as much of the problems of the coming weeks and months as possible and separate out with them the tasks to be dealt with to reduce the feeling of helplessness. We encourage them to talk out the feelings they have, especially the ones they see as unacceptable. We supply them with some psychological tools to deal with the feelings of guilt, anger and failure. We teach them skills in handling their child's physical needs, so that they are again competent in their child's life. We teach them some skills to deal with the hospital system, the community systems, and the social welfare systems.

We offer concrete help around finances, community resources, nursing care, and we work to broaden community resources. We work with the parents' group to enhance their outreach to new parents, and to incorporate their insights into our hospital and clinic program, encouraging them to see themselves as part of the team, to increase their feelings of mastery and control.

How is this at all different from the way it has always been done? First it is planned and self-conscious; it is shared as much as possible with the parents, who feel they have a say in some of the decision-making; the parents, not the child are the priority; and the total team works with the parents' group in what might be called a partner relationship.

With all of this I feel that we are only beginning to scratch the surface of the problem. So far we have talked only about the early weeks and months. The other high-risk periods are the period of gait-training, when the child's differentness becomes highly visible; the period around the first school placement, when separation from the mother is the issue; the later latency years, when the size and weight of the child makes his care at home more difficult for his parents, and when the parents are most apt to ask for residential placement; and of course, the adolescent years when their own aging and the whole future for their child as a handicapped adult faces the parents.

It is my feeling that a developmental task model can be helpful for working with families of children with spina bifida over a number of years. It helps us to see them as ordinary families under extraordinary stress. We need, of course, all the skills and insights that the public health model and the crisis intervention approach offer, but since our families' crises are in effect life-long we need a larger and more comprehensive framework and way of helping that this model provides for this population-at-risk, so that they may go on to manage their *own* lives in a satisfying way.

TABLE 1.

Medical Milestones

New Born	Repair of back, shunt - if needed
	Shunt complications
	Pediatric evaluation
	Orthopedic evaluation
	Urology evaluation
	Physical Therapy evaluation
Infancy	Supervision of urinary tract infections
	Correction of orthopedic deformities
	Occupational therapy work up
	Shunt observations
Early Childhood	Beginning bracing
	Gait training
Pre-school	Continued observation for orthopedic, urologic and neurosurgical problems
	Possible ileal conduit
	Bowel training program
School	Observation for scoliosis
	Continued urologic monitoring
	Bowel training program
Adolescence	Continued orthopedic and G.U. monitoring
	Changing body of adolescence
	Monitoring and/or treatment for scoliosis
	Possible return to wheelchair
	Obesity problems

TABLE 2.

Developmental Tasks of Family*

Readiness to forego immediate sexual and emotional needs because of pregnancy, birth and infant's needs

Working towards maintaining a new sexual and emotional relationship with spouse, separate from role as parent

Continuing to develop as individuals and as a married couple

Accepting and adjusting to stresses and pressures of parenthood

Learning to juggle multiple roles and learn new roles

Reconciling conflicting conceptions of roles and adjusting to new expectations of spouse

Regaining family equilibrium when baby comes home

Celebrating the rituals of birth

Readiness to acknowledge psychological, material, and financial responsibility for infant and sharing this responsibility with spouse

Readiness to be involved in physical care of infant and learning to care for child with competence and confidence

Developing parental expectations of their child

Providing full opportunities for the child's development

Mutually supporting and reconciling the developmental needs and tasks of parents, baby, and siblings in ways that strengthen child and family as a whole

Creating together an atmosphere of love in the home

Creating and maintaining effective communication within family

Beginning to work on a shared value and meaning system as a family

Enjoying a growing family with siblings, teaching a sharing in household, and planning future family

(Father) assuming major responsibility for earning family income

(Mother) giving up income and role as income provider

TABLE 2. (cont.)

(Mother) keeping alive some sense of personal autonomy throughout young motherhood

(Father) maintaining a satisfactory sense of self as an individual, while becoming a "family" man, who "takes care" of his family

Facing and adjusting to changing housing, spending, time and space patterns, needs and rituals, and developing healthful and satisfactory family routines to meet changing needs

Establishing a home within family's income capabilities

Cultivating full potential of relationships with extended family

Accepting, adjusting to, and enjoying independence from family of origin

Sharing responsibilities and struggles of young parenthood with other parents

Exploring and developing a satisfactory sense of being a family within a larger community

Tapping resources, seeing needs and enjoying contacts outside the family

TABLE 3.

Possible Task Complications

Initial abandonment of hopes and plans for child and family

Ambivalence about child's survival and guilt about feelings of anger and flight

Concerns about one's own loss of control and ability to cope

Early separation of parents, of mother from infant, and isolation of mother

Reconciling mother's need to take care of and hold child, to feed and nurse child, with hospital rules and medical procedures

Early "protecting" of mother by relatives and husband, excluding her from decision-making

Accepting one's own or spouse's negative or different feelings about child's problems and facing own prior feelings about handicapped children

Poor communication because each parent concerned about upsetting partner with own feelings

Dealing with grief and loss of "expected" child and immediate need to take on care of "other" child

Difficulty in coming to terms with problem because of indefiniteness of medical picture

Reconciling one's concept of physician as authority, with one's rights as parent

Reconciling father's concept of being one who "takes care" of his family, with inability to make his child well, to protect his wife, or to solve this problem

Difficulty of mother in recognizing own needs and sense of personal autonomy

Role confusion because of demands of time and energy on both parents

Tendency to protect and exclude father from decision-making and concerns at hospital and clinic, paralleling early exclusion of mother

Necessity of living near medical care, or having transportation to it

---

TABLE 3. (cont.)

Managing hidden costs of baby's medical problem (meals out, changed housing needs, etc.)

Father's coping by immersion in job and mother's resultant anger and isolation

Necessity of asking for financial assistance, and dealing with welfare system

Reconciling family needs with job responsibilities, often for both parents

Fear of job or pay loss, and difficulty in finding another because of time needs and insurance problems

Adjusting to change in personal and family life-style, without role models

Postponing of mother's plans for continuing career, if desired

Adjusting community and family rituals of birth to new circumstances

Accepting child with limited potential, without resentment, loss of hope, or immobilizing disappointment

Recognizing the necessity for setting limits on child's behavior, and dealing with relatives' and community's lack of understanding of this need

Differentiating normal infant behavior and fussiness from medical problems

Handling and accepting normal annoyance toward child, and facing community's norm that one must not have anger, rejecting feelings, or a wish to flee

Concerns about ability to meet and reconcile legitimate needs of present and future children, in light of needs of this child

Facing decisions regarding future pregnancies, the chance of a damaged child, or abortion

Impact of genetic implications and "blame" on parents relationship, and on how they see themselves as persons, parents, and sexual partners

Reactivation of old conflicts with grandparents re: dependence/independence

TABLE 3. (cont.)

Ambivalence re: relatives assuming a large role in family's life because of needs

Necessity of placing responsibility for parental chores on friends, relatives, other children

Dealing with child-bearing siblings of parents, and with relatives, who may see this birth as a genetic threat to, or assault on, them

Dealing with grandparents' crisis and fears and need to protect and console them

Difficulty in sharing struggles of young parenthood with other young parents

Dealing with total lack of knowledge of this birth defect in the community

Facing community/family norm that one must place/not place child

Facing friends with healthy new babies and sharing their joy without resentment

Difficulty in exploring sense of family in the community because of isolation and fatigue, and retreat of friends and community in fear and embarrassment

Lack of knowledge of what is expected by the hospital and community

Learning to do battle for self and child in the sophisticated medical system

Struggling to find and retain meaning and a value system in light of these unique experiences

TABLE 4.

Possible Supplementary Tasks of the Family

Learning to acknowledge and live with grief and loss

Learning to use the hospital and clinic as a helping place, part of their support group

Learning to work with, relate to, and trust physicians while retaining sense of one's own rights

Learning to ask appropriate and relevant questions - to speak up

Learning to recognize own rights and needs as person and spouse, vis-a-vis needs and rights of child

Learning to become competent and assured with the infant and his medical and nursing needs

Learning to recognize and live with conflicting and often negative feelings toward infant, hospital, helping persons, and one's spouse

Learning creative ways to anticipate and manage severe stress, fatigue, anxiety, and anger

Making a change to a life style which accommodates to new needs

Finding and using alternate support systems; grandparents, friends, community resources

Learning to use caring relatives and friends, as emotional supports when needed

Recognizing the need for and becoming adept in asking for help when needed

Learning ways to enrich marital life in spite of special demands

Accepting and living with diminished hopes for the child

Learning to reach out to new families

Understanding one's own and one's spouses dependent/independent conflicts relating to the extended family

Enhancing communication in the family

Learning to adjust to shifting roles in the family

TABLE 4. (cont.)

Recognizing the special needs of the siblings of the handi-
    capped baby

Helping the handicapped child to become an integral part of
    the family

Learning the intricacies and subtleties of applying for
    financial aid

TABLE 5.

Possible Tasks of the Systems Around the Family

Hospital
    Supplying medical and nursing care
    Supplying adequate information and communication re:
        medical problems
    Supplying information re: medical resources
    Supplying genetic counseling
    Being open to needs of parents
    Creating of a therapeutic community on hospital wards
    Creating a clinic system that works for parents
    Raising public consciousness regarding the medical
        problem and its physical and social consequences

Social Worker
    Offering crisis intervention services
    Offering counseling services and family life education
    Creating new resources; searching for existing resources;
        referring to and compiling of current resources
    Anticipating problems and crisis periods with parents
    Raising public consciousness regarding social/emotional
        needs of children and parents
    Being resource person to parents' groups
    Referring of parents to parents' groups and other
        parents
    Interpreting to agencies in community the special needs
        of families
    Interpreting families' needs and concerns to hospital
        and staff
    Social research/data collecting

TABLE 5. (cont.)

Community
    Creating and developing of early childhood development
        programs
    Creating and developing concrete social/medical services
        for total family needs
    Making available adequate financial help
    Raising of public consciousness

Friends and Extended Family
    Creating and maintaining of a support group for family
    Including child and family in neighborhood and community
        functions
    Making available financial, emotional, practical help
        when needed
    Assuming some parental roles when needed

Public Health Nurse
    Interpreting home and nursing concerns to hospital
    Acting as liaison between hospital and parent
    Giving emotional support to parents
    Teaching family life skills
    Teaching child care skills

HOSPITALIZATION

Leonard Harris, M.D.

Hospitalization of children with myelomeningocele is a major issue, for we can anticipate multiple hospitalizations over the course of these children's lives. If we can understand something of a child's perception and responses to hospitalization, we can be more helpful and supportive; if we can understand and respond better to those factors that influence the child's perception and responses, then we can make the experience if not exactly enjoyable, at least tolerable. With repeated hospitalizations the child will then be able to develop a tolerance and a relative mastery of the entire process. If we do not understand, the children can and do become increasingly anxious with each episode, until they can become almost panic stricken at the thought of entering the hospital. Essentially we are talking of a traumatic situation which can be dealt with and integrated as compared to a destructive, negatively re-enforcing cycle that can be perpetuating and accelerating.

There are a complex set of interactions that occur when any child is admitted to the hospital. These involve the child, the parent, the medical staff and the hospital itself. I shall attempt to separate out some of the basic issues within each of the component features mentioned, but we must understand that each factor influences and in turn is

influenced by the other. Any separation that I will make is
therefore overly simplistic, but at least I hope it may lead
to a better comprehension of the hospitalization experience
which in turn can aid all of us in being of help to the child
and the parents.

Preparation for hospitalization actually begins the day
the child is born. So much of a youngster's responses to any
stressful situation depends upon the child's prior
experiences in the home during the various stages of development. If a child has a strong feeling of security, stability,
trust in their parents and the general environment, they will
be better able to deal with the stress of a hospitalization
experience. If the youngster has had major developmental
difficulties before hospitalization, no matter how well we
attempt to deal with the situation, these children will have
greater problems both in the hospital and following discharge.
However, these children too can be helped through this period
of stress.

Children have different reactions to hospitalization
depending upon their age and the associated stage of development that they are attempting to master. I shall be discussing the infant and the young child.

Infants and young children have to deal predominantly
with issues of separation from the parent. Although as
infants they may not know or understand what is occurring,
they can sense a difference in the type and style of care
they receive. They also sense a difference in the environment. This can and does lead to anxiety, fretfulness and
crying. This has little to do with the capability of the
caretaking people. Merely the difference in caretaking is
sufficient to trigger off this anxiety. One must also
remember that there are inherent differences in children's

basic personality types. Some youngsters will be little upset by minor changes in their routines; others will be terribly upset and irritable. In this area it is helpful if the hospital personnel can have some understanding of what the youngster's basic routines are and how this child tends to respond to changes in routines, something the parents may very well have noted in their own home.

The older infant who is past the symbiotic phase and has become aware of the mother as a person who ministers to his or her needs still does not have a good internalized image of the parent. After a variable period of time, the child will lose this image. We state that the child has not as yet attained object constancy. Most commonly this is referred to as the stage of separation anxiety. The loss of this internalized security figure (the mother) leads to a feeling of abandonment and severe anxiety. With this you will see a child who will cry severely, almost mourning the loss of the mother. After a period of time many of the children will go into a true depression and withdraw, refusing to eat or drink. These children will whine rather than cry when disturbed. They are often termed "good" babies, because they do not cry and fuss greatly and are not demanding babies. It is only when we look closer at their behavior and often note how slowly they seem to respond to medication and surgery, that we become aware that they are acutely and severely depressed babies.

If the parents can stay with children of this age range, this feeling of abandonment with the attendant anxiety can be alleviated. With many children the mother can transfer her "mantle" of acceptance to someone on the hospital ward or floor. This person can then temporarily act as a surrogate mother. But only temporarily. The mother needs to be with

this age child more than just during the visiting hours once
or twice through the day.

As a child gets older, out of the toddler phase, the
child should have a greater sense of security about the
availability of the mother and can tolerate her absence for
longer periods of time. Progressively therefore, with age,
a child will have less of a feeling of total abandonment but
will still need the mother to be available. If the child is
old enough to have been away from her for protracted periods
of time, such as during the school years, the mother may not
necessarily be needed constantly, but daily visiting is still
imperative. This must be clarified with the child. The
parents may well have to clearly define the times they will
arrive and the times they will leave. If they give the
youngster a time, they should be there at that time.

Compounding this problem of anxiety over parental
absence/loss is the factor of regression under conditions of
stress. And, hospitalization is a stress. The child that
can tolerate separation for longer periods, under stress will
regress and respond as a younger child, with more need for
parental support.

An obvious but often overlooked aspect affecting the
response of a child to hospitalization is the level of the
child's cognitive development. The young infant is not truly
aware of his/her surroundings but is responsive to a gestalt
of the experience. They respond to the differences in the
caring person, noises, smells, the feelings of their clothes,
covers and linen. The somewhat older child is aware of the
difference in the environment, but not necessarily as we
adults tend to perceive these differences. Certainly, the
child is not aware of the reasons for the changed environment.

Something totally strange is anxiety provoking in all. This does not only apply to children. As adults, we would be anxious in a situation that was totally strange, where we do not understand the rationale behind the need for the change, or the situation itself. Fortunately, as adults, we have a large experience of prior episodes that might be seen somewhat similarly. We can draw upon our past in order to help us deal with this new, strange problem. A child does not have this backlog of past experiences.

Children by about four or five do have some ideas about hospitals, but they are distortions culled from their inadequate experiences. The hospital is often seen as threatening and dangerous. Ambulances and hospitals are seen on television as life threatening conditions. Fear and great concern is usually portrayed in the melodramas viewed by the children. Hospitals are places where people are badly upset, Ergo, they must be bad. Family members at home may have spoken in hushed, frightened tones about someone who "had to go to the hospital", an implication of potential danger. Fantasies abound. Usually the child's fantasies are much worse than anything we can or do realistically contemplate. Yet we all too often do not tell the child of impending procedures in words and language they can understand.

Children have a lack of knowledge of their own bodies and internal anatomy. All have an awareness of pain. Brief technical explanations of what is to be done for them (a child will usually see this as being done *to* him) are often distorted and extremely frightening. Few youngsters even receive this minimal amount of information. Frequently all they will acquire are some bits and pieces of information that were told to the parents in the child's presence. They

invariably remember the most frightening aspects of what
they heard.

All surgical procedures are seen as an attack. If one
can explain the procedure and process at the child's level
of understanding, with emphasis on the positive aspects of
what will be hopefully accomplished, the child can better
deal with his fears. It would be unusual for a child, and
no differently than an adult, to *welcome* the procedure, but
they may accept it better. This is not to say that the
children should be given a false picture of hospitalization
or any surgical procedure. They should be told the truth.
However, pain and discomfort need not be dwelt upon and young
children respond quite well to a reassurance that everything
will be done that is possible to make them comfortable. An
additional aspect of a child's perception that influences
their reaction to hospitalization and surgery, is that most
children see pain and discomfort as punishment for real or
imagined transgressions. Some emphasis needs to be made to
the child that the hospital and/or surgery is a necessity,
not a response to misbehavior; that this process is to be
seen as helpful, not punishing.

All children have fears of bodily mutilation. Damaged
children have an even greater fear of further damage or
disability occurring. These aspects apply to all children
requiring surgical procedures. For a child with myelomeningocele, clarification of the surgical procedure is a
necessity, not only to deal with the issues mentioned above,
but to clearly state what is to be hopefully accomplished.
This should be dealt with honestly, for the child, as an
adult, may have totally unrealistic expectations. When these
are not met, the disappointment is hard to bear. Not only
that, but the physician and even the parents will then become

suspect in the child's eyes. Giving false hopes that have to
be dashed, is a cruel thing to do to anyone, even if this is
done inadvertently.

The hospital itself has some built-in problems for all
children. Over and beyond the concern about the strange and
threatening environment, the child has to deal with a
situation wherein she or he has to give up control and
custody of their own being. Others are to once again be
involved in areas that have become self-care areas, issues
that the child has relatively recently mastered. Now, once
again, the child has to permit others to bathe him, turn him,
be involved with his bladder and bowel functions and
possibly even with eating. Children who have recently
recognized a satisfaction and pleasure of feeling competent
in these areas have to yield them. Many children will fight
this regressive pull by the hospital. Their own regression
is enough of a problem to them. This added requirement of
regressive behavior is more than they can tolerate. The look
on some children's faces when they are placed in a crib,
after being in a bed for six months or more, shows how
devastated they can be by this experience. A bed with side-
rails, to a young child, is also perceived as very much like
a crib. There is a feeling that they are not trusted to be
"a big boy or girl". Yet, we ask them to tolerate procedures
like a big boy and girl.

Modesty may or may not be an issue. Hospital personnel
tend to lose sight of this, especially when working with
younger children. Granted, the staff may not be concerned
about a nude or partially dressed child, but what of the
child's feelings?

Hospitals do not present any real opportunity for
children to utilize their most common and helpful defense

against anxiety. This is activity, be it physical or verbal.
Children in hospitals are expected to be quiet and docile.
Disruption is seen as rebellious behavior and is poorly
tolerated. There is good reason for much of this need for
quiet. Excessive activity and noise is disturbing to other
ill patients and disruptive to routines. But it is not helpful for the activity oriented child. It leads to angry
interactions between child, parents and hospital personnel.
Even verbal activity is discouraged, if not overtly at least
covertly. How can a child feel free to be angry and yell at
a nurse who then might be angry with him? If the child is
already uncomfortable over the procedures that are necessary,
how much more uncomfortable can the situation become if the
nurse would be angry at him?

If sufficient pressure is brought to bear, some children
will respond with total rebellion against all routines and
are "bad" patients. Some respond in turn by totally giving
up and acquiescing. They then become totally demanding and
infantile - again - "bad" patients. We really do tend to
give mixed messages to children in the hospital in that we
should like them to be independent in the areas we think are
important and to allow themselves to be totally dependent,
again in the areas we think are important. Unfortunately,
these areas may not necessarily coincide with the child's
list of priorities. If a child's behavior is engendering
some angry feelings, they will recognize this and it does
little but accentuate their own fears of danger and attack
from those who are honestly trying to be of help to them.

All the above operates with children that are in
relatively good physical condition. For a damaged child,
whatever the damage may be, it is even more accentuated.
These children are aware that they have fewer self-resources

to call upon to care for themselves and to defend themselves
against a strange and frightening situation. This applies to
any damaged child, and any ill child is a damaged or weakened
child. Certainly children with myelomeningocele feel even
more insecure. This then will tend to lead to even more
dependency and again a greater need for the parents.

Parents have a major role in assisting the child through
a hospitalization experience. It is much more than just
being available to help the child deal with separation
anxiety. Something we often forget is that children respond
to their families' responses and apply this familial style
of relating. If the mother of a youngster is anxious, tense,
frightened and insecure, the child will tend to respond
similarly. Discussion between professional staff and the
youngster, no matter what the age, will be relatively fruit-
less. The child will perceive the mother's anxiety, respond
to that and in turn will be anxious. If the parent is more
secure and feels that she can trust the physician, the
helping team, the hospital and if she has a positive attitude
toward what is about to be done in the hospital, the child
will be able to accept the issue of hospitalization and whatever procedures are necessary much more readily. Children
respond to the parents' behavior much more than to the
verbalization of either the parents or others.

As children get older they will acquire different views
and attitudes than their parents, but the family attitudes
at a time of stress such as this, will always tend to be
there. Some precociously mature and older children are
amazingly strong and can actually aid their parents through
the process of their own hospitalization and surgery. Many
of us have seen this type of role reversal. Generally, this
is not appropriate. The child has enough of a burden in

dealing with his own internal anxieties and fears without
having to bear their parents' burdens. Remember again, that
an older child might very well regress and respond as a
younger child, once more relying upon parental views and
attitudes and utilizing these as a paradigm for their own
responses and behaviors.

I feel we sometimes lose sight of this aspect of
parenting - the impact of the families' attitudes. As such,
it behooves us to be certain that parents are not seen as
interfering or demanding, but to recognize that the parents
also have needs that must be met. They go through the entire
process of hospitalization with their children and are
anxious and fearful for their own reasons. If we can meet
the parents' needs by understanding this aspect, and respond
by clarifying not only what is going on, but what is to be
done, they will be much more comfortable and more able to
trust their physicians and the entire medical staff they come
in contact with. Their comfort will then be felt by the
child with subsequent relaxation and relative trust in this
new and frightening environment. Information given to the
parents can and should be utilized by them to prepare the
child as much as possible. The greater the preparation for
the procedure, the fewer the unknowns there will be, and the
less anxiety that will be engendered.

I have pointed up some of the issues that children have
difficulty dealing with during a period of hospitalization
and/or surgery. I hope I have emphasized sufficiently the
need of the child for the parents' support. This does not
mean that the parents are to become overly involved and
overly protective of the child. It does mean that the
parents should be an active participant in the child's
hospitalization; that the parents should be prepared for some

of these concerns that their children might be having about
hospital and surgery, in order to be able to understand, to
be supportive, and to help the child to deal with these fears
and anxieties. Hopefully during the hospital stay, the
parents can aid in the care of the child so that they can
feel that they have some important role in concretely helping
the youngster - not feeling that they have given up total
control of their child to others.

To be of support to the child, to prepare the child, to
develop an aura of confidence in the hospital and staff, to
translate to the child the necessity and the meaning behind
the procedures required are roles for the parents. Many
parents will require assistance from team and hospital
personnel in these areas. Limits may well have to be set
upon the children and upon the parents when their own
anxieties become overwhelming. The process of "parentectomy",
severely limiting the mother's contact with her child at a
period of stress, has little to recommend it.

The role of the physician, nurses or other members of
the team working with the child is to be more aware of the
issues and fears children are attempting to deal with during
a hospital experience. They can relate to the children in
their daily contacts in such a way as to attempt to alleviate
as much of their anxiety as possible and to support the
parents in their attempts to be supporting and helpful to
their children.

We must not forget that the parents have needs, fears,
and anxieties that must be dealt with. By helping the
parents we are helping the child. The parents are also a
part of a family unit and although we can see the great needs
of the hospitalized child, there are others in the family who
also need the parents. By overly identifying with the child

who is our patient, we may place an excessive burden on the
parents. They will need our help if for reason of demands
by siblings, or other family members, job or their own intra-
psychic difficulties they cannot offer the optimum involvement with our hospitalized patient. Our role then is to
alleviate some of their guilt and accept what they can do for
the child. Theory does not necessarily match practical
reality situations. We then can define how we can "fill in
for the parents" when they cannot be present.

We must remember that we are *not* better parents than the
parents. Our major role is helping the parents for their
own needs and in order to help them help their children.
Children are not little adults. They have minimal experience,
distorted perceptions, and fewer coping mechanisms than an
adult. Their greatest consistent support has been and should
continue to be their parents. Only in those situations where
parents very obviously cannot be of help to the child should
an attempt be made to usurp this role.

MYELOMENINGOCELE INFANT MAT PROGRAM

Eva Nakos, LPT and Susan Taylor, OTR

The original Infant Mat Program was started January, 1973, with six children enrolled; since then approximately six groups have followed. Of 150 children who are followed in the clinic, 31 children have gone through the mat program.

The program was initiated on the assumption that the child with myelomeningocele appeared to have delayed physical and visual-perceptual development. Psychological testing revealed this at age 4-5 years. There was also a need for the parents to feel comfortable handling their new child, and to provide the stimulation needed for development.

The purpose with the program is therefore twofold:

1. For the child:

    To encourage normal motor, visual-perceptual and social development to his maximum potential within the limitations of his disability.

2. For the parents:

    To receive instructions in normal development and care of the young infant and become acquainted with preparations for future management and concerns. We do encourage *total* family involvement to relieve the mother's responsibilities and worries.

In this area, most newborn myelomeningocele infants are transferred to Children's Hospital for medical care. They

are referred to us from Dr. Oppenheimer, the Director of the
team. The team as a whole decides who will be enrolled in
the program, since this depends on the following considerations:

1. The family's geographical location (distance to
hospital).

2. Means of transportation for the family.

3. Financial situation of the parents.

4. Parent's interest and willingness to learn more
about the disability. (Religion, Cultural, Mentality)

We need a minimum of four children enrolled to start the
program: This allows us to charge a lower group rate based
on the staff and the time involved.

Several different approaches have been tried in terms of
frequency and length of the program. We have found that the
most beneficial approach is to meet every week for two hours
for a period of eight weeks. At the end of the program we
make arrangements to check the children once a month to
follow their developmental progress. On occasion we have
held special sessions in the evening or on Saturday in an
effort to involve the fathers in the program.

The staff involved in the program includes a social
worker, an occupational therapist and a physical therapist.
The social worker initially interviews the parents either at
their home or at the hospital to inquire about their feelings,
their financial status and possible transportation problems,
and their interest in participating in a group program. In
the group, the social worker is the discussion leader and
very often plays a supportive role during the discussions.
The occupational therapist is involved in instruction in
normal development, perceptual and sensory awareness and
feeding management. The physical therapist's involvement is

in normal development; prevention of contractures by doing
range of motion exercises; correct positioning, handling and
lifting; and appropriate brace care. These three disciplines
determine if another discipline has to be called upon for
consultation. (Pediatrician, nutrition, etc.)

We initially focus on the child's status in relation to
normal growth and development. We use the Denver Developmental Screening Test as one of our evaluation tools.
Although it is limited in accurately assessing a specific
developmental level, it does give us a base line of what the
child's abilities are; particularly in fine motor-adaptive
skills.

In some of our population, we have seen some feeding
problems such as oral hypersensitivity, tongue thrust and
poor jaw closure. Interviewing the mother gives some idea if
there is a problem and then leads to further evaluation of
the child.

The purpose of the Physical Therapy evaluation form is
to be able to determine the level of function of the child
with myelomeningocele. The form is used with the infants in
the program and with other children seen in the clinic.

When we do an initial evaluation, we want to determine
the following:

1. The muscle strength, which is tested as a common
manual muscle test adapted to infants. The abdominals are
the first muscle group tested since the level of the lesion
is mostly in the lumbar area.

2. The muscle activity: are the movements controlled,
voluntary or just reflex movements?

3. The sensation is tested with a pinch instead of a
sharp or dull object. We want to determine where the level
of sensation is normal, hypoesthesia or anesthesia.

4.   The range of motion and possible deformities and contractures. The most common deformities and contractures are listed on the form. If others are present we note that also.

Why do we want to know all the above mentioned? This enables us to let the parents (especially parents of infants) know what their child's optimum potential can be in motor development. Other factors influencing the child's development include his intellectual ability, his motivation, and the parents involvement and understanding of their child's problem.

The evaluation of the child is completed during the first group session. The remainder of the group sessions focus on normal development and how each individual child fits into the developmental sequence. Because we attempt to deal with the total child, we find that discussing not only his developmental needs, but also his medical care gives the parent a clearer picture in terms of overall management. Beginning the group with a list of frequently heard medical terms, defined in layman's language, sets the foundation for future discussions.

Major areas of development are covered in discussion and treatment; including gross and fine motor skill, language, and personal-social skills.

A particular area of concern to us has been the visual involvement and how that affects the child's perception and thus, his hand function. It also appears that fine motor function is at a more primitive stage than seen in similar aged non-handicapped children. We frequently see a hand preference even within the first several months of life.

Because of positioning following shunt procedure, the babies often seem to prefer to hold their head to one side.

We have not been able to relate this directly to the shunting as it has not been found to occur consistently to one side more than the other. Our concern has been that development of head control is seemingly delayed in some of the babies following the shunt procedure.

These are a representative sample of some of the specific things we deal with in the group. The method of presentation is talking first about what is expected of a child going through the normal developmental sequence. We make it specific to the individual according to his age. Then we demonstrate what the parents can be doing at home to help the child. And finally, we have the parent try the activity with their child.

SUMMARY

In preparing for today's presentation, we found it necessary to take a critical look at this program in relation to providing optimum services to our MM infant population. We do not have statistical data to scientifically support the program, but we have found that the parent's feedback; the child's progress and our own evaluation of the group have helped us view it in a positive way.

The parents seem to gain an appreciation for the potential of their own child within the limitations of his handicap. They learn that they can do something to help their child to progress along a normal sequence of development. They gain greater insight into the medical management and the many questions regarding the child's future independence are answered.

Another significant aspect is the group dynamics that allow the parents to support one another in their learning to cope with a handicapped child.

It seems that the early intervention affects the child's mobility in general. As he is aware of his own body and his ability to control what he does, he becomes less fearful of movement in space. This later will affect his motivation and ability to ambulate.

The program has not been free of problems. We'd like to share some of those, too. Probably the single factor influencing the group's success is consistent attendance. This is largely dependent upon the geographical distribution of the infant population in relation to our Center. It seems that many of the families are from out-lying areas (Indiana, Northern Ohio or Kentucky). Travel time and expense often prohibit attendance at all, or influence consistency.

A group may originally have five or six children in it and end up with two or three. One group this past year had to be discontinued because of the five participants only one consistently came for the program.

Another frustration for us has been coverage of payment for the therapy services in the group. We must have a minimum of six children to be eligible to charge a group rate, $6.00. Any less than this, has to be charged on an hourly basis which is totally unrealistic. Also, insurance companies are hesitant to reimburse for "parent instruction" rather than "patient treatment", i.e. preventative rather than restorative medicine.

A final concern has been the potential of the parents developing dependency upon the therapist to an unhealthy degree. Although we try to answer their questions, we have found that our accessibility sometimes leads them to contact us when physician contact would be more appropriate. Rather than assume responsibility for information outside of our realm of knowledge, we refer them to the pediatrician or one of the specialists on the team.

At this point, follow-up of the children after the group has ended is rather informal. Some of the children have been followed through the pre-school program. Others have been followed on an individual monthly basis. Presently we meet monthly with the most recent group participants for an hour of discussion. This is more for the parents than the children. If they have particular concerns related to the therapy program, we speak to that, but have found it largely is a time for them to share their feelings. The children are formally re-evaluated approximately every three months.

As we are about to begin another group, we find that we need to refine and "tighten up" the program so that the maximum information is given in the minimum of time. A greater emphasis needs to be placed on parent involvement in carrying out the program from week to week. The possibility of giving specific "assignments" weekly may be feasible in this situation. This would also give us the means of providing consistant, concrete feedback to them about what they are doing with their child. Another consideration is how to involve the fathers more in the program as this largely depends upon those enrolled in the program and their interest and availability.

Although planning meetings have existed for each week's sessions, there is a need to structure ourselves to a greater degree to help the program run smoothly. It almost seems as if we need to write more specific behavioral objectives and implementation plans.

We continue to build and revise on the experience of each group we have. Our ultimate goal is to have a smooth running, high quality program, meeting the needs of each parent and child participating.

A STUDY OF THE SENSORY INTEGRATION
OF CHILDREN WITH MYELOMENINGOCELE

Linda Custis Land, M.S.

INTRODUCTION

Treatment of children with myelomeningocele has recently received much attention. This increased awareness seems to be the result of medical and surgical research providng a more favorable prognosis for these children. Myelomeningocele, a condition once incompatible with life, can now be treated to allow half of the affected children survival into the school years.[2] The most common problems associated with this condition (hydrocephalus, bladder and bowel incontinence, lower extremity paralysis) have been treated with increasingly satisfactory results. Professionals directly involved with the educational and therapeutic management of these children, however, are generally aware of a problem which is not life threatening in nature, but a problem which appears to be related to the perceptual processes.

THE PURPOSE OF THE STUDY

Only recently have a substantial number of children with this serious birth defect survived into the school years. As a result, research into the area of the perceptual processes of children with myelomeningocele is relatively novel and thus far has not produced conclusive evidence. Several factors complicate analysis of research in this area: the

presence or absence of hydrocephalus, the presence or absence
of shunting devices, number of shunt revisions, the presence
or absence of mental retardation as measured by standardized
intelligence tests, level of lesion, normal or abnormal
neurological function of the upper extremities, mobility,
sex, and the degree to which the child's environment has been
stimulating to normal growth and development. This situation
is further complicated by the interdependence of some, but
not all of these factors, in some but not all of the affected
children. Certainly, each of the mentioned factors contribute to the child's perceptual development, yet, control for
all of these variables in any one study would be difficult at
best. It appears that a significant number of studies will
be required; each controlling specific variables and
evaluating various areas of perception in order to produce
conclusive evidence.

Since most research in this area has been concerned with
visual perceptual dysfunction[23, 32, 40, 46] this investigation will also provide information concerning tactile and
kinesthetic perception, motor planning abilities, and
postural, bilateral, and ocular motor integration.

This investigation will consider only children with
intelligence quotients of 80+ so that results will not be
biased by the presence of mental retardation. Indeed, a
score of 80+ on a standardized intelligence test implies
certain capabilities in the perceptual area as well as the
cognitive domain. Yet, the investigator believes that there
is sufficient need to establish the presence or absence of
perceptual motor dysfunction in this select group in order to
add information to the knowledge base concerning the perceptual development of children with myelomeningocele.

The purpose of this research is to determine the

presence or absence of perceptual motor dysfunction as
measured by the Southern California Sensory Integration Tests
(SCSIT) in children with the diagnosis of myelomeningocele,
between the ages of four and nine years, who have demonstrated IQ's of 80+. This study will attempt to provide
additional information regarding the perceptual processes of
children with myelomeningocele, so that conclusive evidence
for the existence or absence of perceptual motor dysfunction,
specific areas of dysfunction, cause, and remediation can
someday be documented.

The primary focus of this study is investigation of the
perceptual development of children with myelomeningocele who
have demonstrated IQ's of 80+.

This study is designed to identify the presence or
absence of perceptual motor dysfunction and will not include
implications of cause or considerations for treatment in any
potentially identified problem areas.

HYPOTHESES

H_0 The mean test scores (on fifteen subtests of SCSIT)
of children with myelomeningocele will not differ
significantly from the mean test scores of a
hypothetical sample derived from the normative data
of the SCSIT standardization.

H_1 The mean test score (on fifteen subtests of SCSIT)
of children with myelomeningocele will differ
significantly from the mean test scores of a hypothetical sample derived from the normative data of
the SCSIT standardization.

.05 will be the criteria for statement of significant differences between groups.

REVIEW OF THE LITERATURE

As a chronic disease causing severe impairment of
locomotion, myelomeningocele is second only to cerebral palsy
in frequency. Because of this prevalence, and the extent of
neurologic manifestations and associated deformities characteristic of myelomeningocele, much literature is available
on this diagnosis and its treatment. Research into the area
of perceptual motor development of children with myelomeningocele, however, has only recently been undertaken. As a
result, literature in this area is scarce.

Tew and Laurence,[46] measured the performance of fifty-
nine children with spina bifida and a matched control group
on psychological and educational tests at five and seven
years of age. The children with spina bifida and no hydrocephalus scored one SD below the British mean score of 105
on the Weschler Pre-School Scale: Verbal, 89.3; Performance
92.3. The children with arrested hydrocephalus demonstrated
a mean verbal IQ of 87.5 and a mean performance IQ of 81.5.
The children with shunts had a mean verbal quotient of 78.1
and a mean performance quotient of 67.1. This distribution
of scores demonstrated that intellectual ability was affected
by the presence or absence of hydrocephalus. The effect of
valve revision on intelligence was also examined; the
difference between the means of those with revisions and
those with trouble free valves was not significant.

The Frostig Test of Visual Perception was administered
to each child. Scores closely resembled the distribution of
IQ scores and correlation between the Weschler and Frostig
tests (p $<$.001) indicated that impairment of visual perceptual functions was strongly associated with low intelligence.

Evaluations of school attainment in reading, arithmetic,
and spelling demonstrated that academic functioning closely

paralleled the distribution of intelligence, but that many of
the children were found to be functioning below expectations
for age and intelligence.

Joanne D. Gressang[23] compared the performance of twenty-
nine children with myelomeningocele on a series of perceptual
motor tests: The Frostig Developmental Test of Visual
Perception, the Beery Developmental Test of Visual Motor
Integration, Ayres Space Test, and the Southern California
Figure-ground Test. She found no significant difference
between the mean test scores of those children with myelomeningocele and hydrocephalus (n=20) and those with myelomeningocele and no hydrocephalus (n=9). She also described
no significant difference between the mean test scores of the
children with the initial shunt and those who had undergone
one, two, or three shunt revisions. The mean test scores of
each group were within the normal range as established by
the respective test manuals, demonstrating no perceptual
motor dysfunction in this sample. Age range was four years,
nine months to nine years, three months; IQ range was 70+.

Sand[40] measured the performance of thirty-seven subjects
with spina bifida manifesta on the Frostig Developmental Test
of Visual Perception. Their results demonstrated that 59% of
the children studied fell below the criterion for deviant
performance. Subtests of eye motor coordination and figure
ground most frequently indicated impaired performance. IQ
range was 68 to 111; age range was four years, zero months to
sixteen years, seven months. The mean perceptual quotient
for the twenty-seven children with hydrocephalus was 82.57
while the mean perceptual quotient for the ten children with
no hydrocephalus was 90.72. This difference was significant
at the .05 level.

Sheila Wallace[51] studied the effect of upper limb

function on mobility of children with myelomeningocele. Two
hundred twenty-five children were assessed by examination of
head circumference, neurological function of the upper
extremities, level of lesion, and degree of mobility.
Dependent upon level of lesion, mobility was considered
adequate in only 50% of the children. Hydrocephalus, whether
treated or not, was associated with a significant increase in
abnormal neurological findings in the upper extremities.
Upper extremity neurological abnormality was significantly
associated with reduced mobility. Wallace further suggested
that functional lower extremity muscles might also be
effected by generalized neurological dysfunction resulting
in inadequate mobility.

Tew and Laurence[47] evaluated the ability and attainments
of spina bifida patients born in South Wales between 1956
and 1962. The mean IQ was measured by the WISC of those
subjects with encephalocele was 51.88. 88.78 was the mean
score for those with myelocele; 93.76 for those with meningocele. A comparison to the full scale IQ's of previous
assessment (1966) showed deterioration of one point for boys
and five points for girls, demonstrating that IQ scores
remain relatively stable.

Of the fifty-eight patients assessed, most showed an
average reading attainment of just more than three years
below chronological age. At least two thirds of the population showed marked evidence of educational handicap, with
females poorer in all skills.

Elizabeth Anderson[2] reported results of the following
investigations in her literature review of cognitive deficits
in children with spina bifida:

Miller and Sethi[37] conducted four experiments on
children with infantile hydrocephalus. These children, some

of whom had spina bifida (no distinction in results is made),
ranged in age from five to fifteen years, and in IQ from 70
to 100. A comparison to a matched control group was made on
the: I, Bender Gestalt Test and the Frostig Developmental
Test of Visual Perception; II, a task involving discrimination of Hindi letters; III, a card sorting task. The results
confirmed that children with hydrocephalus have extremely
poor visual spatial perception, especially in regard to
figure ground discrimination. They also suggested that
children with hydrocephalus were less able to ignore
irrelevant background information.

In experiment IV, Miller and Sethi had the children
match tactile stimuli with the same hand that felt the initial stimuli (uncrossed) and with the opposite hand (crossed).
Their results indicated that children with hydrocephalus
were specifically impaired in the perception of tactile
stimuli and that increased difficulty was encountered in the
crossed condition.

Spain[45] noted differences on results of the subtests
of the Griffith Scale, finding the performance of tasks
involving locomotor components (i.e., eye hand coordination)
was more difficult for children with spina bifida. She also
described deficits in the performance of such tasks as bead
threading, use of a pencil, and building block towers for
two and three year old children. By age three years, only
one third of the children treated for hydrocephalus were
developing normally.

Diller[14] compared the performance of forty-five children
with spina bifida and hydrocephalus, thirty-two with spina
bifida and no hydrocephalus, and fifty-three lower extremity
amputees, on a series of education and psychological tests.
The following WISC scores were demonstrated:

	Full	Verbal	Performance
Spina bifida, hydrocephalus	91.0	92.9	83.3
Spina bifida, no hydrocephalus	96.0	99.7	95.8
Amputees	105.8	108.6	104.2

Verbal scores were better than performance in all three groups, but only in the spina bifida, hydrocephalus group was the difference significant.

No significant difference was demonstrated between the two spina bifida groups on the Frostig Developmental Test of Visual Perception; both groups demonstrated deviant performance. The mean score for the spina bifida, hydrocephalus group was 74.9, the mean for the spina bifida, no hydrocephalus group was 74.6.

Other findings indicated that children with spina bifida and hydrocephalus lag behind other handicapped children in reading, arithmetic, psycholinguistic abilities.

Shurtleff[43] noted considerable delay in acquisition of reading and writing skills in grade school children deprived of erect posture in the three to eighteen month range. He described the myelomeningocele patient as disorganized in space, unable to distinguish d from b, E from 3, or right from left, and he referred to drawings of these patients as poorly organized.

SAMPLE SELECTION

The thirteen children participating in this study included four males and nine females between the ages of four years, six months and eight years, three months. All children received a diagnosis of myelomeningocele at birth and are presently being treated medically by the Cincinnati Center for Developmental Disorders (CCDD). Lesion level ranged from T_{10} to S_2. Seven of the children had VJ shunts,

two had VP shunts, and two had required no shunting devices.
All of the children are presently involved in educational
programs - four are enrolled in pre-school programs, two are
in a pre-school for handicapped children, three are in public
schools, and four are enrolled in a public school for the
orthopedically handicapped.   Independent ambulation was
demonstrated by the entire sample:

ASSISTIVE DEVICES	NUMBER OF CHILDREN
None	2
Bilateral Short Leg Braces	3
Bilateral Short Leg Braces, Quad Cane	1
Bilateral Short Leg Braces, Loftstrand Crutches	1
Bilateral Long Leg Braces, Walker	6
TOTAL	13

All children demonstrated intelligence quotients of 80+ on
either the Stanford Binet or the Bailey Developmental Index.
These IQ scores were obtained from the Cincinnati Center for
Developmental Disorders records for the purpose of determining sample selection.   The mental age determined by each
of these evaluations was converted into an intelligence
quotient by the psychologist administering the evaluation.
IQ's ranged from 81 to 128.   A mean of 96 was determined.

The sample was not randomly selected. Volunteers were
solicited from the population of thirty-three children with
a diagnosis of myelomeningocele, between four and nine years
of age, with IQ's of 80+, treated by the Cincinnati Center
for Developmental Disorders.   The parents of these children
received a letter requesting participation of their child in
this study.   Follow-up telephone calls were made to answer
questions and to learn of the parent's decisions.   The
parents of thirteen children agreed to the participation of

of their child in this study. Procedures, benefits, and
precautions were explained to these parents.

METHODOLOGY

The complete Southern California Sensory Integration
Tests battery with the exception of Standing Balance: Eyes
Open and Eyes Closed was chosen as the evaluation tool.

RESULTS

The null hypothesis investigated in this study was:
There is no significant difference at the .05 level between
test scores on the SCSIT of children with myelomeningocele
and normative data of the SCSIT standardization. Since a
significant difference was demonstrated on seven of the
twenty-one category scores, a portion of this hypothesis is
rejected. Significant differences in mean test scores were
demonstrated on Deisgn Copying, Manual Form Perception (raw),
Crossing the Midline (all items), Crossing the Midline
(contralateral items, only), Bilateral Motor Coordination, and
Motor Accuracy (most accurate hand, accuracy score).

Sample mean scores, standard deviations, t values,
probabilities, and significance are illustrated in Table 1.

CLINICAL OBSERVATIONS

Clinical observations, though not suited to standardization or statistical analysis, are quite valuable in evaluating the nature and extent of sensory integration dysfunction.
These seemingly crude estimates of behavior are especially
important for providing support of the standardized test
results. Table 2 illustrates the results of clinical
observations made on this sample.

Observations of hyperactivity and distractibility were

based on the investigator's concept of "normal", and lack
well established criteria for evaluation. Tactile defensive
behaviors such as slapping or rubbing at the stimuli,
resistance to continuing the evaluation, and restlessness
were noted during administration of the tactile tests. Three
children demonstrated definite behaviors of tactile defensiveness and distractibility.

Diadokokenisis (in this case, alternation of pronation
and supination) and Thumb-Finger Touching were observed first
bilaterally, and then in each upper extremity alone. The
examiner counted the subject's repetitions of the described
behavior during a period of ten seconds. An average for
left, right, and bilateral execution was determined.
Criteria for normal diadokokenisis was considered to be
fifteen or more repetitions, ten or more was considered
slightly deficient, and less than ten was judged poor. The
criteria for thumb-finger touching was established as
follows: twenty-five or more - normal; fifteen or more -
slightly deficient; less than fifteen - poor. Most of the
children fell within the slightly deficient or poor range.

All of the myelomeningocele children demonstrated hyperextension in either all, or some of the MP's, PIP's, or DIP's
and were therefore considered to have hypotonic hands.

Observations of eye dominance were made on the following
activities: looking through a kaleidoscope, a ring made with
thumb and index finger touching, a hole in a paper, and a
telescope. All of the children were consistent with the eye
used on each item and were considered to have established eye
dominance. Observations of hand dominance were made during
writing and drawing. If the preferred hand was also the most
accurate hand as measured by MAC, the children were considered to have established hand dominance. This was not the

case for two of the subjects. Nine of the children demonstrated a right hand preference; four a preference for the
left hand. Three of the children demonstrated a crossed eye-
hand preference.

Each of the children were asked to print their first
name, and to write the numbers 1 to 10. Seven of the ten
older children reversed at least one of these familiar
symbols.

The subjects were asked to follow with their eyes the
eraser of a pencil as the examiner moved it across the midline in a random fashion. Hesitations, irregularity, and
jerking movements were noted. Ten of the children were
considered, by the investigator, to have demonstrated
slightly irregular ocular-motor control.

The children were asked to repeat after the examiner
"door, cup, bird, apple" and subsequently "9, 3, 6, 1, 5".
One omission or reversal was judged slightly deficient, more
than one omission or reversal was considered poor. Seven of
the children demonstrated a slightly deficient response for
four word sequential memory. Eight of the children responded
in either of slightly deficient or poor manner for five digit
sequential memory.

Estimates of choreoathetoid movement, postural changes
of the arms, trunk rotation, head resistance, and discomfort
were made during performance of Schilder's Arm Extension
Test (AET). The test position assumed by this sample was:
seated, eyes closed, arms extended to 90 degrees, fingers
abducted. With forewarning, the investigator rotated the
child's head while the child counted to ten. Seven of the
children demonstrated definite abnormal postural changes of
the arms. The significant difference between the scores of
the hypothetical and experimental samples demonstrated on

seven of twenty-one categories of the SCSIT provides
sufficient information to imply sensory integration dysfunction in the experimental sample. This implication is
enhanced by consideration of the associated clinical
observations (Tables 1, 2).

The SCSIT can assist in identifying four areas of
sensory integration dysfunction: form and space perception,
postural, bilateral, and ocular motor integration, that which
allows the child to be free of tactile defensiveness, and
praxis.

This clustering of test scores appears to indicate
problems in the area of praxis. Clinical observations which
support dysfunction in this area include slightly deficient
scores in diadokokenisis, thumb finger touching, and extra-
ocular motor control (Table 2). Additional evidence is
provided by scrutinizing the results of DC. Frequently
scores of one point were earned by the experimental sample
indicating that the child's problem was not one of visual
interpretation of the design (since the design was reproduced)
but one of precise execution of the reproduction.

Results of this study indicate that children with
myelomeningocele within the normal range of intelligence do
not demonstrate dysfunction in the area of visual perception
of form and space. Difficulty with praxis (planning and
executing motor tasks) was identified. Relating this data
to the findings of previous studies results in the following
conclusions and questions:

A positive linear relationship between intelligence
and sensorimotor proficiency has been frequently documented.
[6,20,22] The mean IQ of 96 demonstrated by this experimental
sample indicates that children with myelomeningocele, even
in the normal range of intelligence, show evidence of

perceptual motor dysfunction.

Deviant hand function demonstrated by children with myelomeningocele[40] could be associated with dyspraxia, since the hand function test employed in that study involves planning and executing skilled non-habitual motor tasks.

Dyspraxia could explain the discrepancy between verbal and performance intelligence quotients[5,14] in children with myelomeningocele and hydrocephalus.

Evidence of visual and spatial perceptual dysfunction in children with myelomeningocele has been documented.[37,40,46] These results could be the consequence of:

1. The positive relationship between the Weschler and Frostig tests - a sample of myelomeningocele children with low intelligence could produce evidence of dysfunction in the area of visual perception.

2. A dyspraxic state since the Frostig tests are not "clean" for visual perception. Responses on the Frostig tests require good motor planning abilities.

Since visual perception is subject to learning,[3] consideration of the obtained data results in the following questions:

1. Do children with myelomeningocele within the normal range of intelligence attack visual perceptual problems through intellectual means?

2. Would children with myelomeningocele and lower IQ's be unable to "reason" the solutions to such problems and therefore demonstrate visual perceptual dysfunction?

3. Are the SCSIT of visual perception subject to cognitive interpretation and solution?

4. Have we "taught" children with myelomeningocele and normal intelligence through our clinical and educational

programs to attack visual perceptual problems on a cognitive
level?

5.   Would children with myelomeningocele and lower
intellectual capacities not be as likely to respond to such
"teaching" and therefore demonstrate visual perceptual
dysfunction?

The investigator speculates that a positive response to
each of the above questions is appropriate. Only with
further research will these and other questions be answered.

Greater confidence could be placed in the results of
this study and its significance in relation to previous
studies if the following criteria had been met: larger
sample size, a standardized testing facility, control for
variables other than intelligence with this multifactorial
condition, myelomeningocele, and a stronger experimental
design. These conditions were not satisfied in this investigation due to limited resources.

IMPLICATIONS FOR FURTHER STUDY

Duplication of this study with a similar sample and a
stronger experimental design would be valuable since:

1.   The general assumption of visual-spatial perceptual
dysfunction in children with myelomeningocele within the
normal range of intelligence has been rejected by the results
of this study.

2.   Confirmation of dyspraxia as a problem area would
allow greater confidence in assuming that motor planning is
difficult for children with myelomeningocele within the
normal range of intelligence.

3.   Once dyspraxia is established as a problem,
clinicians can become involved with activities of remediation.
Subsequently, effectiveness of treatment could be evaluated.

Previous studies indicate that there is a relationship

between high lesion levels, hydrocephalus, lowered intellectual functioning, and difficulties with visual-spatial
perception. Duplication of this study with a sample of
children with myelomeningocele and lower intellectual
quotients could identify whether or not the dysfunction in
this group is truly visual in nature, or again the result of
a dyspraxic state.

This investigation could provide no conclusions concerning the postural, bilateral, and ocular motor integration
of this sample. Certainly a more in depth look at the
sensory integration of children with myelomeningocele in this
area would be valuable.

The area of auditory and language perception was tapped
in this investigation only in the clinical observations of
auditory sequential memory. The slightly deficient responses
by this sample could well indicate dysfunction in this area.
Indeed, auditory-language perception is worthy of further
exploration.

The frequency of shunt revisions has not appeared to
have a significant affect on intellectual functioning[46] or
visual perception.[23] The affect of the number of revisions
on motor planning ability remains unexplored.

Cortically directed visual perception is highly subject
to learning.[3] The question then becomes - are clinicians
and teachers "teaching" children with myelomeningocele to
attack visual perceptual problems through intellectual means?
Directing an investigation toward an answer to this question
would surely be valuable.

SUMMARY

Thirteen children with myelomeningocele, between the
ages of four and nine years, who had demonstrated intelligence

quotients of 80+, completed the Southern California Sensory
Integration Tests[4] with the exception of standing balance.
Results suggest that this sample is developing normally in
the area of visual perception of form and space.[23] No
conclusions were drawn concerning postural, bilateral, and
ocular motor integration since the physical limitations of
myelomeningocele prevented completion of the tests best
suited for detecting dysfunction in this area. Three of the
children studied demonstrated tactile defensive behaviors,
but dysfunction in this area could not be generalized to
include the entire sample. Results of this investigation
indicate that this sample of children with myelomeningocele
is somewhat dyspraxic. Mean score differences between the
experimental sample and the hypothetical sample (derived
from normative data of the SCSIT standardization) were
significant at the .05 level in at least one category of all
subtests involving motor components with the exception of IP.

These results are significant since previous studies
have identified dysfunction in either visual or visual
spatial perception. This study suggests that in children
with myelomeningocele, within the normal range of intelligence, the motor component necessary for response to some
tests of visual perception probably bias those test results.

REFERENCES

1. Allan, L.D., Donald, I., Ferguson-Smith, M.A., Smith,
   E.M. and Gibson, A.A.M.: Amniotic fluid alpha-feto
   protein in the antenatal diagnosis of spina bifida.
   The Lancet, 11:522, 1973.

2. Anderson, E.M.: Cognitive deficits in children with
    spina bifida and hydrocephalus: A review of the
    literature. *Brit. J. Educ. Psychol., 43*:257, 1973.

3. Ayres, A.J.: Sensory Integration and Learning Disorders.
    Los Angeles, Western Psychological Services, 1972.

4. Ayres, A.J.: Southern California Sensory Integration
    Tests Manual. Los Angeles, Western Psychological
    Services, 1972.

5. Badell-Ribera, A., Shulman, K. and Paddock, N.: The
    relationship of non-progressive hydrocephalus to
    intellectual functioning in children with spina bifida
    cystica. *Pediatrics, 37*:787, 1966.

6. Black, A. and Davis, L.J.: The relationship between
    intelligence and sensori-motor proficiency in retardates.
    Am. J. Mental Deficiency, 71:55, 1966.

7. Bunch, W.H., Cass, A.S., Bensman, A.S. and Long, D.M.:
    Modern Management of Myelomeningocele, St. Louis, 1972.

8. Campbell, D.T. and Stanley, J.C.: Experimental and
    Quasi-Experimental Designs for Research. Chicago, Rand
    McNally College Publishing Co., 1963.

9. Carney, A., Newbold, D.B. and Simpson, D.A.: Spina
    bifida in South Australia: Problems in education. *The
    Med. J. Australia, 2*:993, 1971.

10. Carter, C.O.: Polygenic inheritance and common disease.
    The Lancet, 1:1252, 1969.

11. Coffey, V.P. and Jessop, W.S.: The incidence of spina
    bifida. *Irish J. Med. Sci.,* pp. 30, 1955.

12. Davis, J.A. and J. Dobbing (eds.), Scientific Foundations
    of Paediatrics, Philadelphia, W.B. Saunders Co., 1974.

13. Diller, L., Gordon, W.A., Swinyard, C. and Kastner, S.:
    Psychological and Educational Studies with Spina Bifida
    Children. Final Report Project #5-0412, Institute of

Rehabilitation Medicine, New York University Medical
Center, 1969.

14.   Diller, L. and Kastner, S.:   A Developmental Study of
      Reversal Learning in Children with Spina Bifida and
      Children with Congenital Amputations.   Proceedings of
      the 76th Annual Convention of APA, 1968.

15.   Doran, P.A. and Guthkelch, A.N.:   Studies in spina
      bifida cystica.   *J. Neurol., Neurosurg., Psychiat., 24*:
      331, 1961.

16.   Downey, J.A. and Low, N.L.:   The Child with Disabling
      Illness.   Philadelphia, W. B. Saunders Co., 1974.

17.   Farber, S.D.:   Sensorimotor Evaluation and Treatment
      Procedures for Allied Health Personnel.   Indiana Univer-
      sity-Purdue University at Indianapolis Medical Center,
      The Indiana University Foundation, 1974.

18.   Farmer, T.W. (ed.) Pediatric Neurology, Hagerstown,
      Harper and Row, Publishers, 1975, pp. 425.

19.   Field, B. and Kerr, C.:   Potato blight and neural tube
      defects.   *The Lancet, 2*:507, 1973.

20.   Frances, R.J. and Rarick, G.L.:   Motor characteristics
      of the mentally retarded.   *Am. J. Mental Deficiency,
      63*:792, 1959.

21.   Fritzgerald, R.J. and Healy, B.:   The spina bifida
      problem: A longer term review with special reference to
      the quality of survival.   *J. Irish Med. Assoc., 67*:565,
      1974.

22.   Gordon, G.:   Relationships between intelligence, simple
      and complex motor proficiency.   *Am. J. Mental Deficiency,
      74*:373, 1969.

23.   Gressang, J.:   Perceptual processes of children with
      myelomeningocele and hydrocephalus.   *Am. J. Occup. Ther.,
      28*:226, 1974.

24. Haring, N.G. and Stables, J.M.: The effects of gross motor development on visual perception and eye-hand coordination. *J. Am. Phys. Ther. Assoc., 46*:129, 1966.

25. Hide, D.W., William, H.P. and Ellis, H.L.: The outlook for the child with myelomeningocele for whom early surgery was considered inadvisable. *Dev. Med. Child Neurol., 14*:304, 1972.

26. Hunt, G.M. and Holmes, A.E.: Some factors relating to intelligence in treated children with spina bifida cystica. *Studies in Hydrocephalus and Spina Bifida,* suppl. 35 to *Dev. Med. Child Neurol., 17*:65, 1975.

27. Ingraham, F.D.: Spina Bifida and Cranium Bifidum, Cambridge, Harvard University Press, 1943.

28. James, M.C.C. and Lassman, L.P.: Spinal Dysraphism, Butterworth and Company, Ltd., 1972.

29. Klugh, H.E.: Statistics: The Essentials for Research, New York, John Wiley and Sons, Inc., 1970.

30. Kolstoe, R.H.: Introduction to Statistics for the Behavioral Sciences, Homewood, The Dorsey Press, 1969.

31. Koosis, D.J.: Statistics for Self Study or Classroom Use, New York, John Wiley and Sons, Inc., 1972.

32. Lorber, J.: Results of treatment of myelomeningocele. *Dev. Med. Child Neurol., 13*:279, 1971.

33. Marlow, D.R. and Sellew, G.: Textbook of Pediatric Nursing, Philadelphia, W.B. Saunders Co., 1966, pp. 175.

34. Menelaus, M.B.: The Orthopaedic Management of Spina Bifida Cystica, Edinburgh and London, E. & S. Livingstone 1971.

35. Menkes, J.H.: Textbook of Child Neurology, Philadelphia, Lea and Febiger, 1974.

36. Messane, J.M.: Pathology of Infancy and Childhood, St. Louis, The C.V. Mosby Co., 1975, pp. 923.

37. Miller, E. and Sethi, L.: The effect of hydrocephalus
     on perception. *Studies in Hydrocephalus and Spina
     Bifida,* suppl. 25 to *Dev. Med. Child Neurol., 13:*77, 1971.

38. Parsons, J.G.: Assessments of aptitudes in young people
     of school-leaving age handicapped by hydrocephalus or
     spina bifida cystica. *Studies in Hydrocephalus and
     Spina Bifida,* suppl. 27 to *Dev. Med. Child Neurol.,
     14:*101, 1972.

39. Renwick, J.H.:   Hypothesis: Anencephaly and spina
     bifida are usually preventable by avoidance of a specific
     but unidentified substance present in certain potato
     tubers. *Brit. J. Prev. Social Med., 26:*67, 1972.

40. Sand, P.L., et al: Performance of children with spina
     bifida manifesta on the Frostig Developmental Test of
     Visual Perception. *Perceptual and Motor Skills, 37:*
     117, 1973.

41. Sax, G.: Empirical Foundations of Educational Research,
     Englewood Cliffs, Prentice-Hall, Inc., 1968.

42. Shands, A.R. and Raney, B.R.: Handbook of Orthopaedic
     Surgery, St. Louis, The C.V. Mosby Co., 1967, pp. 210.

43. Shurtleff, D.B.: Timing of learning in the meningomye-
     locele patient. *J. Am. Phys. Ther. Assoc., 46:*136, 1966.

44. Smith, D.E.: Spina Bifida and the Total Care of Spinal
     Myelomeningocele, Springfield, Charles C. Thomas,
     Publisher, 1965.

45. Spain, B.: Verbal and performance ability in pre-school
     spina bifida children. *Studies in Hydrocephalus and
     Spina Bifida,* suppl. 27 to *Dev. Med. Child Neurol.,
     14:*155, 1972.

46. Tew, B. and Laurence, K.M.: The effects of hydrocepha-
     lus on intelligence, visual perception and school
     attainment. *Studies in Hydrocephalus and Spina Bifida,*

suppl. 35 to *Dev. Med. Child Neurol.*, *17*:129, 1975.

47. Tew, B.J. and Laurence, K.M.: The ability and attain-
     ments of spina bifida patients born in South Wales
     between 1956-1962. *Studies in Hydrocephalus and Spina
     Bifida*, suppl. 27 to *Dev. Med. Child Neurol.*, *14*:124,
     1972.

48. Tew, B.J. and Laurence, K.M.: The validity of psycho-
     metric studies on children with spina bifida. *Dev.
     Med. Child Neurol.*, *16*:186, 1974.

49. University of Colorado School of Medicine, Birth Defects
     Center, Department of Pediatrics, Department of Physical
     Medicine and Rehabilitation, Symposium on Spina Bifida,
     1969.

50. Vaughn, V.C. and R.J. McKay (eds.), Nelson Textbook of
     Pediatrics, Philadelphia, W.B. Saunders, Co., 1975,
     pp. 1411.

51. Wallace, S.J.: The effect of upper-limb function on
     mobility of children with myelomeningocele. *Studies in
     Hydrocephalus and Spina Bifida*, suppl. 29 to *Dev. Med.
     Child Neurol.*, *15*:84, 1973.

TABLE 1.

SCSIT Data for Thirteen Children with Myelomeningocele

Tests	n	Hypothetical Sample		Experimental Sample		t	P	Significant
		$\bar{X}_1$	s_1	$\bar{X}_2$	s_2			
SV (acc)	13	19.746	2.870	17.077	5.664	1.516	>.1	
SV (adj)	13	16.685	2.510	14.692	4.990	1.286	>.2	
FG	13	13.462	2.113	13.154	5.161	.199	>.5	
PS	13	13.423	3.146	13.692	3.351	-.211	>.5	
DC	13	9.746	4.191	5.000	4.933	2.644	<.02	Yes
KIN	13	64.400	5.374	61.923	17.718	.482	>.5	
MFP (raw)	13	8.654	1.329	6.923	2.660	2.099	<.05	Yes
MFP (adj)	13	7.200	1.194	5.769	2.351	1.956	>.05	
FI	13	10.715	1.150	10.077	2.060	.975	>.2	
GRA	13	13.508	2.318	7.538	4.484	4.264	<.001	Yes
LTS	13	82.485	.960	82.692	5.950	-.125	>.9	
DTS	13	30.723	.789	28.308	4.697	1.828	>.05	
IP	13	11.500	2.565	9.385	4.445	1.486	>.1	
CML	13	18.877	1.997	13.846	6.349	2.725	<.02	Yes
CMLX	13	15.962	3.082	11.385	5.501	2.617	<.02	Yes
BMC	13	6.962	2.590	4.231	2.862	2.551	<.02	Yes
RLD	10	13.010	1.344	11.400	3.688	1.297	>.2	
MAC (most acc; acc)	11	464.182	16.173	444.091	26.399	2.152	<.05	Yes
MAC (most acc; adj)	11	451.636	14.473	436.182	24.070	1.825	>.05	

TABLE 1. (cont.)

Tests	n	Hypothetical Sample		Experimental Sample		t	P	Significant
		$\bar{x}_1$	s_1	$\bar{x}_2$	s_2			
MAC (less acc; acc)	11	444.364	18.943	427.909	36.971	1.314	>.2	
MAC (less acc; adj)	11	433.273	17.153	422.000	35.324	.952	>.2	

TABLE 2.

Tabulated Results of Clinical Observations Made on
Thirteen Children with Myelomeningocele

Age Range	4.6-5.5	5.6-6.5	6.6-7.5	7.6-8.5	Total
n	3	4	4	2	
Hyperactivity					
Normal Activity	1	3	4	2	10
Slightly Hyperactive	2	1	0	0	3
Definitely Hyperactive	0	0	0	0	0
Distractibility					
Normal Attention Span	1	3	3	2	9
Slightly Distractible	0	0	1	0	1
Definitely Distractible	2	1	0	0	3
Tactile Defensiveness					
No Tactile Responses	2	2	3	1	8

TABLE 2. (cont.)

Diadokokenisis					
One or more Definite Responses	1	1	0	0	2
Two or more Definite Responses	0	1	1	1	3
Normal (15↑)	0	1	1	0	2
Slightly Deficient (10↑)	2	1	3	2	8
Poor	1	2	0	0	3
Thumb Finger Touching					
Normal (25↑)	0	3	1	1	5
Slightly Deficient (15↑)	3	1	2	1	7
Poor	0	0	1	0	1
Hand Muscle Tone					
Normal	0	0	0	0	0
Hypertonic	0	0	0	0	0
Hypotonic	3	4	4	2	13
Dominance					
Def. Est. Hand Dom.	3	2*	4	2	11
Def. Est. Eye Dom.	3	4	4	2	13
Reversals					
Letters/Numbers	N/A	4	2	1	7
Eye Movement Across Midline					
Normal	1	0	2	0	3
Slightly Irregular	2	4	2	2	10
Definitely Irregular	0	0	0	0	0

*Two children in this group did not have a well established hand dominance.

TABLE 2. (cont.)

Sequential Memory						
4 Words	Normal	2	2	1	1	6
	Slightly Deficient	1	2	3	1	7
	Poor	0	0	0	0	0
5 Digits	Normal	1	1	2	1	5
	Slightly Deficient	2	2	1	1	6
	Poor	0	1	1	0	2
Schilder's Arm Extension Posture						
Choreo Athetoid	Normal	3	4	4	2	13
	Slight	0	0	0	0	0
	Definite	0	0	0	0	0
Postural Changes of Arms	Normal	0	1	2	0	3
	Slight	0	0	2	1	3
	Definite	3	3	0	1	7
Trunk Rotation	Normal	1	3	2	0	6
	Slight	1	1	2	2	6
	Definite	1	0	0	0	1
Head Resistance	Normal	1	3	2	1	7
	Slight	2	1	2	1	6
	Definite	0	0	0	0	0
Discomfort	Normal	3	4	4	2	13
	Slight	0	0	0	0	0
	Definite	0	0	0	0	0

Part II
NEUROSURGERY

Participants

Fred J. Epstein, M.D.
New York University, New York

W. James Gardner, M.D.
Cleveland Clinic Foundation, Cleveland, Ohio

E. Bruce Hendrick, M.D.
The Hospital for Sick Children, Toronto, Canada

A. James McAdams, M.D.
Children's Hospital Research Foundation, Cincinnati, Ohio

Robert L. McLaurin, M.D.
University of Cincinnati, Cincinnati, Ohio

James E. McLennan, M.D.
University of Cincinnati, Cincinnati, Ohio

Anthony J. Raimondi, M.D.
Northwestern University, Chicago, Illinois

Martin P. Sayers, M.D.
The Children's Hospital, Columbus, Ohio

Luis Schut, M.D.
The Children's Hospital of Philadelphia, Philadelphia,
Pennsylvania

David C. Schwartz, M.D.
Children's Hospital Research Foundation, Cincinnati, Ohio

Kenneth A. Shulman, M.D.
Albert Einstein College of Medicine, Bronx, New York

C. F. Strife, M.D.
Children's Hospital Research Foundation, Cincinnati, Ohio

TERATOLOGIC INFERENCE

ANALYSIS OF STRUCTURAL PRIMORDIAL
RELATIONSHIPS BASED ON POSTNATAL
ANOMALY

James E. McLennan, M.D.

INTRODUCTION

Current knowledge of teratogenesis is synthesized from
two principal sources: 1) studies of static early human
embryos or descriptive reports of unusual postnatal structural defects, and 2) experimental teratogenic models. These
sources have not provided concerted opinions about human
teratogenic mechanisms.[15,19] This is reflected in continuing
controversy about multiple etiologies of such a prevalent
human structural anomaly as the "dysraphic states"; for
example, still under consideration as quite disparate villains
from epidemiologic and experimental viewpoints are the potato
blight virus,[27] oral hormone medications,[9] heavy metals[7] and
fetal-placental hypoxia.[5,11] Even the basic mechanisms of
dysraphic determination, first proposed centuries ago as
either primary neural tube closure deficits[26] or secondary
tube reopening,[22] remain unanswered. Extension of the reopening theory to accommodate "overgrowth and necrosis"[3] or
refinements of the "hydrodynamic hypothesis"[10] to explain
various related conditions further confuse the issue. Static
human malformations do not allow unambiguous reconstruction
of embryologic mechanisms; lower animal models provide

143

information only about distinctly nonhuman developmental
time courses and structural primordial relationships. Reper-
cussion of this confusion is enormous in terms of potentially
misdirected experimental and epidemiologic effort and psychological inuendo for parents that have produced malformed
children.

I present here three brief examples of (spatial and
temporal) reconstruction of early human embryologic (teratogenic) relationships based on statistical analysis of
gestational and postnatal anatomic (pathologic) parameters.
This methodology is inherently powerful in that it provides
a dynamic model of unobservable early human primordial
relationships in "true (nonlinear) developmental time".
Hopefully, extensions of this method will explicate primary
(isolated) and secondary (inductive) anomalous developmental
syndromes and allow improved understanding of the critical
biologic clock for human teratogenic primordial alteration.

TROUBLESOME NOTIONS

A *teratogen*, as used here, is simply the *event* producing
structural alteration. This is probably only rarely an exo-
genous agent, but rather a spontaneous mistake, so to speak,
either at the stage of initial chromosome kinetics (not
reproduced regularly in the next generation), or in the
early development of the zygote. In particular, a teratogenic (primary) "hit" is that moment in developmental time
when the "teratogenic agent" interacts with maximally vulnerable structural primordia. The resultant structural
anomaly is occasionally an isolated one; more often, however,
multiple anomalies co-exist as a consistently recurring
"syndrome".

Although most primary teratogenic states are rationally

explained by alteration of contemporaneously vulnerable structural primordia,[14] it is difficult to deduce just what role "inductive" relationships play in co-existing (secondary) anomaly syndromes. Ideas about induction in the human embryo are derived almost exclusively from (ablation and transposition) animal experiments, generally using lower organisms with vastly differing developmental time courses.[28,33] Observations of recurring multiple anomaly (inductive?) teratogenic states provide meaningful relationships only when structural primordial vulnerabilities are appropriately aligned in developmental time and space by independent evidence. Anatomic (e.g. "electrical") contiguity of some sort would appear necessary for induction effects and no doubt involves the "epithelial nature" of mesodermal tissues.[12] Inductive phenomena are of vastly greater importance at the lower end of the phylogenetic chain, yet these experimental data[1,2,6,16,29] are frequently quoted in etiologic support of human anomalies. Ideas about human teratogenic states are predicated on the presumptive fact of irreversibility of definitive embryologic processes. While this is probably near truth for human development, we are nonetheless aware of the prominence of necrosis and repair providing the substrate for "correction of mistakes" in lower animals.[1]

An important notion in thinking about teratogenic states, particularly in terms of genetic counseling, is the significance of the "familial" epidemiologic spectrum for statistical recurrence of a given defect.[24] If the teratogenic event alters chromosomes directly, it is technically "genetic"; if the alteration involves autosomal DNA, it will have significance for only the affected individual and will not be heritable by Mendelian mechanisms. Evidence for genetic

alteration in a "teratogenic anomaly" may be complicated by
the possibility of suppressed or phenotypically variable
expression rates ("poor penetration"). Much of this ignorance is disguised in the appellation of "polygenic" etiology;[30] this category includes most structural defects
(including dysraphism) that have some measurable recurrence
rate within kinships (and are therefore presumably related
to nucleic acid mechanisms) but are not conveniently correlated with chromosomal events. A possible way to think of
the dysraphic spectrum, for example, is that a "permissive
factor", is operative; it is this "factor" which may be
inheritable (occasionally environmental?) and allows a prevalence of the defect in excess of that expected for a randomly
occuring lesion. Random teratogenic events are those such as
"Streeter's congenital constriction band" anomaly of the
distal extremity[8,17] and Poland's Syndrome;[13] these isolated
entities have no familial recurrence rate and presumably can
only involve autosomes or cell surface interactions.[12] The
following discussion includes both "polygenic" and random
teratogenic events. Perforce, the idea of induction is in-
separable from either.

I. <u>MECHANISM AND SIGNIFICANCE OF HUMAN UMBILICAL CORD</u>
   <u>ECCENTRICITY</u>

     The anatomic position of umbilical cord origin from the
placental surface is noted at parturition to vary from
central to marginal to membranous (velamentous). The latter
end of this normal anatomic spectrum has admitted significance for premature labor and parturitional disaster because
of the precarious fetal blood supply. It is less well known,
but well documented,[18] that a relationship holds between
degree of cord eccentricity from the placental surface and

rate of fetal anomaly, implying perhaps, that cords near the placental margin are associated with intrauterine "fetal asphyxia".[23] The most efficient arrangement is a central cord origin, with radial symmetry of the placental mass. This appears to be Nature's intent. Eccentric cord origin presents adversity for the developing embryo and fetus and is thus a very early teratogenic parameter.

Two principal theories for etiology of eccentric cords have been debated in the literature, namely, 1) determination at the time of fertilized zygote implantation (Fig. 1), and 2) "trophotropism", or a differential wandering of one placental margin later in gestation (Fig. 2). These two possibilities may be distinguished by a simple statistical study, the details of which have been previously published;[20] this serves as an example of distributional analysis providing a model for an early developmental determinant with teratogenic implication.

At the time of implantation, the fertilized human zygote is generally about 7 days old and already polarized in that it is no longer a clump of identical cells (Fig. 3A). A platelike structure with a definite "body stalk" is visable; this stalk will become the future umbilical cord. The *vector* of implantation of this body stalk in relation to the uterine lumen (decidual surface) *determines* the degree of eccentricity of the umbilical cord from the placenta which will develop from interaction of the decidua and zygote (Fig. 3A,B).

This mechanism is verified[20] by proposing a "target" model[4] wherein "Nature" attempts to insert the zygote with the body stalk vector at right angles to the lumen; the "bull's eye" is, however, missed with a predictible regularity (Fig. 4). Velamentous insertions are considered "known events" that miss the target entirely.[4] Eccentricity is

defined (Fig. 5) as the distance (d) between the point of
actual umbilical cord insertion and the centroid of the
placental plane projection. This parameter was measured
from 143 specimens giving a distribution of eccentricities
(Fig. 6A) which adequately reproduces that predicted by the
target model; the distribution was verified from a large
heterogenous population (Fig. 6B).

If the mechanism of trophotropism were significant in
normal singleton gestation, a quite different distribution
would obtain and there should be a (not observed[20]
correlation between the "direction" of eccentricity (angle
of Fig. 5) and the long axis of the placenta (11' of Fig. 5).
This simple analysis has apparently substantiated an embryologic mechanism which has not yielded to descriptive and
experimental investigation.

II. RIB ANOMALIES AND LUMBOSACRAL MYELODYSPLASIA

Rib anomalies, known to frequently accompany spinal
dysraphism (and isolated lumbosacral myelomeningocele),
appear to often occur in the right upper thorax. Since this
implies departure from the attractive idea[19] of *generalized*
very early mesodermal alteration, further verification was
obtained. Chest x-rays of 100 patients with the *primary
index condition* of lumbosacral myelomeningocele disclosed 20
patients with a total of 70 abnormal ribs (Fig. 7A,B). All
these patients had a normal lower thoracic spine and rib cage
between the caudal defect and the abnormal ribs. Rib defects
were graded for "severity" according to rarity in the general
population (bifid $>$ fused $>$ gaps $>$ missing ribs). Anomalous
vertebral bodies co-existed in the upper and middle thorax
in 50% of the patients, but the segment numbers of abnormal
ribs and vertebrae were not necessarily correlated.

Figure 8A shows the total frequency distribution of abnormal ribs and vertebrae by axial position, and Figure 8B confirms peak incidence in the right upper thorax and contiguity of abnormal ribs in 95% of the cases.

This strikingly non-uniform distribution of rib anomalies in association with lumbosacral myelodysplasia may be the result of spatial and temporal alignment of axial structural primordia at the moment of the teratogenic event (Fig. 9). This model is presented only briefly here but discussed at length in another paper.[21] Utilizing a variant of the Log-normal distribution, the theoretical axial distribution of anomalous ribs (i.e. the heavy vertical bars of Fig. 9), codetermined with lumbosacral myelomeningocele, will approximate the observed distribution rather precisely (Fig. 10).

We have thus reconstructed a very early (perhaps pre-somitic) relationship between structural primordial vulnerability and teratogenic event by analysis of defect in the postnatal child. Arguments of both primary mesodermal[19] and neuroectodermal[25] alteration appear less critical as one gains an idea of the true developmental time scale in the 3rd and 4th weeks of gestation (Fig. 11).

III. THE ROLE OF INDUCTIVE MECHANISMS: POLAND'S SYNDROME

The spatial axis of Figure 9 has been generalized to "axial position" to accommodate our ignorance of possible inductive interaction between rib and vertebral primordia. Experimental animal work[16] has not answered the question of interdependence of co-developing axial structures; it has also failed to discover whether or not the anterior and posterior rib segments derive from separate tissues.[16,29]

Analysis of Poland's Syndrome[13] perhaps provides a clue

to inductive forces in rib development. This randomly
occurring teratogenic condition combines absent pectoralis
muscles with ipsilateral hypoplastic hand and syndactylysm
(or polydactylysm); about 10% of these patients, who are
otherwise totally normal, have hypoplastic or missing *anterior* rib segments directly underlying the missing upper
chest wall muscle (Fig. 12). The posterior rib segments are
invariably normal, whereas the defective ribs of myelodysplasia involve both anterior and posterior portions. Thus
one may postulate the following inductive mechansims (Fig.
11): 1) the anterior rib segment requires normal overlying
chest wall muscles for proper development, 2) a posterior
rib segment is necessary for normal anterior rib development.
A rare clinical entity, the "rib gap" defect,[31] indicates
that posterior and anterior rib segments may develop independently yet fail to unite at the lateral rib margin. This
unusual syndrome appears to indicate separate origin of the
anterior (lateral plate) and posterior (somite) portions of
each rib; multiple other defects in these children, however,
make meaningful analysis of etiology impossible. Likewise,
little information accrues from study of rib and vertebral
anomalies in extensive dysraphic conditions (cf. McLennan[21]
case #13). Discovery of primordial relationships is vitiated
by extensive teratogenic disaster (perhaps "prolonged
presence of teratogenic agent"), and inductive effects cannot
be separated from contemporaneous alteration of multiple
structural primordia.

IV.   STREETER'S DYSPLASIA AND SYNDACTYLYSM: EXTENSION
      OF THE DEVELOPMENTAL TIME SCALE

      Hand anomalies (syndactyly and polydactyly) coexist
with abnormal anterior rib segments in Poland's syndrome.

Children with lumbosacral myelomeningocele and abnormal ribs
(posterior and anterior segments) only rarely have associated
upper limb bud anomalies.[21] It is then reasonable to postulate that the period of peak vulnerability for determination
of rib anomalies traverses the largely separate vulnerable
periods for dysraphism (3rd-4th week) and upper limb bud
related defect (6th week) (Fig. 11). It appears further that
the various ribs present a differential vulnerability (non-
uniform distribution of anomaly) throughout this time and
that posterior rib segments probably precede anterior segments in developmental time (Fig. 11).

Analysis of the entity of congenital constriction bands
of the extremities allows extension of our glimpse of developmental time into the 5th and 6th week of gestation. This
anomaly of the distal extremity occurs *randomly*, and, in its
minimal expression, classically[32] produces a ringlike constriction or amputation of a single digit or several fingers
and toes. The teratogenic "hit" appears to occur in the 6th
week when digits are rapidly evolving through the "finger
ray" stage followed by "clearing" to produce individual digits
with radial cartilagenous struts (Fig. 13). Syndactylysm
and polydactylysm accompany Streeter's bands in over 40% of
cases.[8,17]

The frequency of constriction anomaly for given fingers
and toes has been studied by Kino;[17] Figure 14 shows this
distribution for 59 affected patients, plotted according to
digital position. This provides a spatial and temporal
picture of primordial vulnerability akin to that of the 3rd
and 4th gestational week based on rib anomaly. Three of
Kino's patients had associated cleft lip and palate; this
latter defect, probably determined early in the 6th week,
could be used as a primary index condition against which to

align the distribution of defective digits (Fig. 14) just as lumbosacral myelomeningocele provides association for defective ribs (Fig. 11). Figures 15 and 16 show clinical examples of cleft palate and lip associated with syndactylysm and constriction anomaly of the digits; these children were otherwise entirely normal. Coexisting anomalies of anatomically separate embryonic regions are reasonably caused only by contemporaneous primordial vulnerability; any explanation involving inductive mechanisms must be suspect.

The controversy about etiology of the so-called "constrict band" digital and distal extremity defect (often clumped with syndactyly and polydactyly as "Streeter's dysplasia") centers about a primary mechanism of "amniotic bands" encircling the primordia to arrest development.[8,32] Kino[17] states that his observation of the increased anomaly rate in the longer digits implies that these structures protrude furthest from the limb and are most easily injured. He offers experimental evidence that the mechanism of injury is hemorrhage of the primordia caused by vigorous uterine contractions. The amniotic remnants attached to or encircling the defective areas at birth are no doubt adhesions to the injured parts. It is more satisfactory, considering the relative size of the various digital primordia in the 6th week (Fig. 13), the presence of multiple isolated bilateral finger and toe anomalies in the same child, and the prominent association with syndactyly and polydactyly, to recognize that the evidence indicates a differential arrangement of digital primordial vulnerability to *any* teratologic event. In particular the same event might establish cleft lip and palate as the only other defect.

CONCLUSION

Analysis of rib and digital anomalies, aligned against *index events* characteristic of an early developmental stage (LSM-4th week, cleft palate-6th week) has provided an overview of developmental time which is independent of experimental evidence or assumptions based on study of defective human embryos. Numerous overlapping segments of developmental time, investigated by relationships such as these, might be expected to ultimately provide a realistic reconstruction of the vast complex of human primordial interactions in embryonic time and space. It is critical to deemphasize the *nature* of the "teratogen" and focus on the vulnerability -- resistance relationships of the early embryo.

ACKNOWLEDGMENTS

Figures 1A, 2, 5, 6A have been previously published in *American Journal of Obstetrics and Gynecology* (ref. 20).

Figures 9, 10, and 11 are taken from a paper (ref. 21) which will appear in *Biology of the Neonate* and are reproduced with permission of the publisher.

The data of Figure 6B were collected under the auspices of the The Collaborative Perinatal Project of NINCDS.

The author thanks Dr. F.H. Gilles (Associate Professor of Neuropathology, at Children's Hospital Medical Center, Harvard Medical School) for valuable criticism of many of the ideas expressed in this work.

This study was supported in part by funds provided by the United Cerebral Palsy Research and Educational Foundation (R-224-75), by the Program-Project Grant No. NSI-EP, 1P01 NS

09704-01 NSPA, HD, NINCDS, and the Children's Hospital
Medical Center Mental Retardation and Human Development
Research Program (HD 03-0773), NICHD.

REFERENCES

1. Angevine, J.B.: Clinically relevant embryology of the
    vertebral column and spinal cord. *Clin. Neurosurg.,
    20*:95, 1973.

2. Arey, L.B.: Developmental Anatomy. 7th Ed. Philadel-
    phia, W.B. Saunders Co.,1965, pp. 409.

3. Barson, A.J.: Craniospinal dystrophia in the chick
    embryo produced by tissue-specific antibodies. *Dev. Med.
    Child Neurol., Suppl. 27, 14*:17, 1972.

4. Cohen, A.C.: Maximum likelihood estimation of the
    dispersion parameter of a chi-distributed radial error
    from truncated and censored samples with applications to
    target analysis. *Am. Stat. A. J., 50*:1122, 1955.

5. Degenhardt, K.H., Knoche, E.: Analysis of intrauterine
    malformations of the vertebral column induced by oxygen
    deficiency. *Canad. Med. Assoc. J., 80*:441, 1959.

6. DeHaan, R.L., Ebert, J.D.: Morphogenesis. *Ann. Rev.
    Physiol., 26*:15, 1964.

7. Ferm, V.H.: Developmental malformation induced by
    cadmium. *Biol. Neonate, 19*:101, 1971.

8. Field, J.H., Krag, D.O.: Congenital constricting bands
    and congenital amputation of the fingers: placental
    studies. *J. Bone & Jt. Surg., 55A*:1035, 1973.

9. Gal, I.: Risks and benefits of the use of hormonal
    pregnancy test tablets. *Nature, 240*:241, 1972.

10. Gardner, W.L.: Rupture of the neural tube? Clinical
    Neurology. Proc. Congress Neurological Surgeons,
    Baltimore, The William and Wilkins Co., 1967, pp. 57.

11. Grote, W.: Missbildungen des Rumpfskelets nach mutter-
    lichem Blutverlust bein Kaninchen. *Zeitsch. f. Anatomie
    U Entwick., 128*:66, 1969.

12. Hay, E.D.: Organization and fine structure of epithe-
    lium and mesenchyme in the developing chick embryo.
    IN Epithelial-Mesenchymal Interactions, R. Fleischmajer
    and R.E. Billingham (eds.), Baltimore, The Williams and
    Wilkins Co., 1968.

13. Ireland, D.C., Takayama, N., Flatt, A.E.: Poland's
    syndrome: a review of forty-three cases. *J. Bone &
    Jt. Surg., 58A*:52, 1976.

14. Jellinger, K., Gross, H.: Congenital telencephalic
    midline defects. *Neuropadiatrie, 4*:446, 1973.

15. Källén, B.: Early embryogenesis of the central nervous
    system with special reference to closure defects. *Dev.
    Med. Child Neurol., Suppl., 16*:44, 1968.

16. Kieny, M., Mauger, A., Sengel, P.: Early regionaliza-
    tion of the somitic mesoderm as studied by the develop-
    ment of the axial skeleton of the chick embryo. *Dev.
    Biol., 28*:142, 1972.

17. Kino, Y.: Clinical and experimental studies of the
    congenital constriction band syndrome, with an emphasis
    on its etiology. *J. Bone & Jt. Surg., 57A*:636, 1975.

18. Krone, H.A.: Veroffentlichungen aus der Morphologischen
    Pathologie, Heft 62, Die Bedeutung der Eibettstorungen
    fur die Entstehung menchlicher Missbildungen. Stuttgart,
    Gustav Fischer Verlag, 1961.

19. Marin-Padilla, M.: Morphogenesis of anencephaly and

related malformations. *Current Topics in Pathology, 51*:
145, 1970.

20. McLennan, J.E.: Implications of the eccentricity of the
    human umbilical cord. *Am. J. Obstet. & Gynec., 101*:
    1124, 1968.

21. McLennan, J.E.: Rib anomalies in myelodysplasia: an
    approach to embryologic inference. *Biol. Neonate.,
    29*:129, 1976.

22. Morgagni, J.B.: The seats and causes of diseases
    investigated by anatomy. (English translation: Benjamin
    Alexander). London, A. Millar and T. Cadell, 1769.

23. Myers, R.E.: Two patterns of perinatal brain damage
    and their conditions of occurrence. *Am. J. Obstet. &
    Gynec., 112*:246, 1972.

24. Nakano, K.N.: Anencephaly: a review. *Dev. Med. Child
    Neurol., 15*:383, 1973.

25. Padget, D.H.: Neuroschisis and human embryonic malde-
    velopment: new evidence of anencephaly, spina bifida
    and diverse mammalian defects. *J. Neuropath. Exptl.
    Neurol., 29*:192, 1970.

26. von Recklinghausen, F.: Untersuchungen uber die Spina
    bifida. II. Uber die Art und die Entstehung der Spina
    bifida ihre Beziehung zur Ruckenmarks und Darmspalte.
    Virchows Arch. path. Anat., 105:296, 1886.

27. Renwick, J.H.: Hypothesis, anencephaly and spina bifida
    are usually preventable by avoidance of a specific but
    unidentified substance present in certain potato tubers.
    Brit. J. Prevent. & Soc. Med., 26:67, 1972.

28. Roberts, H.: X-ray induced teratogenesis in the mouse
    and its possible significance to man. *Radiology, 99*:
    433, 1971.

29. Seno, T.: An experimental study on the formation of the

body wall in the chick. *Acta Anatomica, 45*:60, 1961.

30. Smith, D.W.: Recognizable Patterns of Human Malformation. Philadelphia, W.B. Saunders Co., 1970.

31. Smith, D.W., Theiler, K., Schachenman, G.: Rib-gap defect with micrognathia, malformed tracheal cartilages, and redundant skin: a new pattern of defective development. *J. Ped., 69*:799, 1966.

32. Streeter, G.L.: Focal deficiencies in fetal tissues and their relation to intrauterine amputation. *Contrib. to Embryol. of the Carnegie Foundation, 22*:1, 1930.

33. Warkany, J., Wilson, J.G., Geiger, J.F.: Myeloschisis and myelomeningocele produced experimentally in the rat. *J. Comp. Neurol., 109*:35, 1958.

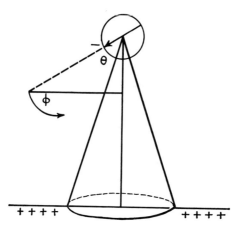

Fig. 1a. Polarized zygote approaches decidual surface and attempts to orient its body stalk vector at 180 degrees to the uterine lumen. "Attractive forces" between zygote and surface are portrayed as electrical. Θ is the angle of the vector in the vertical axis and φ the rotational angle about this axis.

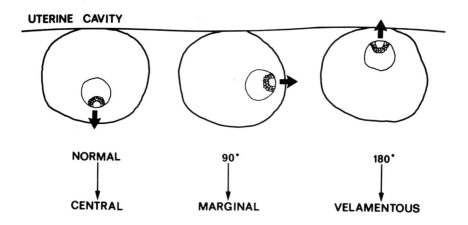

Fig. 1b. Diagram of (7 to 9 day) embryo implanted with its vector properly oriented (left), at 90 degrees to vertical (middle) and "upside down" (right). The latter two instances will produce marginal and velamentous (membranous) umbilical cord insertions respectively.

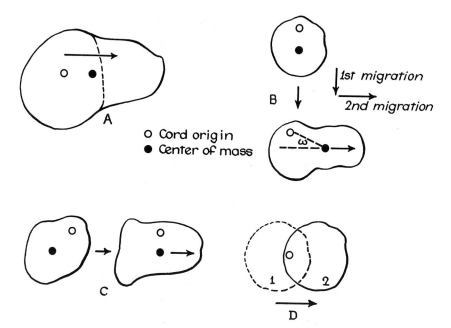

Fig. 2. Possible mechanisms of "trophotropism" or eccentricity of umbilical cord origin arising from differential "wandering" of placental margins. Eccentricity is defined as the distance between the cord origin (○) and the centroid (●) of the placental plane projection at term gestation. A) Elongation of single margin creates eccentric cord from originally central insertion, B) two separate migrations at 90 degrees to each other resulting in eccentric cord origin, C) migration decreases pre-existing eccentricity, D) entire placenta shifts moving originally central cord to the margin; this mechanism is presumably anatomically impossible.

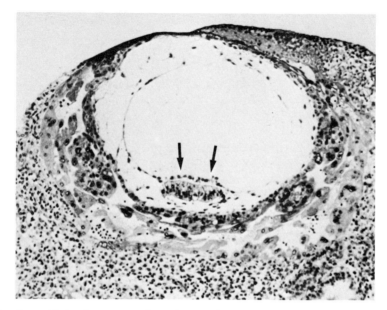

Fig. 3a. 12-day human embryo (arrows) properly oriented into decidual surface at 180 degrees to uterine lumen. (Photomicrograph by Dr. Arthur Hertig.)

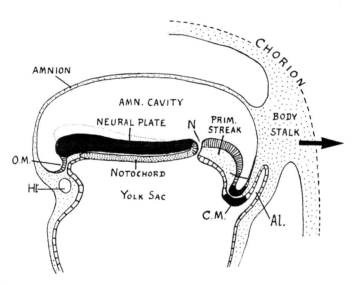

Fig. 3b. Diagram showing recently implanted ("2-3 week") embryo and structural relationship to "body stalk vector" (arrow), amniotic cavity and chorionic membrane. (o.m., oral membrane; c.m., cloacal membrane; Ht, primordial heart; Al, alantosis; N, neurenteric caual.) (Adapted from R. A. Willis, Boarderland of Embryology and Pathology, 1962.)

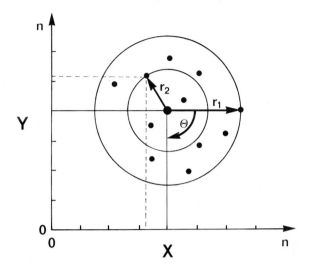

Fig. 4. "Target model" demonstrates "shots," aimed at "bulls eye" but scattering about the center of target with radial (R) symmetry and with a statistically predictable distribution of radial error ($r_1 r_2$). Hits may be characterized by either rectangular (x, y) or polar (r, θ) coordinates.

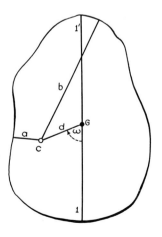

Fig. 5. Diagram of parameters measured or calculated from placental surface (plane projection of placenta removed from uterus). C, cord origin; G, center of mass (centroid); 11', longest axis; a, shortest distance from cord to margin; d, eccentricity; ω, angle between d and 11'.

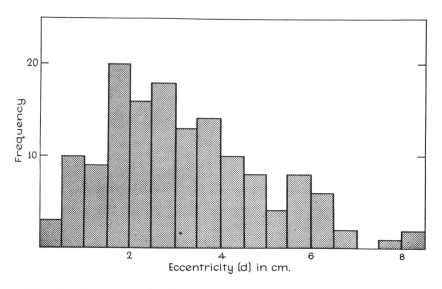

Fig. 6a. Frequency distribution of umbilical cord eccentricity from 142 unselected term gestations.

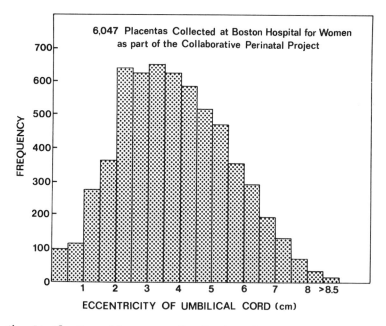

Fig. 6b. Verification of frequency distribution of eccentricity in a large heterogenous population of varying gestational ages (specimens collected as part of the Collaborative Perinatal Project). Both of these populations follow the frequency distribution predicted from the "target model."

Fig. 7. Examples of rib anomalies associated with lumbosacral myelomeningocele.

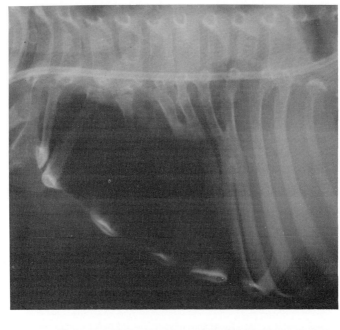

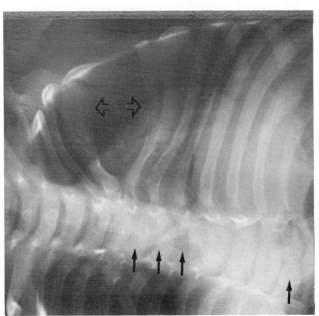

Fig. 7a. Grade 3 defect, large gap (open arrows) between left ribs 4 and 5 with fusion at both margins of gap. Abnormal vertebral bodies are indicated by arrows.

Fig. 7b. Grade 4 defect, multiple contiguous missing rib segments with gap at 2–3 and fusion at lower margin of defect. Vertebral bodies appear grossly normal.

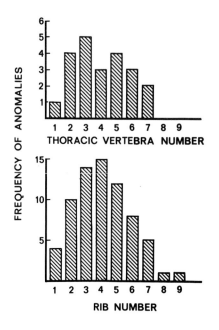

Fig. 8a.   Total axial frequency distribution (right and left) of 70 abnormal ribs and accompanying abnormal vertebral bodies in 20 patients with lumbosacral myelomeningocele.

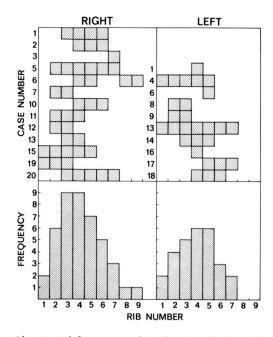

Fig. 8b.   Axial frequency distribution, by hemithorax, of abnormal ribs (bottom panels) and segmental (rib) involvement by case number (top panels).

164

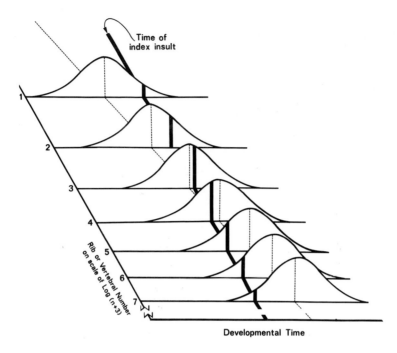

Fig. 9. Three-dimensional model of relationships between axial segment (depth), developmental time (horizontal axis) and primordial vulnerability (vertical axis) at the moment of teratogenic "hit" indicated by the *index insult* (heavy black bar) establishing lumbosacral myelomeningocele. Distributions of segmental primordial vulnerability in developmental time are all portrayed as similar normal distributions for simplicity (see ref. 21 for details of model). The *vertical* black bars at each axial segment correspond to the theoretical spatial frequency of rib anomaly shown in Fig. 10.

Fig. 10. Comparable distribution of theoretical (cross-hatched bars) and observed (open bars) frequencies of anomalous ribs at each axial segment.

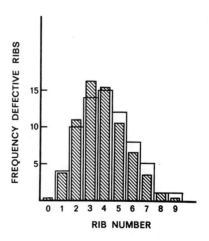

165

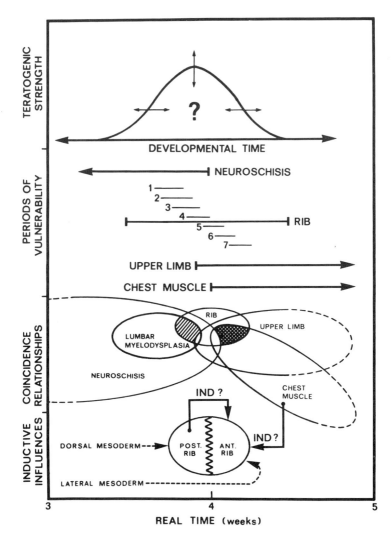

Fig. 11. Overview of some events in developmental time during 3rd to 5th gestational weeks. *Top panel*: teratogenic event characterized as a normal distribution of unknown strength and duration. *Second panel*: estimated periods of vulnerability for determination of neuroschisis, various rib anomalies, upper limb and chest muscle defects showing approximate overlap in developmental time. *Third panel*: Venn diagram of intersection of vulnerable periods–coexistent rib defects and lumbosacral myelomeningocele (cross-hatched, coexistent rib, upper limb and chest muscle anomalies (Poland's syndrome) (strippled). *Bottom panel*: possible inductive influence of posterior rib and chest muscle on anterior rib.

166

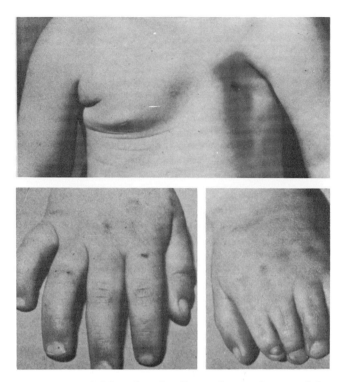

Fig. 12. Child with Poland's syndrome showing left upper thoracic hypoplastic ribs and absent pectoralis muscles with hypoplastic left hand (bottom, right). (Adapted from D.W. Smith[30].)

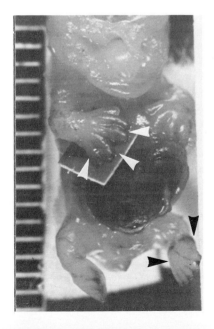

Fig. 13. 6 week (15mm) human embryo demonstrates separate digits on upper limb (white arrowheads) while foot lags in "finger ray" stage (black arrowheads).

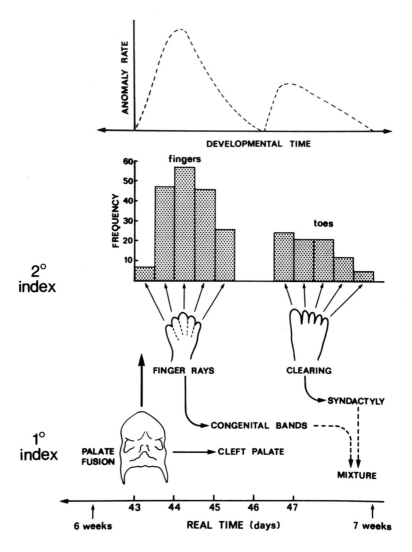

Fig. 14. Overview of developmental time in 6th week of gestation. *Top panel*: estimate of nonlinear developmental time based on anomaly rate of fingers and toes. *Middle panel*: histogram of spatial frequency distribution of anomaly by digital position-data of Kino[17] from 59 patients with constriction band anomalies of fingers and toes—fingers appear to pass through "central clearing" of "finger ray" stage before toes do (cf. Fig. 13). *Bottom panel*: *cleft palate* provides a possible *index anomaly* against which to align finger and toe defects (congenital bands ± syndactyly and polydactyly).

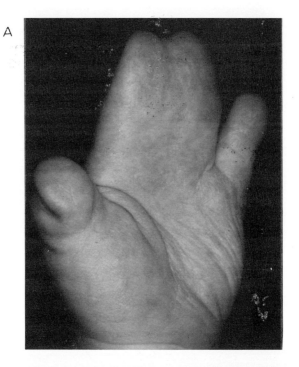

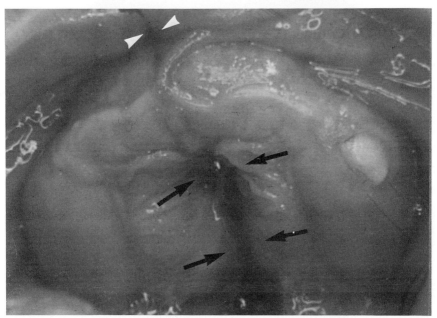

Fig. 15. Otherwise normal child with A) single "mitten hand" (syndactyly) and B) cleft lip (white arrowheads) and palate (black arrows).

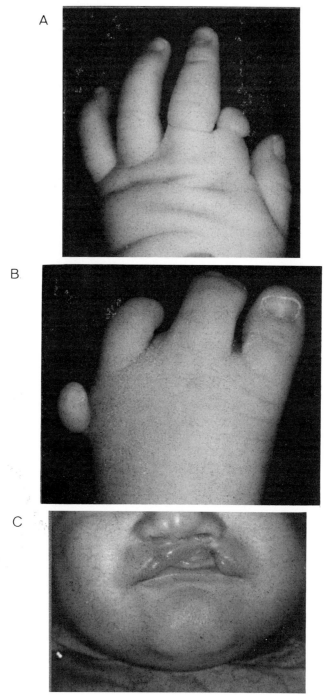

Fig. 16. Otherwise normal child with A) constriction band amputation of the left index finger, B) syndactyly and constriction amputation of left toes, and C) cleft lip and palate.

MENINGOMYELOCELE: A PROGRESSIVE INTRAUTERINE DISEASE

Fred J. Epstein, M.D., Arthur Marlin, M.D.,
Gerald Hochwald, M.D. and Joseph Ransohoff, M.D.

The study of evolving meningomyelocele in human embryos and trypan blue induced dysraphism in the laboratory animal has been the basis of much controversy concerning the basic embryologic genesis of meningocele.[1,2,4,5,6,7]

Some investigators believe that neurulation occurs, but subsequently there is rupture of the hydromyelic spinal cord resulting in the formation of the neural plate. Others believe that neurulation does not become complete, and therefore, the neural tube does not develop, leaving an open neural plate which is later incorporated into the sac of the meningomyelocele.

In an attempt to further elucidate the evolution of meningomyelocele, the authors have constructed a laboratory model in which massive focal hydromyelia occurs. It is based on surgical modification of the hydromyelia which occurs in the chronic hydrocephalic cat.[3] It is the results and implications of this work that is the subject of this report.

METHOD

Eleven adult cats were made chronically hydrocephalic by the intracisternal injection of Kaolin. Four weeks after

the induction of hydrocephalus, the animals were studied by
pantopaque ventriculography which confirmed the presence of
hydromyelia (Fig. 1). Ten days later, the animals were
subjected to a 4-level laminectomy in the lower thoracic
region. The dura was opened, and the wound was closed in
layers leaving only a plegit of Gelfoam over the exposed
spinal cord. A control group of animals, in which there was
no hydrocephalus, was treated by laminectomy in a similar
fashion.

One week later, the ventriculography was repeated,
following which the animals were sacrificed and the spinal
cords removed.

RESULTS

Following surgery, four animals were paraplegic and they
were not included in the study inasmuch as the altered cord
morphology might have been partially due to surgical trauma.
The remaining animals were neurologically intact, and for
this reason, it was assumed that local anatomic alternations
were not the result of trauma.

In all animals in which hydrocephalus and hydromyelia
co-existed, the spinal cord immediately bulged through the
dural incision. Several days later, ventriculography disclosed that the central canal was markedly dilated beneath
the entire laminectomy (Fig. 2), and subsequent pathological
examination confirmed the presence of a focal bulge confined
to the same region (Fig. 3). On sectioning, it was evident
that the central canal was massively enlarged, filling the
entire spinal cord beneath the bulging region (Fig. 4).
This was in contrast to the normal cord in which the radiologic as well as the gross pathological examinations were
normal.

DISCUSSION

Gardner has repeatedly pointed out that the normal embryo undergoes a state of physiological hydromyelia. According to his theory, in the fetus with some element of obstruction to normal spinal fluid pathways, the hydromyelia is exaggerated, and therefore, the spinal cord subjected to a greater hydrodynamic stress which culminates in rupture of the posterior surface of the cord with formation of the neural plate.

On the basis of this study, it is evident that in hydromyelia associated with compensated feline hydrocephalus, it is the intact dural and bony structures which prevent expansion of the underlying, mildly dilated central canal. Following laminectomy and dural incision, the resultant focal hydromyelia bears a physical likeness to foetal myelocele. It is tempting to hypothesize that this animal model is illustrative of prenatal forces that culminate in meningomyelocele. Perhaps in the embryo, hydromyelia coupled with malformation of dural and bony elements underlies the subsequent evolution of massive focal hydromyelia which ultimately causes rupture of the posterior surface of the spinal cord and formation of a neural plate. Therefore, it is possible that spinal dysgraphism is sometimes secondary to an interplay of factors, one being malformation of meso-dermal structures and the other, hydromyelia of the under-lying spinal cord. This combination of anomalies may inter-act to result in focal disruption of neural tissues and plate formation.

Although in the present study actual rupture of the damaged spinal cord did not occur, this was probably because adult animals were utilized. It is likely that the unmye-linated foetal or neonatal spinal cord is more vulnerable to physical stress and, therefore, rupture.

Certainly, this need not be the only developmental sequence in the evolution of this anomaly. It has been well demonstrated that in the developing embryo, the ventral spinal subarachnoid space is often markedly dilated, and therefore, focal pressure from this region may displace the spinal cord posteriorly into the defect where mesodermal elements have not developed. This sustained anterior extrinsic compression may ultimately destroy the terminal cord, forming a similar neural plate to that resulting from disruption of the cord from within.

The actual meningomyelocele plate in the paraplegic neonate most often consists of disorganized remnants of neural tissue, scattered ependymal cells, and fibrovascular stroma. Certainly, functional neural tissue is only rarely present in the lesion. Inasmuch as the severely afflicted children invariably has normal peripheral nerves as well as muscle bulk, and both of these are dependent on the early inductive influence of the intact spinal cord, it would seem that sometime during gestation, normal or near normal cellular elements must have existed in the region of the neural plate. Therefore, it seems likely that the neural plate is the pathological remnant of a progressive disease having as its inception hydromyelia, and only gradually evolving to meningomyelocele.

In support of this concept, it has been noted by Swinyard, that foetal movements of afflicted children were often normal until the last trimester, following which, they declined. This would suggest that occasionally, despite pathological hydromyelia, the foetal spinal cord contains enough normal or near normal elements to induce the growth of normal peripheral nerves and extremity musculature.

However, as gestation continues, the hydromyelic terminal
spinal cord, unsupported by bone, dura, and muscle, undergoes a process of self-destruction which results in formation
of a neural plate.

   Therefore, in conclusion, we believe that meningomyelocele is the end stage of a progressive intrauterine disease
which is initiated by pathological hydromyelia and culminated
by rupture of the unsupported spinal cord as a result of
maldevelopment of associated mesodermal tissues.

REFERENCES

1. Gardner, W.J.: Hydrodynamic mechanism of syringomyelia:
    its relationship to myelocele. *J. Neurol. Neurosurg.
    and Psychiat.*, *28*:247, 1965.

2. Gardner, W.J.: Myelocele: rupture of the neural tube.
    Clin. Neurosurg., *15*:57, 1968.

3. Hochwald, Gerald, et al: Personal Communication.

4. Kallen, B.: Early embryogenesis of the central nervous
    ystem with special reference to closure defects. 1968.

5. Padget, D.: Spina bifida and embryonic neuroschisis -
    A causal relationship. *Johns Hopkins Med. Bull.*, *123*:
    233, 1968.

6. Padget, D.H.: Neuroschisis in human embryonic maldevel-
    opment. *J. Neuropath. Exp. Neurol.*, *29*:192, 1970.

7. Warhany, J.J., Wilson, G., and Gelger, J.F.: Myeloschi-
    sis and myelomeningocele produced experimentally in the
    rat. *J. Comp. Neurol.*, *109*:35, 1958.

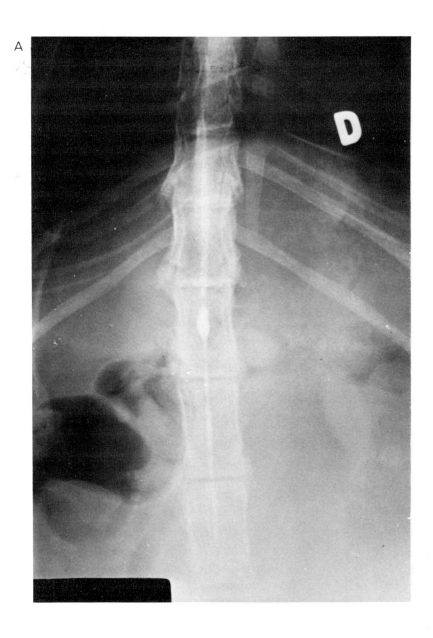

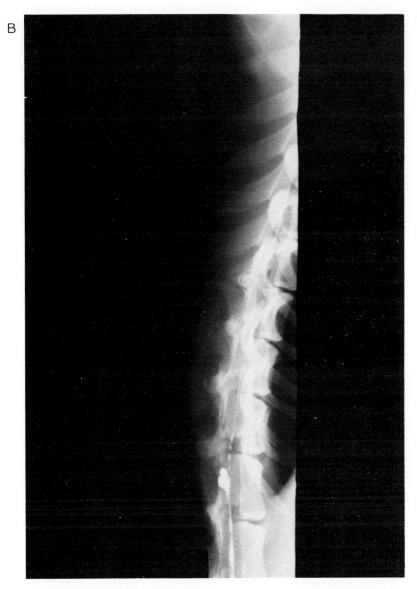

Fig. 1. A & B. Note focal hydromyelia with essentially normal central canal above and below bulge.

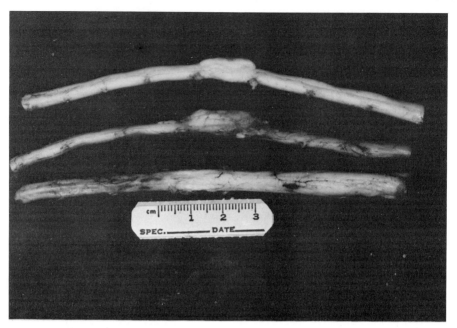

Fig. 2. Note massive focal hydromyelia. This bears some physical similarity to human myelocele.

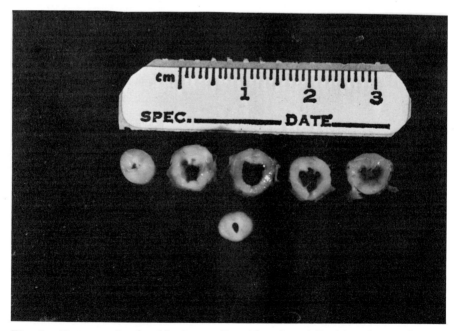

Fig. 3. Note massive focal hydromyelia with only mildly dilated central canal above and below involved region.

INTRACRANIAL PRESSURE IN
HYDROCEPHALUS - NEWER CONCEPTS

K. Shulman, M.D. and A. Marmarou, Ph.D.

Clinical practice defines hydrocephalus as an intraventricular increase in cerebrospinal fluid volume under increased pressure. When it became known that a number of patients with the so-called normal pressure hydrocephalus (NPH) syndrome had normal lumbar spinal pressure, it was thought that perhaps two syndromes of hydrocephalus existed, one of normal pressure in the adult and one of high pressure in infants and children and in adults with obstructive lesions such as tumors. The measurement of steady state intracranial pressure in infants and children with open fontanelle and/or open cranial sutures, during times of active hydrocephalus, have now clearly shown that many such children will have normal steady state intracranial pressure.[11,8,2] Just as in adults with NPH, in infantile hydrocephalus there may be fluctuations in intracranial pressure during the sleep cycle due to a change in cerebral blood volume and perhaps as well a change in the compliance of the cranial contents reflecting an increase in cerebral blood volume. Additionally, experimental studies of hydrocephalus, either with occlusion of the aqueduct, producing a rapid ventriculomegaly,[9] or in the more slowly developing hydrocephalus, caused by instillation of kaolin, silicone, etc. into the

cisterna magna,[13] the experimental animals go through a
period of raised intracranial pressure and then settle down
to normal pressure at a time when there still may very well
be progressive ventricular dilatation. It seems then an
appropriate question: "Does intracranial pressure need to be
elevated in order to maintain ventriculomegaly or to cause
progressive ventricular dilatation?"

It might be argued that pressure need not be elevated if
other volumes are displaced. The law of Weed[15] which is a
reiteration of the Munro-Kellie hypothesis, states that total
intracranial contents are nearly constant so that with
changes of any of the three intracranial volumes, i.e.,
brain, intracranial blood volume (CBV) or intracranial CSF
volume, compensatory changes take place in the other volumes.
Steady state changes in intracranial pressure are due to
uncompensated volume changes in any of these compartments.
Ventriculomegaly can occur theoretically without a pressure
rise if CBV, extraventricular CSF, or brain water are displaced; such changes would allow an increase of about 50 ml
ventricular volume. Beyond this the situation of increased
CSF volume with increased pressure intuitively can be understood but the idea of progressive ventricular dilatation with
normal intracranial pressure requires an understanding of
some newer concepts of intracranial biomechanics, particularly compliance and pressure gradients.

In his thoughtful account of NPH in 1968, Geschwind[6]
discounted the argument of Hakim and Adams[7] that normal intracranial pressure could maintain the ventricles in an enlarged
state because the total force, i.e., pressure times area
increases as the surface area of the ventricles increases.
Geschwind felt that surface area as the only variable could

not account for the behavior even of a very simple system.
He furthermore demonstrated by a series of mathematical
proofs, that the factor which determines changes in pressure
with increasing radius of the ventricle is the structural
properties of the ventricular container. The elastic properties of this container that must be considered are those of
the brain, vascular compartment, dura, and bone. The brain,
dura, and bone taken as individual elements can be described
in terms of an elastic modulus which is the ratio of stress
required to produce a certain strain. Mechanical tests of
these substances by Galford and McElhany[5] showed that the
elastic modulus of dura is 500 times that of brain, and the
ratio of bone to brain approximately 1 million.[14] The
elastic modulus of brain in these studies was measured using
small samples (¼ in. height, ½ inc. diam.) obtained at autopsy
and maintained in Ringer's solution. The elastic modulus of
the entire brain as it is modified by a distributed vascular
network cannot be determined by ordinary methods.

Marmarou and Shulman[10] have chosen to look at the combined action of these elements and describe the distensibility
of the CSF system in terms of compliance, which is the ratio
of CSF volume required to produce a change of CSF pressure
($\Delta V/\Delta P$). Experiments in animals and in man show that compliance of distensibility of the neural tube varies as a function
of pressure. As pressure is increased the compliance is
reduced by an inverse relationship. We have also studied how
compliance is distributed and found that 37% of the total
extensibility of the CNS is provided by the spinal axis.
The remaining 63% of total compliance is contained within the
intracranial space. To express this more simply we have
derived a term, the Pressure Volume Index (PVI) which taken

into account the variation of stiffness with pressure and
allows one to express the distensibility in more practical
terms as the amount of fluid volume required to produce a
ratio of 10 in pressure. The PVI then at least theoretically
can be used to assess the elasticity of the normal periventricular envelope as determined by a distributed vascular
network which is easily compressed. It is intuitively
obvious that with a tight brain less volume will be required
to produce this increase of ventricular pressure. In hydrocephalus, in contradistinction, we postulate that the
compliance of the periventricular envelope is modified due to
the structural and biochemical changes observed; these tissue
changes effect PVI so that the ventricular container becomes
soft and ventricular enlargement can occur without large
pressure rises.

    In both the analytical treatments of Geschwind and those
of Epstein,[3] the brain was modeled as a closed spherical
mass. By such an approach, the analytical relationships of
ventricular pressure, volume and circumferential tension
were confined strictly to wall properties alone. This is
not entirely correct. The mechanisms of formation and
absorption play an important role in determining the stress
on the ependyma as shown in Fig. 1. This figure illustrates
that under steady state conditions, the ventricular pressure
within both spherical models must follow the pressure determined by the product of formation and resistance to CSF outflow. The increase in volume of each container would depend
upon the compliance. If the brain is rigid (low compliance)
as in Fig. 1A, the increase in volume necessary to reach the
pressure level is small. For a soft or highly compliant
brain as shown in 1B, a large increase in volume would be
required.

There is an anatomical limit, beyond which the resis-
ance and compliance mechanisms interact and become mutually
dependent. This condition is realized when volume expansion
of the ventricle compresses the brain surface and increases
the CSF impedance to flow over the convexities. This
increase in resistance to outflow raises the internal pressure level and a vicious cycle is initiated whereby the
ventricular volume would enlarge in attempt to conform to the
higher pressure, resulting in greater compression and further
increase of resistance to CSF outflow. Under these circumstances, the ventricular pressure, ventricular volume, and
compliance become mutually interactive such as to effect a
condition of dynamic pressure instability and progressive
ventricular dilatation.

Shortly following the description of NPH by Hakim and
Adams, Fishman[4] was the first to stress the possibility of
pressure gradients on this basis, theorizing that the
critical pressure for ventricular dilatation is the pressure
gradient from ventricle to subarachnoid space - the trans-
mural pressure gradient across the cerebral mantle. This
when increased results in a loss of lipid and protein from
the adjacent white matter which despite compression has
increased water content. As long as there is free communication between ventricle and surface subarachnoid space there
can be no pressure gradient between them and pressure is
exerted only on the skull. If the subarachnoid space becomes
obliterated, do gradients exist transmurally? Since in the
surgeon's experience, an obliterated dry subarachnoid space
is not observed other possible causes of a pressure gradient
between ventricle and brain are needed. According to the
theoretical studies by Epstein, the ventricular fluid
pressure is not completely balanced by the reactive tension

at the brain surface and a finite gradient of pressure is
continuously aiming to expand the ventricle under steady
state condition. In addition to this constant pressure
difference, transient gradients synchronous with vascular
pulsations must be considered. Bering's[1] observations of the
to and fro movement of CSF in the aqueduct support the notion
of a pulsatile differential in pressure. Our studies have
shown that although the amplitude of CSF pressure pulsation
is uniform throughout the system, small differences in phase
between VFP and subarachnoid pulses can exist and are augmented as the impedance of CSF pathways is increased. These
phase differences might account for the bi-directional flow
found by Bering, and depending upon the viscoelastic properties of tissue could act as a net positive gradient favoring
dilatation of the ventricle at normal pressure levels.

How does the brain parenchyma react to these pressure
changes? Brain tissue pressure does not share in the phasic
pulse pressure phenomena described by Bering. Under normal
conditions brain tissue pressure measured by wick probes is
within the envelope of ventricular fluid pressure slightly
less than the systolic phase of ventricular fluid pressure.
We can therefore look at brain tissue pressure in the para-
ventricular area as equal to or slightly less than steady
state ventricular fluid pressure. There is then a small
pulsatile gradient available for ventricular enlargement
under physiological conditions with maximum circumferential
tension developed at the ependymal surface. Once the ependymal surface is broken in the hydrocephalic process the brain
tissue pressure becomes equal to ventricular fluid pressure
and the gradient disappears. However, in the next adjacent
layer of white matter there is a brain tissue pressure
gradient small but existent, between periventricular brain

tissue and the deeper brain tissue pressure; and this allows
for ventricular expansion by a process, if you would, of
erosion. Finally, brain tissue substances are lost particularly lipid and protein, creating a "vacuum" or volume into
which ventricular expansion can occur. The ventricular
pressure now reflects the added ventricular volume and is in
equilibrium with the large tissue space adjacent to the
ventricle. This increased volume with an unchanged or
expanded compliance results in a normal ventricular fluid
pressure despite the increased ventricular volume (Fig. 2).

It is in our view possible to explain the maintenance of
ventriculomegaly and progression of ventriculomegaly without
increased ventricular fluid pressure by two related biomechanical considerations. First, there occurs a change in
the wall properties of the ventricle. This change is accompanied by a reversible decrease in lipid and myelin with an
increase of water content of the periventricular white matter
and is reflected in compliance changes. The volume-pressure
relationship is modified and since pressure is governed by
formation and absorption parameters, the ventricle must
accommodate by increases in volume in order to preserve equilibrium. The time course of this compliance change can be
described by alterations of the pressure volume index (PVI).
The second mechanism responsible is that of correspondence of
VFP and brain tissue pressure, as ependymal disruption
occurs, causing periventricular tissue pressure to become
identical in its static and dynamic pressures with VFP, with
maximum tension transferred to the next layer of tissue.
A pressure gradient comes into play at the deeper layers of
white matter with the wave of pressure gradually eroding
white matter and bringing with these forces the enlargement

of the ventricle. These advancing tissue changes are
further modifying the compliance and its descriptors, the
PVI.

Restoration of these tissue changes, structural, bio-
chemical and dynamic, results in recession of the hydrocephalic process. When a diversion is created which acts to
remove large amounts of ventricular fluid volume lowering the
VFP below normal, container compliance and pressure correspondence is altered in a beneficial manner permitting the
ventricle which before had enlarged due to conditions of wall
compliance and tissue pressure correspondence, to no longer
enlarge or to actually decrease in size.

REFERENCES

1. Bering, A.E.: Pathophysiology of hydrocephalus. IN
    Workshop in Hydrocephalus, K. Shulman (ed.), Children's
    Hospital, Philadelphia, 1965.
2. DiRocco, C., McLone, D.G., Shimoji, T., and Raimondi,
    A.J.: Continuous intraventricular cerebrospinal fluid
    pressure recording in hydrocephalic children during
    wakefulness and sleep. *J. Neurosurg., 42*:683, 1975.
3. Epstein, Charles. The distribution of intracranial
    forces in acute and chronic hydrocephalus. *J. Neurol.
    Sci., 21*:171, 1974.
4. Fishman, R.A.: Occult hydrocephalus. *New Eng. J. Med.,
    274*:466, 1966.
5. Galford, J.E. and McElhany, J.H.: A visoelastic study of
    scalp, brain and dura. *J. Biomechanics, 3*:211, 1969.
6. Geschwind, N.: The mechanism of normal pressure hydro-
    cephalus. *J. Neurol. Sci., 7*:481, 1968.

7. Hakim, S. and Adams, R.D.: The special clinical problem of symptomatic hydrocephalus with normal cerebrospinal fluid pressure. Observations on cerebrospinal fluid hydrodynamics. *J. Neurol. Sci.*, *2*:307, 1965.

8. Hayden, P.W., Shurtleff, D.B., and Foltz, E.L.: Ventricular fluid pressure recordings in hydrocephalic patients. *Arch. Neurol.*, *23*:147, 1970.

9. Milhorat, T.H.: Experimental hydrocephalus. A technique of producing obstructive hydrocephalus in the monkey. *J. Neurosurg.*, *32*:385, 1970.

10. Marmarou, A. and Shulman, K.: Compartmental analysis of compliance and outflow resistance of the cerebrospinal fluid system. *J. Neurosurg.*, *43*:523, 1975.

11. Shulman, K. and Marmarou, A.: Pressure-volume considerations in infantile hydrocephalus. *Dev. Med. Child Neurol.*, *Suppl. 25*:90, 1971.

12. Shulman, K., Marmarou, A., Shapiro, K.: Brain tissue pressure and focal pressure gradients. Chicago Conference on Neural Trauma, 1975 (In press).

13. Smith, J.W. and Walmsley, R.: Factors affecting the elasticity of bone. *J. Anat. (Lond)*, *93*:503, 1959.

14. Weller, R., Wisneiwski, H., Shulman, K.: Experimental hydrocephalus in young dogs: histological and ultrastructural study of the brain tissue damage. *J. Neuropath. Exp. Neurol.*, *30*:613, 1971.

15. Weed, L.H.: Some limitations of the Munro-Kellie hypothesis. *Arch. Surg.*, *18*:1049, 1929.

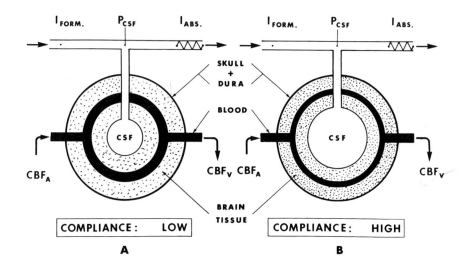

Fig. 1. Mechanical models to illustrate that mechanisms of formation and absorption play an important role in determining stress on the ependyma. Under steady state conditions (I form = I abs), the ventricular pressure within both models must follow the CSF pressure which is a function of the product of formation and resistance to absorption (equal in both models). The increase in volume of each container would depend upon the compliance. If the brain is rigid as in (A), the increase in volume corresponding to the CSF pressure level is small. For a soft or highly compliant brain, (B), a large increase in volume would be required. In the above configuration, the CSF equilibrium pressure is the determining factor to which the volume of the containers must conform. Changing the wall properties affects only the ventricular volume and not the equilibrium pressure.

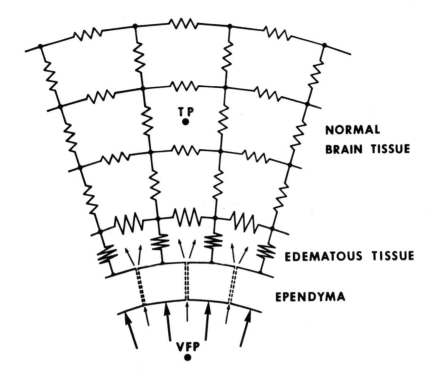

Fig. 2. A schematic model of the brain tissue-ependymal wall configuration. Under normal conditions brain tissue pressure (TP), measured by wick probes, is slightly less than the systolic phase of ventricular fluid pressure (VFP), and compliance of tissue is uniform. In the presence of edema, tissue compliance increases. This softening of the linear layer of tissue permits expansion of the ventricle until pressure equilibrium is required between fluid and tissue. The extension of this process to the next layer of healthy tissue leads to progressive ventricular enlargement with undetectable rise in fluid pressure (N.P.H.).

A TECHNIQUE FOR REPAIR OF
LARGE SPINA BIFIDA DEFECTS

E. Bruce Hendrick, M.D., Harold J. Hoffman, M.D.
and Robin P. Humphreys, M.D.

INTRODUCTION

The purpose of this paper is to present a method for
repair of large spina bifida defects. It has presented a
technical problem with the elimination of philosophical and
social concepts.

For many years the closure of the small myelomeningocele
with a pedunculated presentation has presented no problem
from the surgical standpoint. The *Bete-Noir* of the pediatric
neurosurgeon, orthopedic surgeon and plastic surgeon has been
the large cessile myelomeningocele with a large skin defect
and associated neural elements presenting on the surface.
Very often compounding this problem is the presence of huge
protuberant shark-tooth-like, bony excrescences on either
side of the midline or in some patients a gibbous deformity
of the involved spinal area with hemivertebra and protrusion
of the bone posteriorly. Even with adequate skin closure in
the latter two problems, the bony prominences themselves will
deprive any skin graft no matter how carefully rotated, of
its blood supply leading to subsequent breakdown and
secondary infection. It is our purpose to describe a combined technique using multidisciplines to achieve adequate
skin closure of these defects (Fig. 1).

191

Because of what we thought was a difference in technique amongst the staff neurosurgeons at the Hospital for Sick Children in relation to myelomeningocele closure, a survey was carried out by one of our plastic surgeons, Dr. Hugh Thomson. Each patient when admitted was carefully charted as to size of myelomeningocele and type of wound closure. The purpose of the project of course, was to be a comparison of wound healing in using 3 different techniques. It turned out, however, that the techniques were not all that dissimilar varying only in minor points. The major similarity, of course, was adequate dissection of the dura off the lumbar fascia and a tight and adequate dural closure. There was very little difference in technique of closure of the fascia as an extra book-type support to give a secondary water tight membrane. The major differences occurred in skin closure with one individual using membrane skin and 2 others preferring to swing full thickness rotation flaps. The most important consideration, which applied to all wounds, was that the edges of the skin, no matter what type, would be closed without tension. In some patients, this involved the use of stainless steel sutures and buttons to take the tension off the wound edges. In other patients by massive undercutting and stripping of skin, the wound could be closed with interrupted silks or Dexon in the subcutaneous tissues and through the skin itself.

At the end of the survey, which dealt only with the large cutaneous defects, it was apparent that we were able to divide the cases into 3 groups.

Group I healed without complications within 2 weeks. Group II healed with minor complications such as minimal CSF leak, infection or wound necrose of 2 weeks. Group III was

delayed in healing which was interpreted as being over 2
weeks. In the group of patients surveyed there were 31
patients, 24 of which fell into Group I and Group II and 7
fell into the delayed group.

It became obvious that wound healing was not directly
influenced by: 1. the size of the lesion (ranges from 3.0-
10.5 cm in the crossed diameters). 2. the direction of
closure (axial, transverse, & oblique). 3. the presence of
hydrocephalus. 4. the use of a muscle fascial flap. 5.
suture material.

CONCLUSION

The wound healing was delayed when membrane skin was
used in closing and some alternative method of closure should
be used if the lesion can only be closed using membrane skin.

BONY DEFECTS

Following this survey of large cutaneous defects, we
have been faced with the problem of not only the large
cutaneous defect, but the patient who in addition, had a
marked bony spike or deformity presenting underneath the
skin. Very often these patients were not seen as newborns
but were referred some months later from another hospital,for
definitive surgery. Often these patients required some delay
or procrastination in their treatment to allow the child to
grow sufficient skin area over his buttocks and lumbar area
to enable a satisfactory plastic closure of the defect.
Each patient was carefully screened by neurosurgery,
orthopedic surgery and plastic surgery concerning the best
method of treatment. Unfortunately, our experience has been
limited in this type of case to approximately 5 patients. In
each case however, the patients presented with a total

paraplegic at or below the site of the lesion so no major
attempt was made to preserve nerve tissue. The neurosurgical
part of the procedure consisted of careful dissection of the
dura and dura remnants free of the bony canal, which is laid
open like a tulip with a broad bony base. In 3 of the
patients because of the marked gibbous deformity, the
remnants of the nonfunctioning cord or cauda equina were
amputated and the proximal end of the amputated dura closed
into a water tight sac. The orthopedic surgeons then removed
the keystone of the arch of these deformities and in 1 case,
removed 2 vertebrae. The remaining vertebrae were then
allowed to drop back into normal alignment and fastened by
various means. In 1 patient, by Harrington hooks and rods
and in another patient by slot grafting on the anterior
aspect of the vertebral bodies and wiring posteriorly.
Various forms of skin closure have been carried out but the
most satisfactory had been the double sickle flaps with the
use of buttons and wires to take up the tension. Occasionally,
the denuded area following the swing of the full thickness
flap has been so large that a split thickness graft has been
required.

The results to date, although limited in number, has
been most gratifying and illustrate again, the requirement
for cooperation amongst all pediatric surgical specialities
in the handling of major congenital deformities.

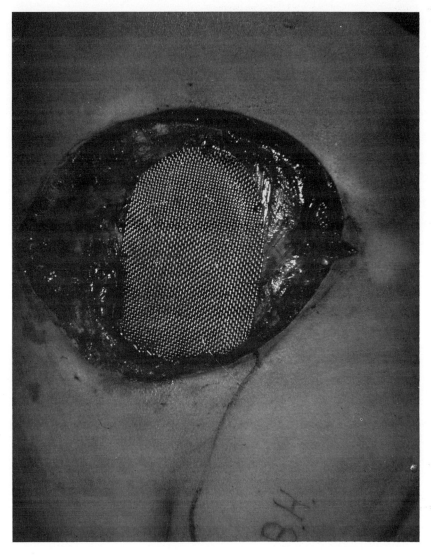

Fig. 1. Metallic (steel mesh) prosthesis for bony defect in myelomeningocele.

THE ARNOLD-CHIARI MALFORMATION:
PATHOLOGY AND DEVELOPMENTAL
CONSIDERATIONS

A. James McAdams, M.D.

In this description of the pathology of the AC malformation my considerations are largely limited to what I
believe to be its essential features. In essence, the
Arnold-Chiari malformation is an elongation of the hindbrain
(Fig. 1). Notwithstanding the superficial variability that
can be found within any population of cases, the malformation
is remarkably constant in kind. A part of the extended
brain stem, the medulla and sometimes the pons, resides in
the cervical spinal canal, as does a portion of the cerebellar
vermis, the so-called dorsal tongue. The recognizable extent
of the cerebellar tongue is the most variable expression of
the AC malformation, but there is always an extended caudal
velum which then constitutes the roof of an elongated 4th
ventricle. At the caudal end of the dorsal velum is the
choroid plexus (Figs. 2 & 3).
    Intimately related to the malformation is a reduction
in the size of the posterior fossa, an enlarged foramen
magnum and, what I consider the key to understanding the
malformation, an enlarged cervical spinal canal. My evidence
here is anecdotal and I am not aware of great emphasis having
been placed upon the large cervical spinal canal. For many
years, in addition to a large foramen magnum, we have

described cranialization of the cervical spinal canal understanding this to mean that it is the residence of a portion
of the brain that is normally intracranial. Some observers
describe this differently, speaking of the posterior fossa
as being small and conical in shape (Fig. 4).

Without taking too much liberty, it can be stated that
the Arnold-Chiari malformation in childhood is invariably
associated with some form of myelomeningocele. In the case
of myelomeningocele we encounter much variability in site
and expression in contrast to the remarkably constant
features that characterize the Arnold-Chiari malformation.
I am not going to discuss the developmental basis for
myelomeningocele but I would agree with the opinions of
teratologists favoring multifocal causes. I do not, however,
believe this to be true of the Arnold-Chiari malformation.
What connection then do I, as a pediatric pathologist, see
between the two?

Returning to the hindbrain malformation, the dorsal
vermian tongue and malposition of the choroid plexus has been
interpreted by others, and convincingly so, as evidence of a
developmental disturbance in the formation of the vermis.
A conceivable basis for this is that the nodulus and choroid
plexus are affixed by the too long brain stem preventing the
normal approximation of the nodulus to the fastigium.
Embryologically, the normal position is attributed to a
greater growth of the mid-vermian structure so that the
nodulus is, in effect, tucked in (Figs. 5,6). Obviously,
underdevelopment of the vermis could contribute to this and
it is notable that cerebellar hypoplasia is invariably
present in the Arnold-Chiari malformation.

The smallness of the posterior fossa can be related to

2 factors: The hypoplasia of the cerebellum and the fact
that a part of the hindbrain is developmentally within the
spinal canal. This is not a herniation in the usual sense.
In keeping with practical experience and supported by
experimental evidence, growth of the boney structure accommodates the contained object. The spinal canal is enlarged
because the medulla has developed there.

To explain the elongated brain stem and its developmental location within the spinal canal it seems necessary to
invoke a hydrostatic mechanism. In the original hydrostatic
theory, the hydromyelic, it was conceived that failure of
formation of the median aperture of the 4th ventricle, the
foramen of Magendie, was the primary event, the neural tube
being forcibly reopened. A serious obstacle to such a
mechanism is the observation of lumbosacral spina bifida
cystica in a 5.5 mm human embryo described by Lemire. This
is at a gestational time very close to that of normal closure
of the posterior neuropore and well in advance of choroid
plexus or median aperture formation.

It seems highly likely to me that an open neural tube is
the primary event and that the Arnold-Chiari malformation
occurs later and should be regarded as a secondary malformation. Evidence that the Arnold-Chiari malformation does
occur at a later time, developmentally, than myelomeningocele
can be seen experimentally in rats as shown by Warkany.
This can be inferred also from some human embryo specimens
but is not explicitly stated.

Of the suggested explanations for the elongated brain
stem, I find the most attractive, the one implicating an
interference with formation of the pontine flexure and this
is where I would invoke a hydrostatic mechanism. My

suggestion is that a closed neural tube is necessary for
the existence of a hydrostatic force essential to pontine
flexure formation. One of the questions I would ask
embryologists is how certain are we that the cervical flexure
defines the junction of brain and spinal cord? Is it
possible that the future medulla must ascend from the
cervical spinal column and will do so only as a consequence
of pontine flexure formation?

I have ignored many of the other findings in the central
nervous system in Arnold-Chiari malformation because I believe they have tertiary explanations. I would, however,
like to comment further on the dorsal deformity at the
junction of medulla and spinal cord. When severe this is
actually an S-shaped deformity - a doubling back. If it is
correct that the medulla is developmentally within the
cervical spinal canal, it would seem inevitable that such a
deformity would occur. This would in part be due to the
continued growth of the medulla and in part because there is
no well defined aperture comparable to a foramen magnum
between the cranialized and non-cranialized portion of the
cervical canal. There is also a practical consideration
here. The fetus *in utero* is in cervical flexion and one
could expect additional crowding of the hindbrain would be
inevitable upon birth with straightening of the neck. How
important this may be in accelerating hydrocephalus after
birth is difficult to assess. Of 26 patients with sufficient
data for analysis, 13 did show accelerated enlargement of
the head after birth. Nine of these had prompt surgical
closure of the myelomeningocele after birth. However, 5 of
the 13 who did not show accelerated enlargement also had
prompt surgical myelomeningocele closure.

It may be appropriate to reconsider some form of surgical decompression. It may be that only a delamination is necessary, possibly with release of one or more of the denticulate ligaments. The delamination would have to fully encompass the region of the dorsal deformity. Consideration could also be given to removal of the dorsal tongue when it is possible (Figs. 7,8,9). I would advocate that a trial of decompression should precede surgical closure of the myelo-meningocele.

REFERENCES

1. Barry, A., Patten, B.M., Stewart, B.H.: Possible Factors in the Development of the Arnold-Chiari Malformation. *J. Neurosurg.*, *14*:285, 1957.

2. Benda, C.E.: Dysraphic States. *J. Neuropath.*, *18*:56, 1959.

3. Brocklehurst, G.: A Quantitative Study of a Spina Bifida Foetus. *J. Path.*, *99*:205, 1969.

4. Brocklehurst, G.: The Development of the Human Cerebro-spinal Fluid Pathway with Particular Reference to the Roof of the Fourth Ventricle. *J. Anat.*, *105*:467, 1969.

5. Daniel, P.M., Strich, S.J.: Some Observations on the Congenital Deformity of the Central Nervous System Known as the Arnold-Chiari Malformation. *J. Neuropath.*, *17*: 255, 1958.

6. Gardner, W.J.: Rupture of the Neural Tube. *Arch. Neurol.,* *4*:1, 1961.

7. Holtzer, H.: An Experimental Analysis of the Development of the Spinal Column. Part I: Response of Pre-Cartilage Cells to Size Variations of the Spinal Cord.

J. Exp. Zool., *121*:121, 1952.

8. Lemire, R.J., Loeser, J.D., Leech, R.W., Alvord, E.C., Jr.: Normal and Abnormal Development of the Human Nervous System. Harper and Row, 1975.

9. Lemire, R.J., Shepherd, T.M., Alvord, E.C., Jr.: Caudal Myeloschisis (Lumbo-Sacral Spina Bifida Cystica) in a Five Millimeter (Horizon XIV) Human Embryo. *Anat. Rec.*, *152*:9, 1965.

10. Levick, R.K., Emery, J.L.: Displacement of the Brain Stem Arteries in Children with Hydrocephalus and the Arnold-Chiari Deformity. *Ann. Radiol.*, *10*:141, 1967.

11. Lichtenstein, B.W.: Atresia and Stenosis of the Aqueduct of Sylvius with Comments on the Arnold-Chiari Complex. *J. Neuropath.*, *18*:3, 1959.

12. McCoy, W.T., Simpson, D.A., Carter, R.F.: Cerebral Malformations Complicating Spina Bifida. Radiological Studies. *Clin. Radiol.*, *18*:176, 1967.

13. Peach, B.: The Arnold-Chiari Malformation. Morphogenesis. *Arch. Neurol.*, *12*:527, 1965.

14. VonHoytema, G.J., Van den Berg, R.: Embryological Studies of the Posterior Fossa in Connection with Arnold-Chiari Malformation. *Devel. Med. Child. Neurol.*, *Supp.#11*:61, 1965.

15. Warkany, J., Wilson, J.G., Geiger, J.F.: Myeloschisis and Myelomeningocele Produced Experimentally in the Rat. *J. Comp. Neurol.*, *109*:35, 1958.

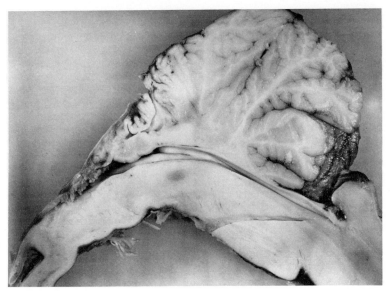

Fig. 1. Midsagittal section of hindbrain in Arnold-Chiari malformation. Note the tectal beak on the right, the elongated pons and medulla ending in an S-shaped deformity with the spinal cord on the left, and the elongated fourth ventricle. The malformed vermis shows no well defined uvula or nodulus being extended in a caudal velum to end with choroid plexus, on the left, as the posterior roof of the fourth ventricle (the dorsal tongue).

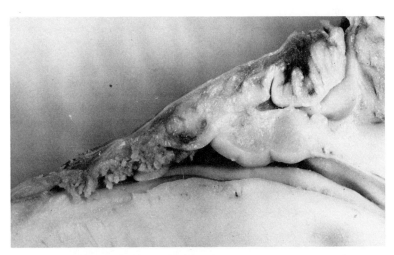

Fig. 2. A closer view of the posterior roof of the fourth ventricle in Arnold-Chiari malformation to show the anomalous caudal velum ending in choroid plexus.

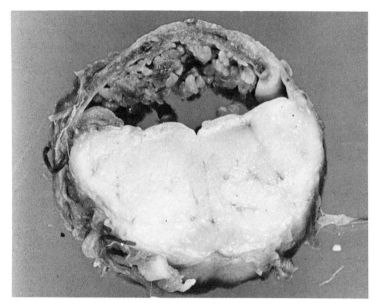

Fig. 3. Transverse section of elongated medulla in Arnold-Chiari malformation showing the dorsal tongue. Note the abnormal caudal velum and choroid plexus which form the roof of the fourth ventricle.

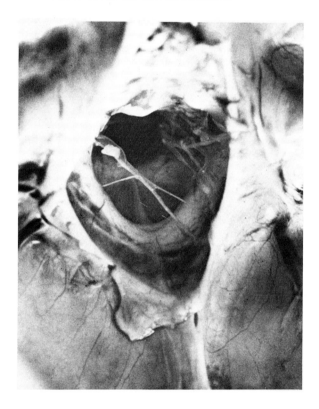

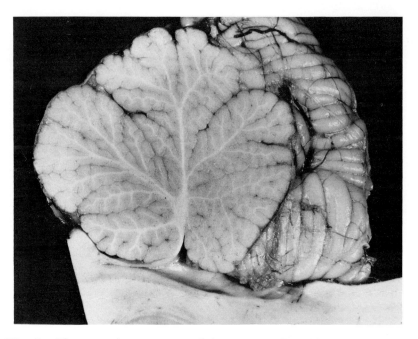

Fig. 5. The normal appearance of the vermis. The nodulus apposes the fastigium. Pons left, medulla right.

Fig. 4 (left, on facing page). View of posterior fossa in Arnold-Chiari malformation from anterior (top)—posterior (bottom) axis. The opened tentorial leaflet of the very small posterior fossa is seen center, near the bottom, lying in the extended middle fossa. The rim of the posterior margin of the large foramen magnum is seen opening into a very large upper cervical canal. Note the cruciate-like ligament between the rim of the foramen magnum and the arch of the atlas representing an attenuated posterior occipito-atlantic ligament. The strands of tissue crossing the foramen represent adhesions.

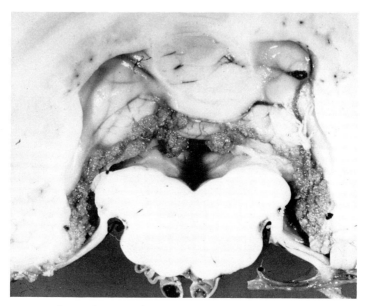

Fig. 6. View of a moderately enlarged fourth ventricle in transverse section at the level of the nodulus to show the normal arrangement of the choroid plexus. Leukemic patient with adhesive arachnitis.

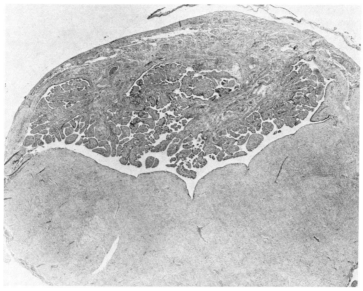

Fig. 7. Dorsal tongue in a 5-day old infant with Arnold-Chiari malformation. Surgical resection would appear to be feasible.

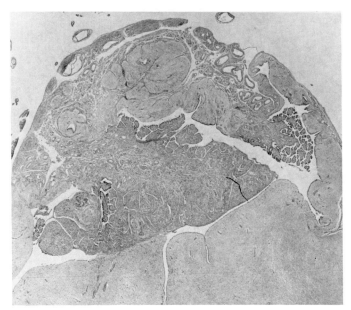

Fig. 8. The dorsal tongue in a 1½-month old infant with Arnold-Chiari malformation. The adhesion to the floor of the fourth ventricle seen to the left of center may prevent surgical resection.

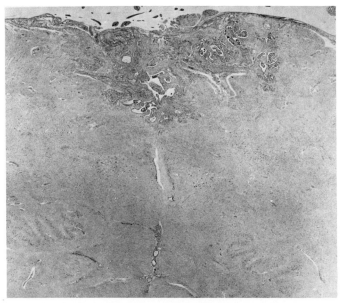

Fig. 9. In this 4-month old infant with Arnold-Chiari malformation the dorsal tongue is inextricably, perhaps secondarily, bound into the floor of the fourth ventricle.

THE ARNOLD-CHIARI MALFORMATION - ITS
RELATIONSHIP TO SYRINGOMYELIA

W. James Gardner, M.D.

The Arnold-Chiari malformation (ACM) constitutes the
most common anatomic substrate of syringomyelia. This fact
was an accidental discovery which came about as follows.
During the 1930's at the Cleveland Clinic, pneumoencephalography began to be performed on patients with suspected
brain tumor[14] for the following reasons. A small room with
an upright Bucky diaphragm, designed for chest films, was
available immediately adjacent to the surgical pavilion and
was found to be satisfactory for pneumoencephalography.
For ventriculography, however, the air injection was performed in surgery after which the anesthetized patient was
transported down eight floors, across 100 yards of tunnel,
then up one floor to the outpatient x-ray department where
films could be made with the patient horizontal. Should
resusitive measures become necessary this arrangement made
ventriculography hazardous. Therefore, in patients with
suspected brain tumor, pneumoencephalography became the
preferred technique although in the presence of papilledema,
a precautionary trephine was made to tap the ventricle
should need arise. With growing confidence, pneumoencephalography was employed even in patients with suspected
cerebellar tumor, and the pneumocephalographic picture of
posterior fossa tumor gradually emerged.[9] It consisted of

lack of air in the ventricles, the shadow of a hindbrain
hernia in the cisterna magna and air outlining the midline
supracallosal sulcus.

In one such patient with posterior fossa signs, and
with this pneumoencephalographic picture, the subsequent
craniotomy for cerebellar tumor disclosed a congenital
hindbrain hernia below which the spinal cord was cystic.
The postoperative diagnosis was syringobulbia with asymptomatic syringomyelia. Six weeks later a patient was seen
with classic syringomyelia but with no posterior fossa signs.
Pneumoencephalography and subsequent operation disclosed the
identical findings. With improving technique, the collapsing cord sign enabled the surgeon to differentiate syringomyelia from cerebellar tumor[15] (Fig. 1 A,B). It was
pneumoencephalography, therefore, that established that the
cause of syringomyelia is not in the spinal cord but in the
hindbrain, and with proper technique, this remains the best
diagnostic procedure.

ACM of adulthood with associated hydromyelia was
described by Chiari as his Type 1.[6,7] His specimens were
examined after removal from the skull so that he failed to
see the downward dislocation of the tentorium that is always
present in his Type 2 of infancy. However, he did recognize
that the herniation must have developed "with the growing
of the cerebellum".

In 1965, the operative findings in 74 consecutive cases
of syringomyelia were described[11] (Fig. 2A-F). In none was
pantopaque myelography employed, and pneumoencephalography
was required in only 46. In the remaining 28, the clinical
diagnosis of syringomyelia was obvious from the history and
neurological findings together with frequent roentgenographic evidence consisting of scoliosis, basilar impression,

Klippel-Feil fusion or an abnormal widening of the cervical canal. In three of these 28 patients, the diagnosis had been established by a prior cervical syringotomy performed elsewhere. In every patient in whom it was possible to expose the floor of the fourth ventricle at surgery, there was disclosed a funnel-shaped opening of the central canal beneath the obex large enough to accept a plug of muscle or a double knot of number 2 silk suture material (Fig. 2 B,C). Similar patency is never present in the normal hindbrain. In one early case, in order to demonstrate this communication with the syrinx, pantopaque was introduced into a lateral ventricle and manipulated into the fourth ventricle. The resulting film (Fig. 3A) showed that no pantopaque had escaped into the subarachnoid space but some could be seen entering the central canal to come to rest opposite the 10th thoracic vertebrae. The pantopaque also outlined a finger-like pouch extending caudally from the fourth ventricle similar to that described by Blake[4] in fetuses of lower mammals in which the foramen of Magendie does not perforate. Peach[18] has described a similar Blake's pouch in the ACM associated with myelocele of infancy (Fig. 3B).

Of these 74 patients, the partial obstruction of the foramen magnum was due to ACM in 68, to a Dandy-Walker malformation in 3, and in the remaining 3 there was a congenital loculated cyst obstructing the foramen of Magendie (Fig. 2E). These transparent so-called "arachnoid" cysts develop in the unperforated lower portion of the double-layered rhombic roof, i.e. Weed's area membrancea inferior, shown in figure 2D. Because its inner ependymal layer is more permeable than its outer piaglial layer, the ventricular fluid pulsations may drive fluid between these

two layers to form a cyst. Their fluid content resembles
CSF but unfortunately, the cyst wall is seldom examined
microscopically for the presence of ependyma. When
encountered in the infant with the classical evidence of
Dandy-Walker malformation, the posterior wall of a similar
loculated cyst may be mistaken for a posterior bulging of
the double layered rhombic roof. In this case, however, it
arises from Weed's area membrancea superior.[14]

In the 68 cases of syringomyelia with ACM the herniation
consisted chiefly of the tonsils rather than the vermis as
is the case in the severe infantile form of this malformation. In 28 instances, the herniated tonsils were cone
shaped and bound down to the medulla by thick vascular
arachnoid-like tissue which has been described as "arachnoiditis"[1] (Fig. 2F). However, true arachnoiditis is not
vascular, whereas brisk arterial bleeding is encountered
when this tissue overlying the herniated tonsils is incised.
This tissue is in fact, the tissue which would have formed
the fibrous and vascular elements of the choroid plexus had
it been invaginated into the ventricle in the ordinary
course of development.[8] This posterior choroid plexus is
nourished by a branch of the posterior inferior cerebellar
artery. This explains why, not only the anlage of the choroid plexus may be protruded with the herniated cerebellum,
but the hernia may also include a loop of one or both
posterior inferior cerebellar arteries (Fig. 2B). Observations of the hindbrain during operation for syringomyelia
have frequently disclosed an abnormally low position of the
obex. In some cases, the everted nodulus may protrude
through the foramen magnum together with the tonsils which
may be bound down by the so-called "arachnoiditis". In
these cases, the floor of the fourth ventricle may be

exposed only by incising the vermis, since attempts to
incise the tough covering of vascular tissue may result in
troublesome bleeding and bulbar symptoms.

THE CAUSE OF ARNOLD-CHIARI MALFORMATION

 In syringomyelia as in myelocele, the ACM develops in
fetal life because the posterior fossa is too small to
accommodate the growing hindbrain. This smallness in
myelocele is the result of an abnormally low tentorium[3,13]
which, in turn, results from the pressure of a hydrocephalic
forebrain in fetal life (Fig. 4). In syringomyelia, a
lowlying tentorium is probably also present though seldom
sought. In many cases the overcrowding of the posterior
fossa can be accounted for by the associated basilar
impression. The latter has been explained on the basis of
a too heavy head resulting from mild, perhaps unrecognized
hydrocephalus in infancy.[12] The severe Arnold-Chiari Type II
is almost universally present in the infant with myelocele.[5]
In the latter, the caudal rupture of the neural tube (myeloschisis) has permitted the CSF pulsations imparted by the
embryonal posterior choroid plexus to escape freely into the
amniotic sac. Since the posterior migration of the tentorium results from the competition between the expanding
effects of the large anterior plexus versus that of the
smaller posterior plexus,[12,13] the explanding effect of the
anterior plexuses is no longer opposed by the latter. As a
result, the anlage of the tentorium is pushed much too far
posteriorly. Since the vermis develops earlier than the
tonsils, this is the part of the cerebellum that is extruded
in myelocele.

 In the adult form of ACM, the hydrocephalus of the
lateral ventricles usually has become compensated in fetal

life so that the neural tube does not rupture.[14] For this
reason, the smallness of the posterior fossa is less severe
than in cases of myeloschisis. However, prior to this
compensation the posterior fossa may have been sufficiently
reduced in size by the enlarging lateral ventricles so that
the later developing tonsils protrude through the foramen
magnum. The nodulus of the growing vermis is also displaced
caudally but only rarely does it accompany the tonsils
through the foramen magnum. In addition to the cerebellar
protrusion, the brain stem and upper cervical cord are
frequently dislocated downward resulting in telescoping of
the cervicomedullary junction. In the infant with myelocele
this telescoping is sufficient to kink off the dilated
central canal whereas in syringomyelia, the telescoping is
milder and therefore is not sufficient to do so.

In only 28 of the 74 surgical exposures of the hindbrain,
did the surgeon describe the readily overlooked caudal dislocation of the obex. This dislocation, however, has been
demonstrated on postoperative films in the cases in which a
small metallic marker was applied to the bit of muscle
plugging the upper end of the central canal. In at least
36 cases the second cervical nerve roots pursued an upward
course to their foramens of exit, indicating that the
cervicomedullary junction was also dislocated downward. A
telescoping and posterior bulging of this junction was
described in 18 cases and is illustrated in figures 2 A,D and
E. This telescoping, however, was never severe enough to
occlude the central canal as happens in the infant with
myelocele. In 24 cases the foramen of Magendie was found to
be enclosed by an intact membrane whose attachment to the
taenia indicated that it represented an unperforated rhombic
roof (Fig. 2D). In two young syringomyelic patients, this

membrane was lined by ependyma and in one of these it
contained choroid plexus. This failure of perforation of the
rhombic roof indicates that it had been compressed in the
hindbrain hernia prior to the stage at which it normally
perforates. This same failure, at times resulting in a so-
called Blake's[4] pouch, occurs also in the infantile form of
ACM[18] (Fig. 3A,B).

The neurosurgeon has the opportunity not afforded the
neuropathologist to observe the pathology in the living.
When he exposes the normal hindbrain with the patient in the
sitting position, he sees the intact arachnoid pulsating
with each cardiac systole, whereas the cerebellum remains
as still as in a cadavar. Contrary to popular belief, the
brain is a non-pulsating organ because its large pulsating
arteries are not within its substance but in the subarachnoid space. The pulsations seen when the forebrain is
exposed at operation are transmitted from the CSF. When,
with the patient in a sitting posture this fluid is allowed
to drain from the cisterna magna, all pulsations cease
unless there is a hindbrain hernia which interferes with the
escape of the pulsating CSF into the distensible spinal
subarachnoid space. The protruding cerebellum in the
syringomyelic patient is impacted further into the foramen
magnum with each systole and restracts during diastole.
This impaction creates a degree of subarachnoid block during
systole that is relieved during diastole. The foramina of
Luschka, are located above the level of the foramen magnum
block and therefore, even when patent, they cannot freely
discharge their fluid into the distensible spinal sac during
systole. This intermittant impaction exaggerates the
amplitude of the intracranial subarachnoid fluid pulse wave
and superimposes it upon the ventricular fluid pulse wave.

The amplified ventricular fluid pulse wave in turn, is
directed into the funnel-shaped entrance of the central
canal so that the syrinx pulsates synchronously with the ACM.
By age 30, this pulsation has occurred more than 1.2 billion
times. As in the old cockney adage, "Hits not the 'eavy
'awling that 'urts the 'osses 'oofs, hit's the 'ammer,
'ammer, 'ammer on the 'ard 'ighway". In the more severe ACM
in the infant with myelocele, the central canal remains
hydromyelic[2] but does not distend further because its cephalic
end has been closed off by telescoping in the severe down-
wardly displaced cervicomedullary junction. However, in one
3 year old hydrocephalic child with ACM, but without myelocele[17] such closing off had not occurred and the result was
spectacular. This hydromyelic central canal was segmented,
its appearance suggesting the haustrations of the bowel
(Fig. 5A,C). This exact appearance was first demonstrated
in a case of adult syringomyelia by Heinz et al[16] and it is
also illustrated in a postmortem specimen of syringomyelia
which appears on page 147 of a monograph on syringomyelia.[2]
The present author believes that this unusual form of overdistention of the central canal is evidence that it occurred
during the somite stage of embryonic life shortly after
neural tube closure. At this stage, the dense bordering
somites (Fig. 5B,D) obviously will offer more resistance to
the distending force than the less dense intervals between
them. Therefore, the "haustra" develop at these yielding
intervals. This unusual and bizarre form of hydromyelia
constitutes one more anatomic feature that is common to the
ACM of infancy and that of the adult with syringomyelia. It
has not been described in myelocele, in which case rupture
of the neural tube during the somite stage has relieved the
increased pressure in the central canal.

CONCLUSION

The patient with syringomyelia may have in lesser degree all of the CNS anomalies that one finds in the infant with myelocele. The sole exception being an open neural tube.

REFERENCES

1. Appleby, A., Bradley, W.G., Foster, J.B., Hankinson, J., and Hudgson, P.: Syringomyelia due to chronic arachnoiditis at the foramen magnum. *J. Neurol. Sci.*, *8*:451, 1969.

2. Barnett, H.M.F., Foster, J.B., and Hudgson, P.: Syringomyelia. Philadelphia, W.B. Saunders Co., 1973, pp. 318.

3. Barry, A., Patten, B.M., and Stewart, B.H.: Possible factors in development of Arnold Chiari malformation. *J. Neurosurg.*, *14*:285, 1957.

4. Blake, J.A.: The roof and lateral recesses of the fourth ventricle considered morphologically and embryologically. *J. comp. Neurol.*, *10*:79, 1900.

5. Cameron, A.H.: Arnold Chiari and other neuroanatomical malformations associated with spina bifida. *J. Path. & Bact.*, *73*:195, 1957.

6. Chiari, H.: Uber Veranderungen des Kleinhirns infolge von Hydrocephalie des Grosshirns. *Deutsche med. Wchnschr.*, *17*:1172, 1891.

7. Chiari, H.: Uber Veranderungen des Kleinhirns, des Pons und der Medulla oblongata in Folge von congenitaler hydrocephalie des Grosshirns. *Denkschr. Acad. Wiss. Mathnaturw Kl.*, *63*:71, 1895.

8. Daniel, P.M. and Strich, S.J.: Some observations on congenital deformity of central nervous system known as

Arnold-Chiari malformation. *J. Neuropathol. Exp. Neurol., 17*:255, 1958.

9. Gardner, W.J. and Nosik, W.A.: Experiences with encephalography in cerebellar tumor. *Am. J. Roentgenol., 47*:691, 1942.

10. Gardner, W.J.: Anatomic features common to the Arnold-Chiari and Dandy-Walker malformations suggest a common origin, *Cleveland Clin. Quart., 26*:206, 1959.

11. Gardner, W.J.: Hydrodynamic mechanism of syringomyelia: Its relationship to myelocele. *J. Neurol. Neurosurg. Psychiatr., 28*:247, 1965.

12. Gardner, W.J., Smith, J.L. and Padget, D.H.: The relationship of Arnold-Chiari and Dandy-Walker malformations. *J. Neurosurg., 36*:581, 1972.

13. Gardner, W.J.: Anomalies of the craniovertebral junction. IN Neurological Surgery, Vol. I, J.R. Youmans (ed.), Philadelphia, W.B. Saunders Co., 1973.

14. Gardner, W.J.: The dysraphic states: from syringomyelia to anencephaly. IN Excerpta Medica, Amsterdam, 1973, pp. 201.

15. Greenwald, C.M., Eugenio, M., Hughes, C.R., and Gardner, W.J.: The importance of the air shadow of the cisterna magna in encephalographic diagnosis. *Radiology, 71*: 695, 1958.

16. Heinz, E.R., Schlesinger, E.B. and Potts, D.G.: Radiologic signs of hydromyelia. *Radiology, 86*:311, 1966.

17. James, H.E. Shut, L. and Pasquariello, P.P.: Communication of hydromyelic cavity with fourth ventricle shown by combined pantopaque and air myelography. Case report *J. Neurosurg., 38*:235, 1973.

18.   Peach, B.:   Cystic prolongation of fourth ventricle; an anomaly associated with the Arnold-Chiari malformation. *Arch. Neurol., 11*:609, 1964.

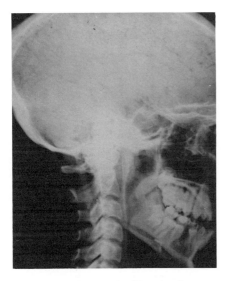 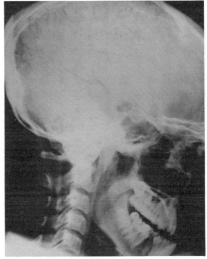

Fig. 1A.   This early film discloses an absence of air in the ventricles, a hindbrain hernia and a swollen cord.

Fig. 1B.   The cystic cord has collapsed and the negative pressure in syrinx, transmitted to the ventricles, has caused the hindbrain hernia to be retracted through the foramen magnum.

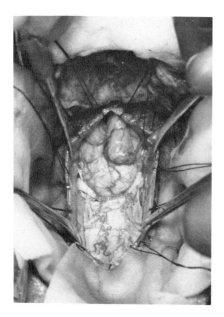

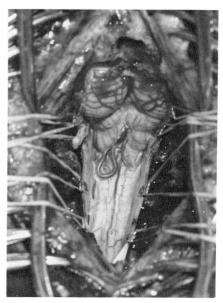

Fig. 2A.   The tonsils are herniated through the foramen magnum and cover the upper portion of the telescoped cervicomedullary junction. The C2 nerve roots course upward. The cystic cord has collapsed. (Patient in sitting position.)

Fig. 2B.   A loop of one or both posterior inferior cerebellar arteries may be herniated with the tonsils.

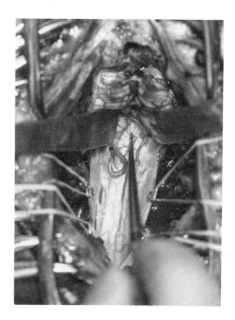

Fig. 2C.   Retraction of the tonsils discloses the obex at a lower level than normal. A nerve hook is impacting a muscle plug into the dilated upper end of the central canal.

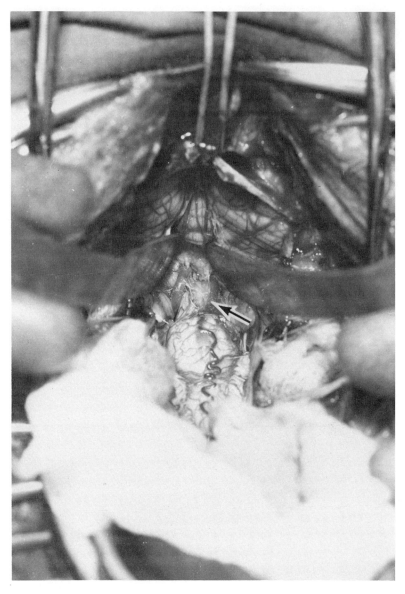

Fig. 2D. The arrow points to a dense membrane attached to taenia. This is constituted by Weed's area membrancea inferior located below the posterior choroid plexus. It is the site of the foramen of Magendie that failed to perforate.

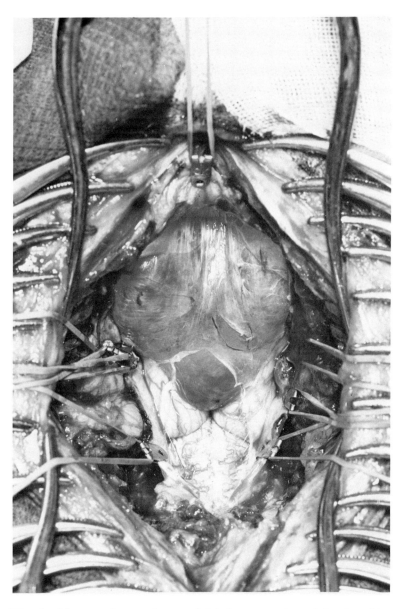

Fig. 2E.   In this case, the two layers of this lower portion of the rhombic roof shown in Fig. 2D have been dissected widely apart to form a huge loculated cyst. The herniated tonsils preclude the possibility of Dandy-Walker malformation. Injected indigo carmine did not escape from the cyst, establishing its loculation.

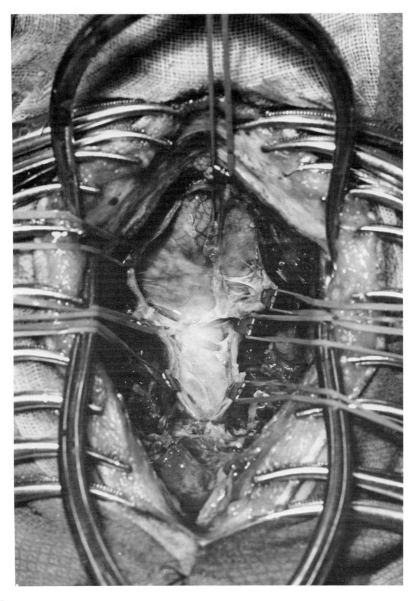

Fig. 2F. In this case, the dense so-called arachnoiditis entirely conceals the hindbrain hernia.

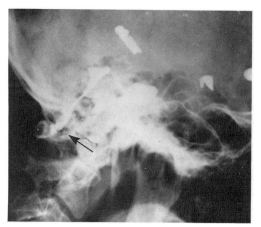

Fig. 3A. Arrow indicates pantopaque in the central canal. Posterior to this it has filled a caudal diverticulum of the fourth ventricle which is constituted by a bulging of the unperforated rhombic roof. This represents a pathologic form of Blake's pouch.

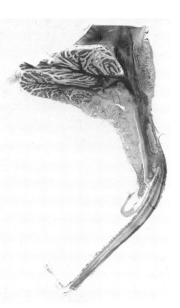

Fig. 3B. Blake's pouch in the infantile form of A.C.M. (Reproduced from Peach[18] —with permission of author and publisher).

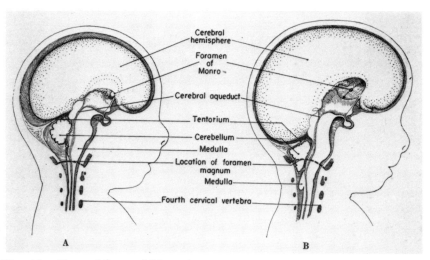

Fig. 4A. Normal fetus of 18 weeks.

Fig. 4B. Arnold-Chiari malformation in fetus of same age. (Reproduced by courtesy of authors[3] and publisher).

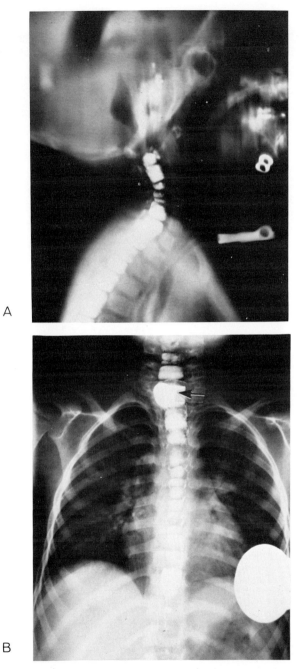

Fig. 5A, B. The enormously dilated and haustrated central canal in a 3-year old child with A.C.M. (Reproduced from films kindly furnished by the authors[17]). The arrow in B indicates the tracheostomy tube.

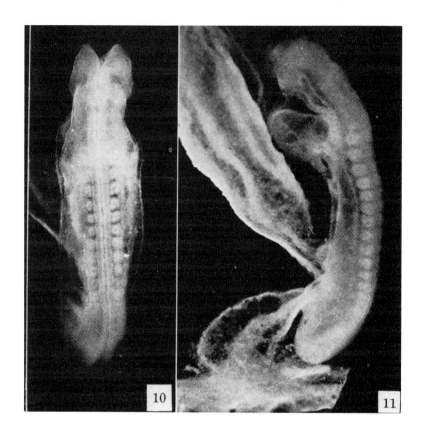

Fig. 5C. The increased density of the bordering somites is well shown in this early human embryo. (Reproduced from Streeter, G.L. Developmental Horizons in Human Embryos. Embryology Reprint Vol. 2, Carneg. Inst. Wash., Washington, D.C. 1951).

THE NEURORADIOLOGICAL EVALUATION OF
THE ARNOLD-CHIARI MALFORMATION

Leonard Cerulla, M.D. and Anthony J. Raimondi, M.D.

ABSTRACT

This study consists of a general description of the characteristics of the vertebral basilar system in the Chiari II malformation. A description of the changes in form, location and size of the dural sinuses of the posterior fossa are also presented by studying carefully the course and form of the various branches of the vertebral basilar system. One may diagnose the Arnold-Chiari II malformation and identify the degree of cerebral-cerebello-medullary deformity. Study of the dural sinuses permits one to determine whether opening of the dura of the posterior fossa may be performed safely.

The Arnold-Chiari malformation is a complex derangement of anatomical interrelationships between individual cerebral-cerebello-medullary structures and the craniospinal axis which envelops them. In addition to this, the cerebral-cerebello-medullary structures are displaced, deformed, and, in some instances, destroyed. These macro- and micro-anatomical changes result in varying degrees of neurodys-function.

Hydrocephalus is associated with the Arnold-Chiari II malformation in 78% of the patients treated at the Children's Memorial Hospital between the years 1962-1975. For the sake of simplicity, the classification of hydrocephalus in these children with the Arnold-Chiari II malformation has been: 1) Communicating hydrocephalus; 2) Aqueductal stenosis or occlusion; 3) Constriction of the basal cisterns. In this paper, no attempt is made to describe or discuss the various forms of hydrocephalus, its pathology, or its pathogenesis.

The most common anatomical changes of the brain stem, cerebellum and upper cervical cord are illustrated in Fig. 1. The forward displacement of the thalami with widening and elongation of the postero-inferior portion of the third ventricle as it tapers into a deformed, constricted and elongated aqueduct of Sylvius is well illustrated as is the relative bulbar deformity of the upper portion of the fourth ventricle. The hypertrophy of the collicular plate, in this instance more marked posteriorly than anteriorly, is quite typical of this anomaly as is the lengthening and flattening of both the mesencephalon and pons varolii. The kinking, or buckling, of the medulla oblongata within the floor of the fourth ventricle is also well illustrated as is the dysplasia and destruction of the tonsils of the cerebellar hemispheres

and the elongation of the tonsils with their extension into
the cervical spinal canal. Of particular interest is the
horizontalization of the cerebellum and the flattening of its
superior surface with relative increase in size of the quadrigeminal and superior cerebellar cisterns. One notes also
the posterior displacement of the medial surfaces of the
temporal lobes and the inferior displacement of the hippo-
campus and medial portion of the occipital lobe so that they
come to rest lateral to the cerebellar hemisphere. This
occurs commonly, since there is very often a dysplasia of
the tentorium of the cerebellum.

Since the arterial structures of the posterior fossa are
attached to the surfaces of the medulla oblongata, the pons
varolii, the mesencephalon, the peduncles, the cerebellar
vermis and the hemisphere, the tonsils, and the quadrigeminal
plate, it is reasonable to assume that angiography may provide considerable information concerning relative displacement, deformity and destruction of each of these structures.
In addition to this, the posterior communicating, posterior
choroidal and posterior cerebral systems may be expected to
provide information concerning downward displacement of the
cerebral hemisphere, displacement and deformity of the
thalami, downward displacement of the inferior surfaces of
the temporal and occipital lobes and the medial surface of
the occipital lobe.

Fig. 2 illustrates the very characteristic folding of
the vertebral arteries upon themselves at the cranio-vertebral
junction and the lengthening of the basilar trunk, both of
which result from stretching of the brain stem and dislocation of the posterior fossa contents into the upper cervical
canal. It also illustrates the downward course of the
posterior inferior cerebellar artery to the level of the

second cervical vertebra and then its hairpin curve upon
itself to return to the foramen magnum. One should note that
the superior cerebellar arteries, in this child, course
directly posteriorly from the basilar artery, which continues
its vertical course to extend almost directly into the
posterior cerebral arteries, which run postero-superiorly at
approximately a 45 degree angle, giving off medial and
lateral posterior choroidal arteries which themselves are
verticalized. The posterior communicating artery is well
filled, showing evidence of downward herniation of the cerebral hemisphere, as indicated by a sharp kink at its mid-
portion. This results from incarceration of the third
cranial nerve, rather than tenting by the thalamo-tuberal
branch of the posterior communicating artery, which, in this
instance, courses posteriorly. The increased distance between the posterior cerebral and superior cerebellar arteries
is a very common observation in the Chiari II malformation,
indicative of downward displacement of the cerebellar hemispheres and hypertrophy of the tectum and tegmentum of the
midbrain.

Another example of folding of the posterior inferior
cerebellar artery upon itself and inferior extension of the
posterior inferior cerebellar artery is shown in Fig. 3.
Here also the basilar artery is lengthened. One notes,
however, in this child that the space between the superior
cerebellar and posterior cerebral arteries is not remarkably
increased and that, to a greater or lesser degree, these two
systems parallel one another, thereby indicating lesser hypertrophy of the tectum and tegmentum of the midbrain and greater
inferior displacement of the temporal occipital lobes into
the posterior fossa. The mesencephalic portion of the
posterior cerebral artery as well as the posterior cerebral

proper follow an almost vertical course, giving off the
medial and lateral posterior choroidal arteries, which, in
turn, also run directly superiorly. These changes are
expressive of anterior displacement of the thalami and
dilation of both the quadrigeminal and superior cerebellar
cisterns.

When the occipital temporal lobes are dislocated almost
completely into the posterior fossa which may be funnel
shaped to a greater or lesser degree, the changes in the
posterior cerebral arteries are quite characteristic (Fig. 4).
The point of continuity of the posterior cerebral into the
internal occipital artery is folded with the latter vessel
curving downward along the medial surfaces of the temporal
and occipital lobes. The apex of the curve formed by the
posterior cerebral and internal occipital arteries indicates
the point of origin of the quadrigeminal branches of the
posterior cerebral system, which are anchored to the collicular plate, which, in turn, is displaced anteriorly. This
same figure illustrates rather remarkable deformities of the
anterior inferior cerebellar arteries, resulting from inferior
and anterior displacement of the ventral surfaces of the
cerebellar hemispheres and the descent of the posterior
inferior cerebellar artery and its "switch-back" course upward from the level of C3 through the foramen magnum and into
the posterior fossa is also well shown. If one reviews this
figure carefully, he may visualize the forward displacement
of the thalami and midbrain, the lengthening of the brain
stem, the dislocation of the medulla oblongata and cerebellar
tonsils into the upper cervical canal, the movement of the
temporal occipital lobe into the posterior fossa, and corre-
late these with the anatomical photograph shown in Fig. 1.

An extreme example of verticalization of the brain stem
with remarkable stretching from the superior surfaces of the
thalami superiorly to the floor of the fourth ventricle
inferiorly is illustrated angiographically in Fig. 5. Note
the medial and lateral posterior choroidal arteries superiorly with the lateral posterior choroidal artery curving
smoothly over the pulvinar and the characteristic figure of
the appearance of the medial posterior choroidal artery being
deformed. The posterior cerebral arteries themselves follow
a directly vertical course whereas the superior cerebellar
arteries run perpendicular (in a posterior direction) to both
the basilar and posterior cerebral arteries. The cerebellar
tonsils are dislocated downward to the level of the fourth
cervical vertebra, as indicated by the well-visualized loops
of the posterior inferior cerebellar arteries.

Careful study of the AP projection (Fig. 6) permits one
to interpret a narrowing effect which stretching, flattening
and compression have upon the brain stem. Superiorly, one
notes that the posterior cerebral and superior cerebellar
arteries course upward immediately they take origin from the
basilar artery and that they then loop upon themselves to
course inferolaterally, describing a narrow arch as they
adhere snugly to the ponto-mesencephalic surfaces. These
vessels are displaced medially by the downward herniation
of the medial surfaces of the temporal and occipital lobes.
Similarly, one notes inferiorly that the course of the
vertebral arteries, once they have entered the subarachnoid
spaces and proceed superomedially to join forming the basilar
artery, appears to be a mirror of the posterior cerebral
superior cerebellar systems. In sum, at the upper end,
constriction is resulting from stretching of the brain stem
and downward herniation of the temporal occipital lobes

whereas at the lower end, constriction is resulting from
stretching of the ponto-medullary junction and downward
herniation of the cerebellar hemispheres and vermis. The
posterior inferior cerebellar arteries descend vertically in
a paramedian plane, whereas the anterior inferior cerebellar
arteries ascend vertically in the identical plane. The quadrigeminal branches of the posterior cerebral system indicate
compression of the tectum.

Fig. 7 permits one to look carefully at the internal
occipital branches of the posterior cerebral system bilaterally and to study the quadrigeminal vessels, thereby
appreciating fully the compression of the brain stem which
occurs very often in the Chiari II malformation. It should
be compared with subsequent illustrations of just the opposite: increase in circumferential volume of the brain stem
resulting from hypertrophic or gliotic changes.

An excellent example of these latter anatomical changes
is illustrated in Fig. 8 where one notes that the posterior
cerebral arteries sweep widely and gently around the midbrain, whereas the superior cerebellar arteries describe a
triangular form. This wide sweep of the posterior cerebral
arteries as they run through the mesencephalic and ambient
cisterns to approach the quadrigeminal cisterns, where they
course vertically, is indicative of an increase in volume of
the midbrain, which, anatomically, results from either hypertrophic or gliotic changes. Similar changes occur in the
colliculi.

Apart from any clinical or anatomical considerations,
careful retrograde jugular venographic studies designed to
visualize completely the jugular, sigmoid, and transverse
sinuses, one is advised to insist upon such studies prior to
undertaking decompressive craniectomy of the posterior fossa.

The relative downward displacement of the cerebral-cerebello-
medullary structures is accompanied by a similar dislocation
of the dural sinuses. The net result is that the transverse
sinus often rests upon the inferior surface of the squamous
portion of the occipital bone with the sigmoid and jugular
sinuses being converted into minimal vertical or lateral
extensions of the transfer sinus. Therefore, following
craniectomy of the squamous portion of the occipital bone,
the surgeon may open into the transverse, sigmoid or jugular
sinuses, which would be located within the dural sheaths
immediately posterior to the cerebellar hemispheres and
tonsils. In addition to this, the Arnold-Chiari II malformation is associated with abnormal labyrinth dural sinus formations which cover the posterior fossa.

In Fig. 9, a lateral retrograde internal jugular venogram, one notes that the transverse sinus rests upon the
inferior surface of the squamous portion of the occipital
bone and that the sigmoid and jugular sinuses represent an
uncinate deformity of the transverse sinus. The superior
petrosal sinus is remarkedly dilated. Fig. 10, a retrograde
jugular venogram in the half-axial projection, illustrates
clearly the downward dislocation of the transverse sinuses,
the dilation of the petrosal sinus, the presence of a plexi-
form abnormal system of sinuses over the dura in the posterior
fossa, and the remarkable dilation of the angular sinuses
surrounding the foramen magnum. These changes in location,
form, communication and size of the dural sinuses make opening of the dura in the posterior fossa exceedingly difficult
and dangerous.

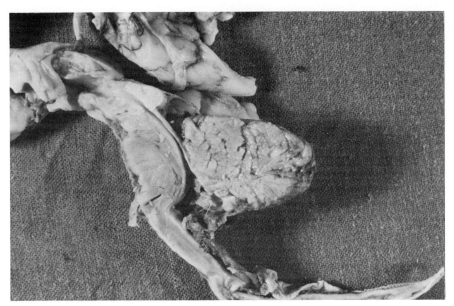

Fig. 1.

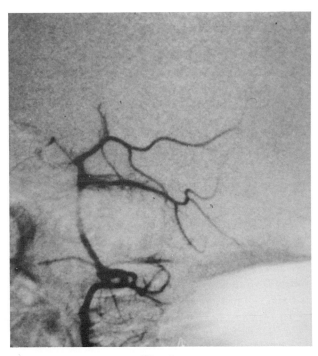

Fig. 2.

235

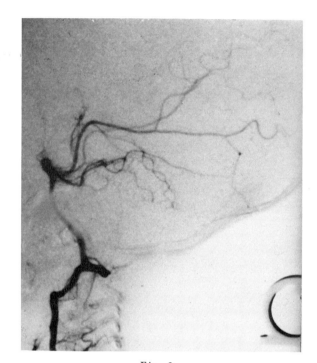

Fig. 3.

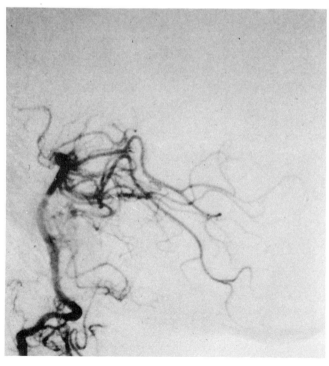

Fig. 4.

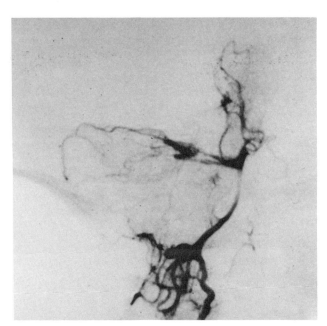

Fig. 5.

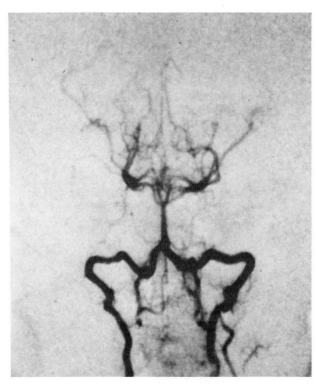

Fig. 6.

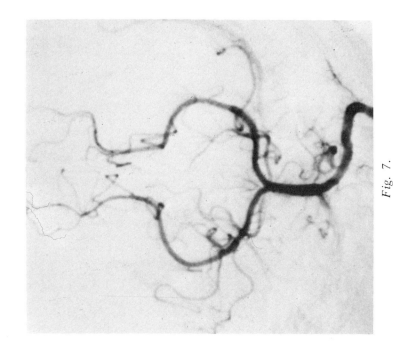

Fig. 7.

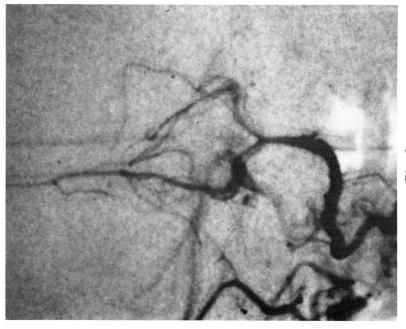

Fig. 8.

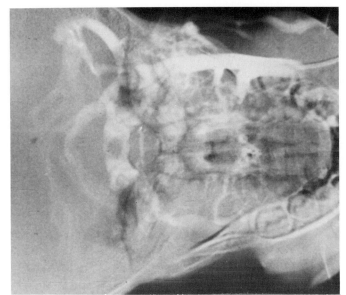

Fig. 10.

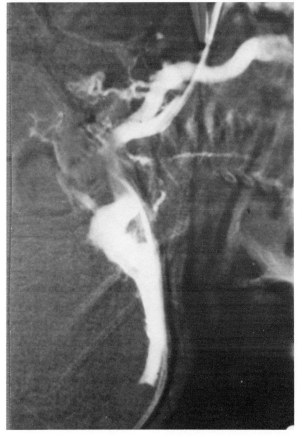

Fig. 9.

THE SIGNIFICANCE OF THE
ARNOLD-CHIARI MALFORMATION

Martin P. Sayers, M.D.

The Arnold-Chiari malformation[1,2,3] is present to some degree and at some time in the course of 85% of children with myelodysplasia. The condition is often clinically manifest in the newborn period. In our series of 655 infants with myelomeningocele approximately 15% (82 patients) had weakness of feeding, crying or breathing, hypotonia or spasticity related to the malformation. The condition led to early mortality in about one-third of these patients though fulminating infection might be the terminal event.

These babies vary greatly in the severity of their neurologic impairment. Some are so weak that they are able to make only a few gasping respirations in the delivery room. Others breath relatively well for a few days before manifesting the familiar crowing respirations of laryngeal nerve weakness. In these children the vagus nerve is hardly larger than a horse hair, the medullary nuclei are often sparse and distorted. Yet if they can survive a few months of labored breathing, the vocal cords regain adequate nerve supply and if other factors are favorable respiration may never again be a problem.[4]

We have felt that the extremes of brain stem weakness constitute a contraindication to early surgical treatment of myelomeningocele, but of those babies that develop late

laryngeal stridor 26 of 38 or about two-thirds steadily
gained strength and later progress to normal speech. If the
neonatal hydrocephalus is shunted and sepsis can be avoided,
the brain stem and cerebellum appear to gain a new lease on
life. We have not found it advisable to attempt surgical
treatment of the Arnold-Chiari malformation in the neonatal
period. Tracheostomy in this stage of development should be
avoided to the point of absolute necessity as it subjects the
patient to prolonged morbidity and high mortality rates.

Suboccipital craniectomy and upper cervical laminectomy
in the neonate is a high risk procedure and is followed by
such rapid bone regeneration that the period of decompression
may be only a few weeks in duration - the cerebellum and
brain stem are then locked in again as tightly as ever.

We apparently induced a decompensation of posterior
fossa dynamics in 4 of 36 of our patients subjected to spine
ostectomy for severe kyphosis between ages 2-4 years. The
spine was straightened and shortened, the dura was not
specifically opened, the cord was not transsected. What then
was the cause?

In effect we had partially untethered the cord and dura.
There may have been some bruising of or bleeding from subarachnoid structures and inadvertently the children were less
active and in the horizontal position almost continuously.
One of them died at home in respiratory failure before the
family or physicians realized that the problem existed. The
shunt was functioning adequately, ventricles were small.
Why did she die? At this time I believe that the prone
position with excessively long periods of neck extension, i.e.
the "turtle" position, reduces the space for already crowded
posterior fossa structures and may have been one of the
primary factors. The mechanism would be impaired blood

circulation in the brain stem.

To understand how this can happen we should analyse the sequence of events during early post natal brain growth. It is probable that the first crowding and downward displacement in the posterior fossa occurs early in pregnancy during an initial period of in utero hydrocephalus. This hydrocephalus tends to compensate toward the last trimester by virtue of circulation through developing subarachnoid spaces and semipermiable membranes and through the central canal into the amniotic fluid. However, at birth the environment for CSF dispersion again becomes unfavorable with loss of channels into the amniotic fluid, loss of maternal hormones, increased secretory pressure and inflammation.

Again the hydrocephalus tends to recur, and further compression of the posterior fossa results from the odd bubble like manner with which the soft fetal brain expands first at the sites of least resistance (the La Place or boiler plate principle). Possibly this is the cause for the relatively high rate of aqueduct stenosis in children with myelomeningocele. At any rate this new threat is usually avoided by the early and first shunt.

Now as the excessive CSF is conducted off from the lateral ventricles we have a congenitally crowded subtentorial space and a loose floppy supratentorial area in which the pressure is maintained only by the peripheral resistance of the shunt. Assuming that rehydration and growth will occur at approximately the same rate in both areas, it is apparent that there is plenty of room above, but that the tentorium must be stretched upward to accomodate expansion of the cerebellum and stem. This is easier to state than to accomplish apparently, the lateral sinuses are fixed to the bone and therefore probably some of the posterior fossa

expansion takes place into the upper spinal canal even at
this stage. But the skull and meninges are relatively soft
and expansible and compensation is satisfactorily maintained.

However, the cerebrum normally outgrows and is a larger
structure than the cerebellum post-natally. This will
eventually become the key to secondary decompensation of the
Arnold-Chiari anomaly. During early shunting the skull
probably closes more rapidly and the bone thickens excessively
due to the relatively diminished growth pressure against the
inner table while the existing "dead space" caused by the
dilated ventricular system is being filled by expanding
cerebrum. We see the same phenomenon in the skull overlying
"congenital hemicerebral atrophy" but confined to the damaged
atrophied side.

The shunt continues to function, the rapidly growing
cerebrum fills the intracranial space, the skull is excessively thick, the sutures are excessively unyielding. It is
probable that some of the excessive skull thickness is a
normal physiological response to early excessive distention,
as it also frequently occurs over untreated infantile subdural hematoma. Now both the supra and the infratentorial
structures want to grow, the calvarium is excessively unyielding and the result can be very small lateral ventricles
and excessive downward thrust on the tentorium further
herniation of the cerebellum and brain stem and buckling of
the cord.

How does this look to us clinically? Most often the
wonders of nature somehow absorb the shock and the somatic
manifestations are remarkably subtile. The foramen magnum
has enlarged to incorporate the upper spinal canal into the
cisterna magnum and C_1 almost always remains or becomes bifid
and very thin (Fig. 1). Head and neck movements become

cautious. Stretching of the cranial and upper spinal nerves which gradually are pushed further away from their exit foramena results in gradual atrophy of the facial, neck, tongue and shoulder muscles, hearing is diminished and coordination becomes ragged. Accessory muscles become more important in respiration. Unfortunately EMG's have been unrewarding - audiometrics are more quantitative. X-rays of the foramen magnum and upper cervical spine confirm that the anatomical features are present. Respiratory tidal volume is diminished, the rate gradually more rapid.[5]

Weakening voice, excessive use of the accessory muscles of respiration and thinning of arms and hands denote a far advanced stage of the chronic decompensation process.

Sudden or acute decompensation must be linked to impaction or obstruction of the subarachnoid spaces, and is one of the most compelling emergencies in pediatric neuro-surgery. Some of the features of chronic progressive hernia-tion may have been present for weeks or months prior, but we have seen this syndrome occur with no prior warning. The patient complains of headache, may experience brief fugue or trance-like states and manifests 5-20 second periods of head retraction without full loss of consciousness. There is no papilledema, the shunt is functioning normally and supra-tentorial ventricular tap shows small ventricles and normal pressure.

This is much different from the posterior fossa obstruction by tumor or aqueduct stenosis which tends to be relieved by ventricular drainage. It is temporarily relieved by hypertonic solutions. The tight posterior fossa must be treated by posterior fossa and upper cervical decompression. If allowed to continue untreated, a grand mal convulsion will ensue. This may be the "coup de grace" for the brain stem,

and one of our patients remained apneic following the convulsion. On our service the combination of headache, trance-
like episodes and head retraction in a myelomeningocele
patient with small ventricles and functioning shunt is
indication for emergency decompression day or night.

Some other conditions such as hydromyelia, (Fig. 2)
arachnoid cyst, chronic hydrocephalus, or multiple pulmonary
emboli can simulate chronic Arnold-Chiari syndrome, but few
other conditions produce the above picture of acute
decompensation.

The subject of this paper does not include the specifics
of diagnosis and treatment but does encompass experiences and
speculation about the destiny of the patient with the Arnold-
Chiari malformation. We have performed decompression
operations on 31 patients for the condition. Preoperatively
two died on the ward and one died at home. Four progressed
gradually to death in spite of decompression and two are
hopeless invalids with very little reserve after treatment.[6]
The remainder have returned to routine activities including
school and are living comfortably with minimal evidence of
progressive loss of function. At this time their outlook for
the future is indefinite, but it is clear that 10 years or
more of good quality survival is possible after decompression.

How many of the presently asymptomatic cases will later
decompensate? It would appear that the period of growth and
particularly from age 4 to 16 years carries the greatest
risk. Possibly the incidence will fall off sharply after
age 20. On the other hand it is possible that changing
dynamics, shunt failures, arteriosclerosis, arachnoiditis,
and future surgery may precipitate the condition as in our
spine ostectomies. At present the incidence of decompressions
in our series is 31 of 544 cases or 5%. There has been no

operative mortality, but 4 have died and 2 are very weak.
Three died before decompression while we were learning to
understand the condition.   These statistics suggest that
until we develop better treatment techniques we may expect
a 15 to 20% mortality in the patients who develop advanced
late symptomatic Arnold-Chiari syndrome.   Nineteen of the 31
decompressed cases were in the category of patients who were
born with marked kyphosis in the thoracolumbar spine.   This
kyphosis is known to be an unfavorable prognostic indicator
and by some surgeons is listed as a relative contraindication
to early repair.   On the other hand some of these children
thrive and develop normal mental capacities.   Their problem
constitutes one of the most complex and disturbing ones that
we face in the treatment of myelodysplasia.

SUMMARY

The Arnold-Chiari malformation is estimated to occur in
85% of children with myelomeningocele.   In our experience it
caused disabling symptoms in about 15% at birth but tended
to subside in treated patients.

The late advanced symptomatic form of the affliction
manifested during the growing years in spite of adequate
shunting in about 5% of the repaired cases.   It has been
lethal or totally disabling in about 20% of these advanced
cases.

REFERENCES

1.   Arnold, J.: Myelocyste Transposition von Gewebskeimen
     und Symbodie. *Beitr. path. Anat., 16*:1, 1894.

2. Chiari, H.: Ueber veranderunger des Kleinhirns infolge
    von hydrocephalie des gross hirns. *Dtsch. Med.*
    Wochenschr., 17:1172, 1891.

3. Chiari, H.: Ueber veranderunger des Kleinhirns, des
    pons und der medulla oblongata in folge von congenitaler
    hydrocephalie des gross hirns. *Denschr. Akad. Wiss.*
    Wein, 63:71, 1896.

4. Hoffman, H.J., Hendrick, E.B. and Humphreys, R.P.:
    Manifestations and management of Arnold-Chiari malforma-
    tion in patients with myelomeningocele. *Child's Brain,*
    1:255, 1975.

5. Krieger, A.J.: Measurement of respiration in Arnold-
    Chiari malformation. *Child's Brain, 2*:31, 1976

6. Sayers, M.P.: Shunt complications. IN Clinical
    Neurosurgery, Vol. 23, Baltimore, Williams and Wilkins,
    1976, pp. 393.

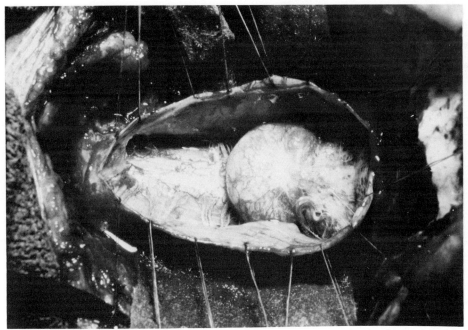

Fig. 1. Funnel-shaped enlargement of the upper cervical spinal canal with Arnold-Chiari malformation.

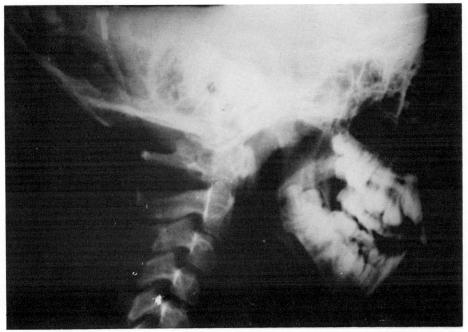

Fig. 2. Cervical hydromyelia with Arnold-Chiari malformation.

LATE COMPLICATIONS OF THE ARNOLD-CHIARI MALFORMATION

K. Shapiro, M.D. and K. Shulman, M.D.

Valve regulated control of hydrocephalus has prolonged survival in a significant percentage of selected myelomeningocele patients. As this population increases one of the critical issues in survival will be the treatment of the Arnold-Chiari hindbrain malformation as it presents in later life. Although the Type I malformation usually is associated with adulthood presentation, Gardner[3] has treated several non-myelomeningocele adult patients with varying degrees of caudal displacement of the vermis associated with hindbrain impaction in the foramen magnum (Type II). This would suggest that some of the symptoms and signs seen in adult Arnold-Chiari patients may be associated with the myelomeningocele population when it survives to adulthood. However a significant portion of the myelomeningocele population will be distinguished by iatrogenic changes in CSF dynamics induced by shunting. The following case illustrates this combined pathogenesis.

M.C. is a 14 year old girl born with a lumbosacral myelomeningocele. Hydrocephalus was managed by right choroid plexectomy at 3 months of age. At 2 years of age the myelomeningocele was repaired and at the same time she had a lumboperitoneal shunt. When she began to walk at age 2 it was apparent that there was a marked inversion of both feet

with a slight foot drop. This was corrected at age 7 by
muscle transplants with gait improvement. However, by age 9
she became unsteady in walking which progressed over the next
2 years. In addition she developed urinary frequency and
urgency. These progressive changes in her neurological
status prompted admission under our care for the first time
at age 13 years. Myelography demonstrated a narrowed sacral
sac with a compartment outside the confines of the bony canal
extending posteriorly which probably represented the repaired
meningocele. Although the contrast material was run up into
the cervical region the thoracic cord was not well visualized
because the study was done in the prone position.

A lumbar laminectomy was performed to explore the previously repaired myelomeningocele site. At operation the
cord extended down to L5. At this level there was an acute
angulation of the cord due to bony overgrowth on the left
side of the canal. Numerous adhesions and thickened arachnoid fixed the spinal cord at multiple levels. Full vessels
were seen above L4. At L4 there was a band which had interrupted the dorsal vasculature of the cord leaving a pale
area below the conus. The filum terminale was isolated and
sectioned (Fig. 1). Post-operatively she had lower motor
neuron signs as manifest by increased weakness of her legs,
depressed knee reflexes and an atonic bladder requiring
urecholine for adequate micturition.

Gradually over the next few months the lower motor
neuron signs were replaced with those of spasticity of the
lower extremities and a spastic bladder. These signs were
suggestive of a lesion above the previous surgery. Myelography was performed at age 14 years and demonstrated an
arachnoid cyst extending from T5 to T7 which filled only

when she was placed in a lateral or supine position. The contrast was run up to the foramen magnum showing the cerebellar vermis at the level of C1 confirming the diagnosis of Arnold-Chiari malformation. She had a thoracic laminectomy from T8 through T5. The dura was distended and upon opening the dura a large translucent cyst was exposed in the right posterolateral aspect of the canal splaying the dorsal and ventral roots and displacing them downward. The cyst tore on attempted dissection releasing a clear colorless fluid with a protein of 17 mg%. Several large strips of the wall were removed, but the upper limits of the cyst were not visualized.

Post-operatively her spasticity was reduced and she steadily improved for 2 weeks. Her neurological status plateaued for another week and she then gradually deteriorated to her pre-operative status with a sensory level at T4. Two months post-operatively she had no useful function of her legs. At this time she began to complain of headaches and vomited several times. Funduscopic examination showed fresh flame shaped hemorrhages in the right eye. Myelography was repeated and showed pooling of the contrast material in a cystic space extending above the previous laminectomy region. The lumbar puncture done did not demonstrate increased pressure, but the spinal fluid protein was 2 gms%. Repeat thoracic laminectomy extended from T5 to T1. At the upper level the cord was normal and residual cyst was totally excised from T5-T1 (Fig. 2).

On the night of surgery she was noted to be breathing deeply and complained of a pressure sensation in her chest. She became progressively more lethargic and had irregular respirations. She was intubated but her breathing became more irregular with periods of gasping respirations followed

by apnea. Tachycardia and hypertension accompanied these
changes. Her neurological status was as follows: ocular
bobbing with jerky nystagmus on all fields of gaze; inter-
nucelar ophthalmoplegia; no oculocephalic responses; no
reaction to cold calorics; left sided weakness with decreased
sensation on the left; retained ability to follow simple
commands.

A right ventricular tap was performed with an opening
pressure of 120 mm of water. The fluid was clear with normal
protein. She was maintained on ventricular drainage as well
as on assisted ventilation for the next 3 days, at which time
she was alert and following commands. She no longer had the
internuclear ophthalmoplegia or the ocular bobbing, but she
continued to have nystagmus in all fields of gaze. She had
moderate cerebellar signs; neck movements produced numbness
and weakness of her upper extremities. Gag reflexes were
depressed; she talked in a whisper with dysphagia. Her eye
grounds did not change. On the 6th post operative day a
suboccipital craniectomy with removal of the arches of C1
and C2 was performed. The cerebellum extended down to C1
and was covered with a milky, thickened arachnoid. The obex
of the fourth ventricle extended down to C2. The right side
of the clava was hyperremic (Fig. 3). Indigo carmine was
placed in the right lateral ventricle but did not pass into
the cisterna magnum confirming internal obstruction; a
ventriculo-pleural shunt was performed. Post operatively
she did well until about 6 P.M. when there was an abrupt
change in her vital signs. She became less responsive as
before with tachycardia, hypertension and gasping respirations. She was re-intubated and ventilation was assisted.
At the time of intubation both vocal cords moved well. The
wound was re-opened expressing a small collection of blood

but her general condition did not improve. Because of the
gasping respirations she was paralyzed and ventilated mechanically for the remainder of the night. A tracheostomy was
performed after the exploration. During the next week her
neurological status was similar to the early syndrome:
internuclear ophthalmoplegia; nystagmus in all fields of
gaze; weakness of both arms; moderate cerebellar signs;
absent corneal reflexes; depressed gag responses; difficulty
swallowing; intermittent episodes of hiccups and irregular
gasping respirations.

During the next 2 weeks she had intermittent episodes of
slowed respirations and hypertension. Pulmonary function
studies showed decreased respiratory rate when breathing
room air and decreased minute ventilation breathing 5% CO_2
(Table I). Eventually she died. At autopsy, the lower
quarter of the medulla extended below the foramen magnum.
There was moderate cerebellar herniation on both sides of the
medulla. Microscopic examination showed cell loss and glio-
sis of the inferior olives as well as the lower cranial nerve
nuclei. The cervical spinal cord was normal including the
orientation of the roots. The thoracic spinal cord was
necrotic and showed secondary tract degeneration.

DISCUSSION

The symptomatic late complications of the Arnold-Chiari
malformation are conveniently divided into three presenta-
tions. The most common manifestation is laryngeal palsy
associated with stridor which usually affects infants and
those in the first decade of life. Whether adults are
usually spared because patients prove to develop this
complication are selected out at earlier ages or the brain
dynamics change in later life is not certain. Inspection of

brains in patients dying from this complication reveals two
pathologic findings. In all patients the bulbar and spinal
nerves course upward; in the minority of patients these
findings are coupled with intramedullary hemorrhages.[5] Onset
of stridor may be insidious or present precipitously; all
patients with medullary hemorrhages have abrupt onset of
stridor. Although many of the reported cases were associated
with bulging fontanelles or progressive hydrocephalus, other
instances are cited where stridor has occurred in the
presence of a functioning shunt.[8] Since spontaneous improvement has occurred without any form of surgical intervention,
the etiology of laryngeal dysfunction cannot be generalized.[7]

Although the tenth nerve deficit is the most common and
often most dramatic deficits involving the third, fifth,
sixth, seventh, eighth, ninth, eleventh and twelfth cranial
nerves have also been reported (Fig. 4). Penfield and
Coburn's report also shows anatomic evidence of stretching
of all the true cranial nerves.[6] This case is of major
interest because of th cephalad course of all the cranial and
spinal nerves extending from T2. This patient interestingly
had a high thoracic meningocele repaired during childhood.
Although caudal traction is usually discounted as a cause of
the Arnold-Chiari malformation, it is possible that in certain isolated cases, the tethering of the spinal cord may
produce secondary traction on the lower brain stem as differential growth occurs. As noted in our case it is possible
that traction at the repair was present and that tethering
may have occurred in later life.

The second abnormality associated with the Arnold-Chiari
is respiratory embarrassment apart from stridor. This
complication often presents precipitiously as episodes of
apnea. Although usually found in early infancy, these

episodes have been reported in older patients with Arnold-
Chiari as seen in our illustrative case. Wealthall et al
reported that respiratory malfunction usually occurs during
sleep, heralded by periodic breathing and coinciding with
bursts of active eye movement.[9] EEG correlation and cerebral
blood flow abnormalities have not been studied in these
patients. Although stridor may be associated, apnea can
occur independently and appears to be a function of insensi-
tivity to carbon dioxide similar to that found in the Pick-
wickian Syndrome. As seen in our case decreased minute
ventilation followed breathing 5% CO_2.

Alterations in CSF dynamics characterize the third group
of late complications of Arnold-Chiari malformation. In the
present case decompensation occurred after surgery on the
arachnoid cyst. The release of fluid inferiorly probably
caused a significant increase in the pressure differential
between the closed intracranial cavity and the spinal canal.
This did not result in an immediate impaction of the medulla
but it did cause further impairment in the cerebrospinal
fluid circulation as evidenced by the headaches, vomiting
and hemorrhages in the right fundus. The resultant medullary
impaction occurred after the second laminectomy. This delay
in medullary compromise may be related to the conversion of
a communicating hydrocephalus to a noncommunicating type
between operative procedures. The present case illustrates
a most unusual association that of an extramedullary arachnoid cyst; the decompensation following operation must be
related to iatrogenic alterations in CSF dynamics.

All three types of delayed complications share one
common abnormality: the Arnold-Chiari hindbrain malformation. The severity of the malformation, including the degree

of hindbrain impaction, neuronal abnormalities and spinal
distortion, may vary markedly from one patient to the next.
Various forces may act on the basic Arnold-Chiari malformation, perhaps contributing to the delayed clinical presentation of the Arnold-Chiari malformation.

As shown by Emery upper brain stem deformities and
aqueductal shortening beyond the basic Type II malformation
may be induced by CSF diversion procedures.[1] These abnormalities may place further traction on the lower brain stem
which has been impacted within the foramen magnum and may be
incapable of ascending. Should traction result, relative
ischemia or impairment of venous outflow may follow. The
Sheffield group has also demonstrated vascular distortions
consisting of downward looping of the vertebral arteries into
the spinal canal with displacement of the basilar artery
origin beneath the foramen magnum.[2] A threefold descent of
the posterior inferior cerebellar arteries accompanied lumbosacral myelomeningoceles while thoracic meningocele patients
had up to tenfold descents of these arteries. Whether these
arterial dislocations occur in patients with adequate treatment of hydrocephalus is not clear, nor is it apparent that
these abnormalities result from the hindbrain malformation or
changes in CSF dynamics. The latter may be at least a contributing factor since similar, although not as marked,
distortions of posterior fossa vascular structures are
described in non Arnold-Chiari patients harboring intracranial masses.

A final common pathophysiologic finding can be found in
brain stem compression. The impacted hindbrain of the Type
II malformation is predisposed to any mechanism which further
comprises its functional integrity. In these settings the
additive effects of vascular and CSF factors discussed above

may contribute to the total neurologic picture. The pulsatile force of the CSF may increase the degree of impaction, especially when differential changes in CSF pressures are induced even by well intentioned therapeutic endeavors. One may attribute progressive impaction to the combined effects of the patient's growth and secondary tethering of neural structures, but usually the onset of symptoms does not coincide with growth spurts. A feature not described to date would be the contribution of basilar impression, an entity often found in Arnold-Chiari patients.

From the foregoing discussion certain points emerge. Adequate control of hydrocephalus is not an assurance that late complications of the hindbrain malformation will not occur. Further, decompression of the hindbrain malformation has not uniformly resulted in improvement, so that pressure and local compression are not the only causes of these late complications.[8] The self-limited nature of the deficits in some patients indicates that some complications may result from transient phenomena, perhaps of a vascular etiology.

If the cause of these complications is multifactorial, then caution must be exercised when dealing with patients at risk. Cranial nerve function must be assessed fully and sequentially. Respiratory evaluation must include ventilatory response to CO_2 in order to anticipate sleep-induced apnea described above. Finally the surgeon must have delineated the full extent of the abnormalities in any patient so that operative manipulation of one segment of the Arnold-Chiari malformation does not precipitate decompensation of another component. Of particular importance is the maintenance of an adequate CSF diversionary procedure during and after any operative intervention.

REFERENCES

1. Emery, J.L.: Deformity of the aqueduct of Sylvius in children with hydrocephalus and myelomeningocele. *Dev. Med. Child. Neurol. Suppl. 32, 16*:40, 1974.

2. Emery, J.L. and Levick, R.K.: The movement of the brain stem and vessels around the brain stem in children with hydrocephalus and the Arnold-Chiari deformity. *Dev. Med. Child. Neurol., Suppl. 11, 8*:49, 1966.

3. Gardner, W.J.: Hydrodynamic mechanism of syringomyelia: its relationship to myelocele. *J. Neurol. Neurosurg. Psychiatr., 28*:247, 1965.

4. Kirsch, W.M., Duncan, B.R., Black, F.O. et al: Laryngeal palsy in association with myelomeningocele, hydrocephalus and the Arnold-Chiari malformation. *J. Neurosurg., 28*: 207, 1968.

5. Morley, A.R.: Laryngeal stridor, Arnold-Chiari malformation and medullary hemorrhages. *Dev. Med. Child. Neurol., 11*:471, 1969.

6. Penfield, W. and Coburn, D.F.: Arnold-Chiari malformation and its operative treatment. *Arch. Neurol. Psychiat., 40*:328, 1938.

7. Rullen, A.: Associated laryngeal paralysis. *Arch. Otolaryng., 64*:207, 1956.

8. Sieben, R.L., Hamida, M.B., and Shulman, K.: Multiple cranial nerve deficits associated with the Arnold-Chiari malformation. *Neurology, 21*:673, 1971.

9. Wealthall, S.R., Whittacker, G.E., and Greenwood, N.: The relationship of apnoea and stridor in spina bifida to other unexplained infant deaths. *Dev. Med. Child. Neurol, 16, Suppl. 32*:107, 1974.

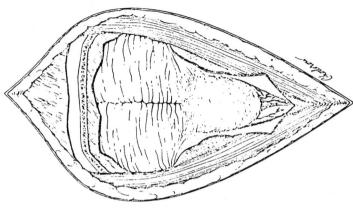

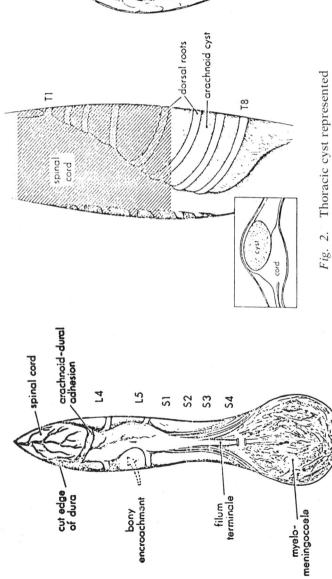

Fig. 1. Lumbar laminectomy findings. Spinal cord extended to L5 and was angulated by bony overgrowth from the left side of the canal. Arachnoid adhesion at L3–4 rendered the caudal segments of the cord ischemic.

Fig. 2. Thoracic cyst represented as composite from two operative explorations. The shaded area depicts the portion of the cyst encountered during the second operation. The dorsal roots were splayed and depressed by the cyst. Insertion shows the right postero lateral location of the cyst.

Fig. 3. Suboccipital craniectomy exposure with removal of the arches of C_1 and C_2. The cerebellar vermis is depressed; the obex extends down to C_2.

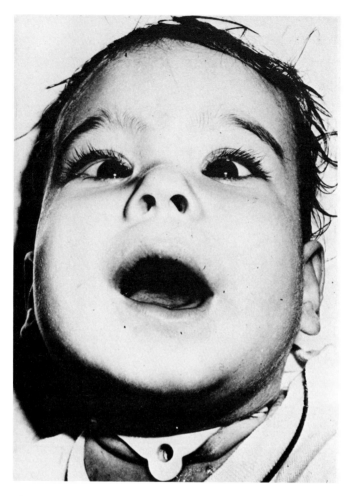

Fig. 4. This patient has bilateral VIth cranial nerve palsies accompanied by VII, IX, X, XI and XII cranial nerve deficits. Tracheostomy was placed after severe inspiratory stridor developed.

	After Laminectomy	Room Air After Posterior Fossa	1 Month Later
Minute Ventilation (liter/min)	7	6.7	3.2
Rate	26	11	12
Tidal Volume (cc)	270	611	270
$PaCO_2$ (mm Hg)	27	42	40
		5% CO_2	
Minute Ventilation	29	19.4	10
Rate	31	23	18
Tidal Volume	940	843	565
$PaCO_2$	40	51	45

Table I. Changes in ventilation breathing room air and 5% CO_2. Pulmonary function studies show decreased ventilatory response to CO_2.

THE USE OF THE CT SCANNER IN THE
PATIENT WITH MYELODYSPLASIA

K. Shulman, M.D., N. Leeds, M.D.,
T. Nadich, M.D., and K. Shapiro, M.D.

With the development of computerized axial tomography
and its availability in the United States during the past 18
months, predictions were made that this diagnostic mode would
revolutionize neurosurgical diagnosis and subsequent care.
These predictions have been fulfilled in the area of brain
tumor, vascular disease of the brain including subarachnoid
hemorrhage and in head injury. The usefulness of the technique in the pediatric patient and specifically in the patient
with myelodysplasia is still undergoing assessment. Location
and availability of CT scanning units is expanding as these
units have been useful to screen large numbers of out and in-
patients, and it is predicted that most major medical centers
will have such equipment available if not now then in the
near future. In a review of our experience in the past year
at the Montefiore Hospital and Medical Center and the Albert
Einstein College of Medicine, it would appear that although
the CT scanner is of definite use, its effectiveness in
myelodysplasia is still being evaluated. The questions to be
raised in this presentation are two: 1) Is the CT scan useful in the early management of the child with myelodysplasia
in the attempt to provide an earlier diagnosis of progressive
hydrocephalus or to demonstrate other congenital malformations

of prognostic significance with regard to mental development, and, 2) In the follow-up of children with myelodysplasia and hydrocephalus, what is the proper interval for repeat scans to provide optimum management of hydrocephalus and associated mental retardation? This latter question would also apply to many other pediatric neurosurgical conditions.

In contrast to the cooperative adult, most infants undergoing CT scanning must be anesthetized in order to reduce the movement artifacts of the study. Our attempts to obtain scans in the sedated or semi-awake infant have generally not been successful. This has required then the admission of each child to hospital for CT scanning at least for the day of the study and the preceding evening. Immediately then, a restriction is raised on the frequency of studies by the need for hospitalization.

With regard to the first question, the early diagnosis of specific brain defects, it has not been generally possible to discern the characteristics of the Arnold-Chiari malformation in the children with myelodysplasia. Although it has been possible in the older child with congenital hydrocephalus on the basis of aqueductal stenosis or Dandy-Walker malformation to characterize the posterior fossa site of obstruction utilizing the CT mode, the smallness or largeness of the head size in the infant with myelomeningocele makes it impossible to obtain adequate images of the posterior fossa to either see the Arnold-Chiari malformatiɔn or to diagnose aqueductal stenosis. The currently used water bag makes low imaging of posterior fossa impossible. These diagnoses then still remain for air study. The CT has confirmed what has been known clinically for some time that the head circumference does always indicate advancing hydrocephalus in the child with myelodysplasia so that nearly all children with

high lesions and marked paralysis will have distended
ventricles on CT scan. This is in contrast to the infant
with the low lesion and good leg function whose ventricular
dilatation during the first three weeks of age will be considerably less. The demonstration of ventricular dilatation,
however, does not solve the management question as to the
need for a shunt. Other forms of treatment such as expectant
care, head wrapping and medical management, however, are made
easier if a repeat CT scan can be performed to assess the
value of the therapy applied. In this sense then, the CT scan
both theoretically and pragmatically has decreased the number
of shunts early in the management of myelodysplastic patients.
The demonstration of other congenital malformations such as
polymicrogyria or large heteratopias, cerebral atrophy, etc.,
conditions which would predict in a definitive manner the
presence of mental subnormality and therefore select out a
child for treatment has not been realized in our experience
using the CT mode. The current 160 matrix allows the dis-
cernment of pathology of 1 cm diameter or less if it has
proper density features. The newer CT 10-10 with no water
bag may allow lower posterior fossa sections; the body
scanner should show us the spinal cord.

The answer to the first question then on the early
management and selection out of patients and the earlier
diagnosis of hydrocephalus must be then qualified as discussed. The hoped for total understanding of mental potential
has not been realized. The major use seems to be at the
present time to allow a more conservative management awaiting
for compensation of the hydrocephalus.

In the large clinics with a considerable myelodysplasia
population who are actively being followed, is it useful to
obtain a CT scanner on each of these patients when the

scanner becomes available as an attempt to predict mental function and to assess adequacy of treatment of the hydrocephalus? This is an important issue. Such children being cooperative are easier to scan and out-patient scans are possible in some children in this group. The cost of the procedure of some $250 to $300 is however a consideration.

Our approach has been for selective CT scans on these children when real clinical questions are posed or instead of the shunt survey at age 3-4 years. We have found the scan useful in assessing the need for a shunt in a child whose school performance was less than adequate after a shunt had been removed perhaps at an earlier age for infection. Certainly mantle size and width can be determined easily by this mode. In the past, ventricular size has been measured on air study by assessing the thickness of the frontal part of the brain parenchyma on lateral view. Echoencephalography has also been used. On the CT scan the body of the ventricle can always be seen. Lindgren's index which is the distance between the lateral walls of the anterior horns divided by the largest internal skull diameter, a/b, can be used for sequential studies.[1] Lateral to third ventricle ratios are less useful. Illustrative cases with legends follow. Twenty-one illustrations.

REFERENCE

1. Lindgren, E.: Encephalography in cerebral atrophy. *Acta Radiol.*, *35*:277, 1957.

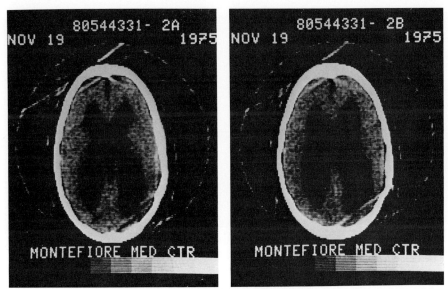

Figs. 1 & 2. Scan on 6-year old child thought to have compensated hydrocephalus showing symmetrical ventricular dilatation. Shunt reinstituted.

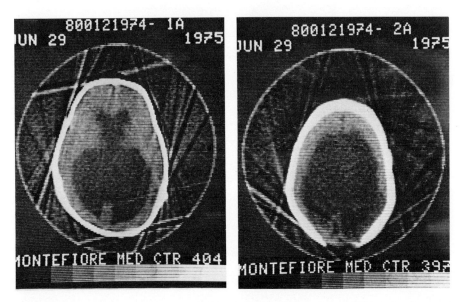

Figs. 3 & 4. Scan at age 1 of a child who had shunt removed for infection at 6 months.

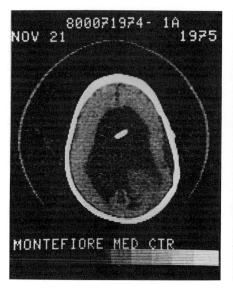
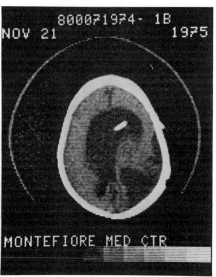
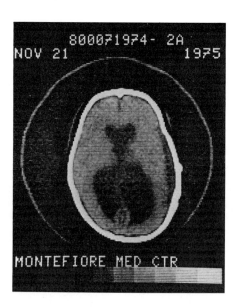

Figs. 5, 6 & 7. New shunt placed in frontal location. Note decrease in ventricular size and presence of subdural collection on right communicating with porencephaly.

268

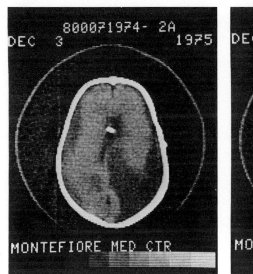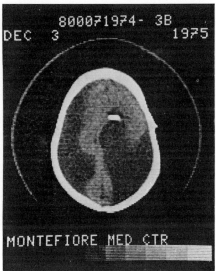

Figs. 8 & 9. Same child. Subdural collection on left as well as on right due to collapse of very thin cortical mantle.

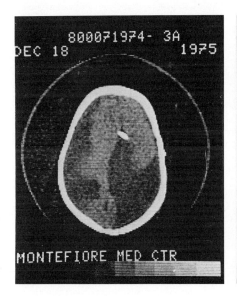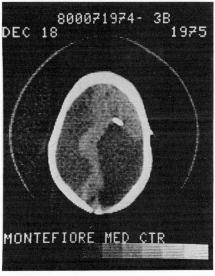

Figs. 10 & 11. Persistence of collections despite repeated taps.

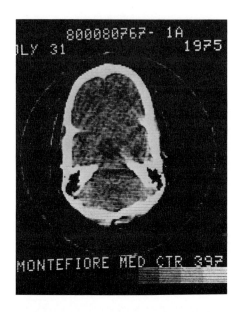

Fig. 12 (left). 8 year old with high lesion. Low cut in attempt to see the Arnold-Chiari malformation.

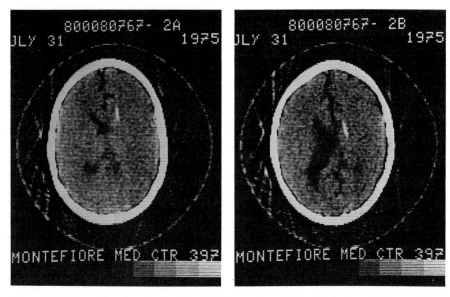

Figs. 13 & 14. The shunt tube in right lateral ventricle showing collapse of that ventricle.

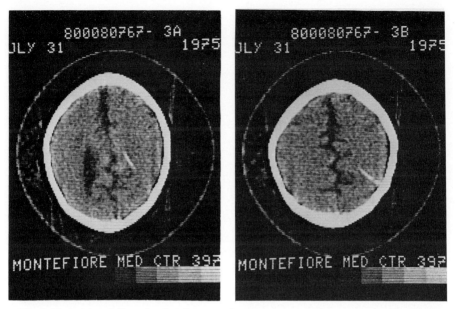

Figs. 15 & 16. Dilated sulci frequently seen in post shunt myelodysplastic patients.

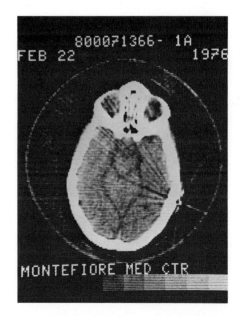

Fig. 17 (right). 11-year old with enlarged cerebellar vermis.

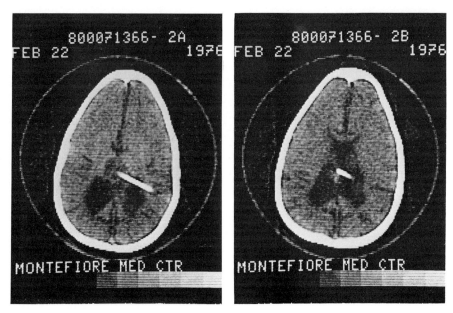

Figs. 18 & 19. Same child showing shunted symmetrical ventricles and enlarged cortical sulci.

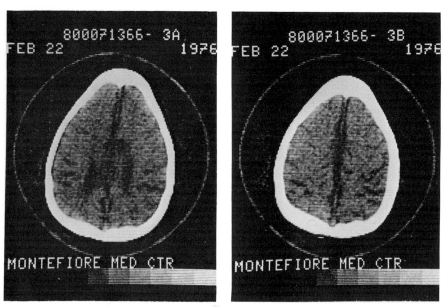

Figs. 20 & 21. Higher cuts demonstrating prominent sulcal pattern.

RADIOLOGIC PROBLEMS IN PATIENTS
OPERATED FOR HYDROCEPHALUS

H.J. Globl, L. Schut and H.J. Kaufmann

This is a preliminary report on all patients shunted for hydrocephalus at The Children's Hospital of Philadelphia from January 1, 1969 to December 31, 1971. 477 such shunts were performed in 262 patients. In 152 this was the first shunt, in 325 a revision due to complication was needed. The annual complication rate of shunts has been estimated at 9%.

Radiology has a role in the pre-operative diagnosis as well as in the post-operative follow-up in hydrocephalics. Different types of operations have been devised; the one most frequently used is the ventriculo-vascular shunt.[2] During recent years, ventriculo-peritoneal shunts have become increasingly important.[1] Sub-arachnoid-peritoneal shunts and diversion of the cerebro-spinal fluid into the pleural space, the middle ear, the ureters and even the Fallopian tubes are occasionally used. Knowledge of these and the different inserted valve systems is basic for proper evaluation.

Most commonly used are the valve systems of Spitz-Holter, usually combined with a Rickham reservoir, Pudenz-Heyer and Ames.

At post-operative examination the position of the proximal and distal catheter must be judged. In some cases

the proximal tubing was not in the ventricle but in the
subdural space. In ventriculo-auricular shunts, the distal
tubing is placed within the right atrium under electro-
cardiographic control. Misplacement in the right ventricle
causes insufficient drainage due to the local high pressure.
The position of the distal tip in the superior vena cava, an
inevitable result of growth of the patient, may be complicated
by fibrinous blockage. Occasionally the distal catheter can
get into the azygos, the sub-clavian, the axillary or hepatic
vein.[3]

In order to avoid a revision during growth, the distal
catheter was placed deep in the inferior vena cava. However,
such catheters frequently curled and slipped back up. This
happened to one patient who presented with respiratory
difficulties, seven weeks following the insertion of a
ventriculo-vascular shunt. Chest films showed a curled
distal tubing and massive cardiomegaly. Autopsy revealed a
perforation of the right auricular appendage (Fig. 1).

Tsingoglou and Eckstein reported 10 cases of pericardial
tamponade. Either forceful introduction of the distal
catheter during a shunt revision or an overly long distal
catheter were assumed to be responsible for cardiac
tamponade.[9] Respiratory difficulties or cardiac failure
combined with an enlarged heart following a ventriculo-
auricular shunt are indicative of a pericardial tamponade.
Diagnosis can be made by injecting contrast material into
the valve, pumping the valve briefly and taking a chest film.

Besides malposition of the shunt tubings, separation,
fracture or kinking of the proximal or distal catheter is
not uncommon. Reconnection of the proximal tubing does not
cause major difficulties in most cases. If a distal catheter
gets disconnected and slips away, catheterization has to be

applied. In four patients William Rashkind removed the distal tubing, using his own technique.[8]

Radiologic changes of the skull may follow a successful shunt. If intracranial pressure drops too quickly, epidural and subdural hematoma may develop, due to rupture of bridging veins and overlapping of the cranial sutures may occur. Further sequelae may be thickening of the diploic portion of the vault (Fig. 2). Following the occlusion of sutures, demineralization of the sella may develop in patients with unsatisfactory functioning of the shunt and chronic increased intracranial pressure.[3]

In rapid decompression of a large hydrocephalus, congestive heart failure has been reported.[4] We found this complication just once. A very frequent and major complication in ventriculo-vascular shunts is the thrombo-embolisation of the involved veins, the heart and the lungs.

The presence of polyethylene or silicone tubings stimulates the production of thrombi on the surface of the tube or on the traumatized adjacent areas.[10] This mechanism is favored by chronic infection of the cerebro-spinal fluid and the shunt system and the contents in coagulation factors of the cerebro-spinal fluid. The following may result:

1. Cases with complete obstruction of the jugular vein, or superior vena cava. It is impossible to recanalise such veins. Ventriculo-peritoneal or ventriculo-pleural shunts are an alternative. In two cases direct insertion of the distal catheter into the right atrium was done.

2. Thrombo-embolism with pulmonary hypertension(s) (Fig. 3).

3. Calcification of thrombi of the superior vena cava. This condition is only rarely reported in the literature.[6] We have seen four such patients (Fig. 4).

COMMENTS ON VENTRICULO-PLEURAL SHUNTS

Ingraham and coworkers (1945) could demonstrate in their experiments that dogs are able to absorb normal saline through the pleural surface.

Six of our patients had a ventriculo-pleural shunt, one patient with an arachnoid cyst had a cysto-pleural shunt. Except for the cysto-pleural shunt, the diversion of the CSF into the pleural space was a repeat operation due to malfunctioning of previous shunts. These have been present for 6 weeks to 6 years.

In five cases the ventriculo-pleural shunt was left in only for 2 to 8 weeks, in one patients for 15 months and in one case for 4 years. In all cases the ventriculo-pleural shunt had to be removed after shunt revisions and thoracocentesis were performed several times. Because of these unsatisfactory results ventriculo-pleural shunts have been largely abandoned (Fig. 5).

COMMENTS ON VENTRICULO-PERITONEAL SHUNTS

Two major advantages have helped to propagate the ventriculo-peritoneal shunt:

1.   The lack of cardio-vascular and pulmonary complications.

2.   The use of well tolerated silicone tubings with a slit valve at the distal end, preventing reflux of fluid into the shunt system.

Here again infection, plugging of the ventricular catheter and separation of the parts of the drain system may occur. Due to infection, the peritoneum may lose its absorptive capacity, but may fully recuperate.

A 2½ year old patient showed the clinical signs of an Ileus. After two earlier shunts a ventriculo-peritoneal shunt had been inserted 5 months prior to the present admission. Radiographically an abdominal mass was demonstrated (Fig. 6). The distal end of the ventriculo-peritoneal shunt and about 400cc CSF were removed and a new left ventriculo-auricular shunt inserted.

A further 1½ year old patient was seen with an abdominal mass in the right lower quadrant. After a repair of meningomyelocele at birth several shunt operations were necessary. Two weeks prior to admission a right ventriculo-peritoneal shunt was performed. Radiographically there was a right lower quadrant mass. Barium enema was suspicious for adhesions involving the distal ileum.

Diagnoses discussed were infected shunt, a collection of cerebro-spinal fluid or a ruptured appendix.

The patient was treated with antibiotics. Four weeks later a pelvic abscess drained through the rectum.

Finally the possibility of perforation of parts of the tubing into the bowel must not be overlooked. One such patient was seen.

It was the purpose of this report to demonstrate some of the many possibilities of complications after shunt operations. A further, more detailed study is under way to determine the actual incidence of the different radiologically recognizable complications in a larger material, since it can be anticipated that we will have to deal with increasing numbers of such iatrogenic complications in the future.

REFERENCES

1. Ames, R.H.: Ventriculo-peritoneal shunts in the management of hydrocephalus. *J. Neurosurg.*, *27*:525, 1967.

2. Blatt, C.J. and Shulman, K.: X-ray manifestations of
    the Holter valve in hydrocephalus. *Radiol., 92*:1517,
    1969.

3. Cohen, W.N.: Roentgenographic manifestations of
    complications secondary to cerebral ventricular-cardiac
    atrial shunts. *Amer. J. Roentgenol., 98*:689, 1966.

4. Emery, J.L. and Hilton, H.B.: Lung and heart complica-
    tions of the treatment of hydrocephalus by ventriculo-
    auriculostomy. *Surgery, 50*:309, 1961.

5. Friedman, S., Zita-Gozum, C. and Chatten, J.: Pulmonary
    vascular changes complicating ventriculovascular shunting
    for hydrocephalus. *J. Pediat., 64*:305, 1964.

6. Gabriele, O.F. and Clark, D.: Calcified thrombus of the
    superior vena cava, complication of ventriculoatrial
    shunt. *Amer. J. Dis. Child., 117*:325, 1969.

7. Kurlander, G.J. and Chua, G.T.: Roentgenology of
    ventriculoatrial shunts for the treatment of hydrocepha-
    lus. *Amer. J. Roentgenol., 101*:157, 1967.

8. Rashkind, W.J.: A cardiac catheter device for removal
    of plastic catheter emboli from children's hearts.
    J. Pediat., 74:618, 1969.

9. Tsingoglou, S. and Eckstein, H.B.: Pericardial tamponade
    by Holter ventriculoatrial shunts. *J. Neurosurg., 35*:
    695, 1971.

10. Strenger, L.: Complications of ventriculovenous shunts.
    J. Neurosurg., 20:219, 1963.

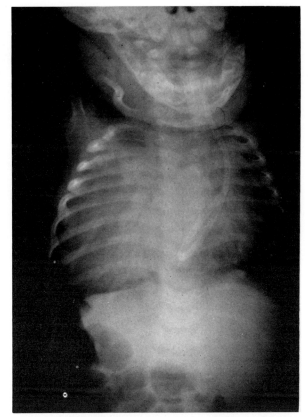

Fig. 1. Pericardial tamponade caused by perforation of
an overly long distal tubing.

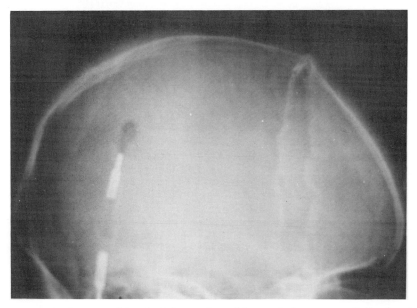

Fig. 2. Thickening of the diploic portion of the vault in a successfully shunted
child.

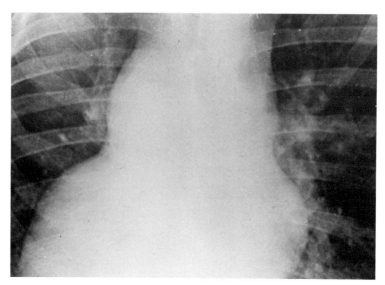

Fig. 3. Cardiomegaly, marked dilatation of the pulmonary artery and scanty peripheral pulmonary vasculature in an 11-year old child with pulmonary hypertension following ventriculo-vascular shunt at age of 4 months.

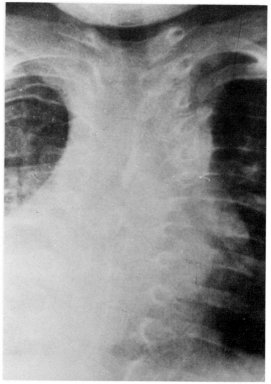

Fig. 4. Calcification at the distal end of the tubing within the superior vena cava.

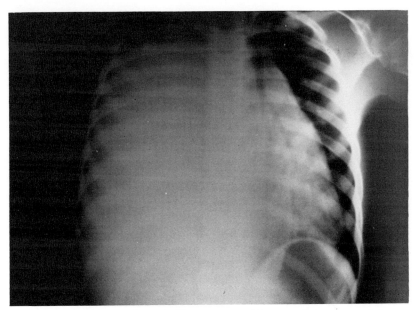

Fig. 5. Massive pleural effusion caused by nonabsorption of the cerebro-spinal fluid in a child with ventriculo-pleural shunt.

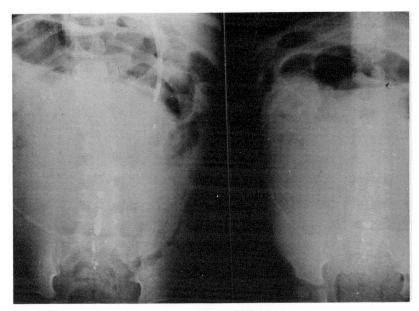

Fig. 6. Displacement of bowel loops by an "abdominal mass" due to failure of the peritoneum to absorb the cerebro-spinal fluid in a ventriculo-peritoneal shunt.

COMPLICATIONS OF VENTRICULO-PERITONEAL SHUNTING PROCEDURES

Joe Sam Robinson, M.D., Keiichi Kuwamura, M.D.
and Anthony J. Raimondi, M.D.

ABSTRACT

The complications of ventriculo-peritoneal shunts were analyzed as two separate chronological groups, 1968-73 using the three piece system and 1974-75 using the one piece system, identifying morbidity and mortality in both groups. All complications are listed in the tables. It appears that infections represent the highest morbidity and that shunt related infections the only cause for death in both series being reported. There is a direct relationship between shunt failure and shunt infection, and also between number of shunt revisions and incidence of infection in a given child or group of children. The one piece has a significantly lower morbidity and failure rate.

Since the days of Hippocrates, efforts have been undertaken to decompress the intracranial space and control hydrocephalus.[9] With the advent of suitable anesthesia and
surgical sterility the first primitive efforts took a more
realistic turn. Zenner in 1886 implanted the first internal
ventricular drainage system. In 1893, Miculicz of Germany
implanted the first internal shunt. Watson, Cheyne, Bellanie
and Andrews all were soon advocating their own techniques
for connecting the ventricles with either the subarachnoid
or subdural spaces, using gold or platinum tubes.[5] In a
famous 1898 report, Ferguson related his technique for shunting cerebrospinal fluid from the lumbar subarachnoid space to
the peritoneal cavity.[15] In 1905 Kausch, of Germany, used a
small rubber tube to shunt cerebrospinal fluid from the
lateral ventricle to the peritoneal cavity. Payr in 1908
shunted ventricular cerebrospinal fluid into the circulatory
system.[23] Additional papers reported ventriculo-pleural and
ventriculo-ureteral shunts.[9]

Following these initial procedures, however, enthusiasm
for shunting waned. The favorable experiences of Ingram with
plastic shunt tubing stimulated Cone of Montreal to repopu-
larize shunting procedures.[26] Sparked by these advances, a
number of innovative shunting procedures were undertaken
using widely diverse physiological areas as absorptive targets
for shunted cerebrospinal fluid.[22,34,37,47]

By the late 1950's, silastic ventriculo-atrial shunts
had proved to be the most effective and widely performed of
shunting procedures.[27,34,44] Unfortunately, as experience
accumulated with this shunting procedure, a rather high rate
of morbidity and mortality came into evidence. New alternatives were sought. We began to shunt routinely into the
peritoneal cavity in 1963 and reported on a simplified

technique for this in 1967.[45] At the time, we reasoned that
the peritoneal ends of shunt systems, since they were invariably open-ended tubes, were being plugged with omentum and
that, accordingly, the Pudenz slit valve would obviate this
form of occlusion. This proved to be true. In a 1967 paper,
Ames published his experiences with silastic catheters in
ventriculo-peritoneal shunts.[2] Many centers have now elected
to use ventriculo-peritoneal shunting systems. While a
number of reports detail the complications of ventriculo-
atrial shunting procedures, rather less data is available
concerning the use of ventriculo-peritoneal shunting procedures. This paper reports our experiences with ventriculo-
peritoneal shunts and external ventricular drainage in infants and children, specifying complications and their
incidence. It also offers preliminary reports of the results
obtained with the single-piece ventriculo-peritoneal shunt.*

CLINICAL MATERIAL

The results of 849 insertions, removals, and revisions
among 231 patients were analyzed and complication rates
ascertained at the Children's Memorial Hospital, Northwestern
University, Division of Neurosurgery. The shunting procedures
were undertaken only after angiographic evidence of hydrocephalus had been obtained. This portion of the present
study is a retrospective review of all patients shunted at
our institution from 1968 to 1973 whose medical records were
obtainable. The procedure of choice was a ventriculo-peritoneal shunt. This procedure was carried out 598 times. A
recent history of peritonitis or ureterostomy was the only
contraindication to a ventriculo-peritoneal shunt. Ventriculo-

*Unishunt

atrial procedures undertaken as a secondary choice were
performed 40 times. Lumbar subarachnoid peritoneal shunts
were performed 4 times, Dandy-Walker and posterior fossa
cysts were shunted directly on 16 occasions. Subdural fluid
collections were treated with subdural-peritoneal procedures
in 33 cases. External ventricular drainage was instituted
148 times (Table 1).

The second portion of this study reports data upon the
161 patients shunted 297 times with single-piece ventriculo-
peritoneal shunts between July 1, 1974 and December 31, 1975.

Operative Techniques

In children under the age of two years, a ventriculo-
peritoneal shunt was performed under local anesthesia.
Following a 10-minute scrub with Povidone-Iodine scrub solution and an application of Povidone-Iodine paint, the cephalic
incision was made in the area of the parietal prominence.
Under fluoroscopic control, the ventricular portion of the
shunt was placed in the lateral ventricle anterior to the
choroid plexus. Access to the abdominal cavity was obtained
by use of an abdominal trocar. All patients were catheterized
to guard against the danger of puncturing the bladder.[44]
Ventriculo-atrial shunts were done under general anesthesia.
Proper placement of the atrial portion of the shunt was
assured by fluoroscopic control. All patients were closely
observed in the hospital for 10 days following the operative
procedure. If there was any evidence of shunt malfunction
or infection, the child was taken to the operating room
immediately and the shunting apparatus revised. On discharge,
all patients were closely followed in the outpatient clinic,
and the parents of the patients were encouraged to bring
their children back to our service for further evaluation if

there were any suspicions or evidence of shunt infection or malfunction.

Prior to July, 1974, a three-piece shunting apparatus was used. After that date, a presterilized, one-piece shunting system was inserted.

METHODS AND RESULTS

The total of 231 patients shunted between 1968 and 1973 ranged in age from newborn to 16 years. Any time a shunt was inserted, removed or revised, it was counted as a procedure. A computation of complications was made by a retrospective chart study. There were a total of 160 complications divided among 91 patients. The majority of these complications were infections, predominantly ventriculitis. We diagnosed ventriculitis when cerebrospinal fluid cultures following a shunting procedure were positive.

There were no operative or post-operative deaths. Our 6 shunt-related deaths were all attributed to ventriculitis. The complications found in using ventriculo-peritoneal shunts were itemized in their own groupings (Tables 4,5,6). Additional correlations were formulated by comparing the complications of shunting procedures with the indications for the shunting procedures (Table 7). A statistical comparison was also made between the complication rate, sex and age of the patient at the time of the first shunt (Table 8). The results of single-piece ventriculo-peritoneal shunts are compared with three-piece ventriculo-peritoneal shunts by general diagnostic category and result (Table 9).

DISCUSSION

A number of factors should be entertained before any discussion of complications is undertaken. It should be kept

in mind that, in many cases and centers, the indications for
shunting procedures and revisions are still subject to debate.
In any case mix, a number of patients hover between a diagnosis of rather "generous" ventricles with a dysplastic
mantle and hydrocephalus. Even when the nature of the
patient's defect is established, as in the case of Dandy-
Walker cysts, posterior fossa cysts, subdural hematoma,
hydrocephalus in the presence of myelomeningocele, many
different treatment regimens exist. The policy each center
adopts upon such issues obviously will influence each center's
reportable shunting complications. Moreover, the cultural
dispositions, native language, age, and mobility of each
neurosurgical center's referral population will influence
reported results. And, finally, the subjective inclinations
and reportive techniques of the center will influence the
patterns of complication results.

An extraordinary number of collected studies reveal in
great detail the complications involved in ventriculo-atrial
shunts.[3,6,7,8,17,18,19,25] They emphasize the dangers of
shunt infections and sepsis.[40,42,52,53,56] Rarer complications include thrombosis of the superior or inferior vena
cava[18,25,38,40,56] occlusion of the pulmonary artery and/or
pulmonary emboli,[3,13,14,18,19,20,38,50,55,57] migration of
the catheter into the pulmonary artery,[18,25,33] cardiac
tamponade,[3,12,18,28,56,58] and subdural hematoma.[18,19,25,40]

Ventriculo-peritoneal shunting results and complications
are less well documented. Regretably many authors have had
the tendency to lump complications of ventriculo-peritoneal
and lumbar-peritoneal shunting procedures. Scott et al and
Jackson et al in 1955 each reported rather unfavorable results
using non-silastic shunts for ventriculo-peritoneal and
lumbar-peritoneal procedures.[29,54] In Ames' 1967 report, he

cites 120 ventriculo-peritoneal procedures done over a 9 year
period, with 4 deaths (all due to infection), and one case
in which the peritoneal cavity lost its absorptive ability.
Of the 24 cases operated between December, 1965 and April,
1967, when his operative technique was "perfected", only 2
revisions were necessary, and there was one death caused by
infection.[2]

Weiss, writing in 1969, advocated ventriculo-peritoneal
shunts as easier and quicker procedures with fewer untoward
complications than ventriculo-atrial shunts. Of his 22
patients -- though only followed for a few months -- there
were no shunt-related deaths but there were 3 shunt infections.[60] In 1971, Hammon, writing from Walter Reed, urged
ventriculo-peritoneal as the procedure of choice in children
and infants. After detailing the many complications of his
use of ventriculo-atrial shunts, he reported upon 52 patients
receiving either lumbar-peritoneal or ventriculo-peritoneal
shunting procedures. Over an 18 month period he reported
one shunt-related death, 8 revisions, and 3 cases of shunt
infection. In a sub-series of 43 cases whom he followed
from 17 to 35 months post-operatively, he reported 72% to be
complication free.[21]

Little *et al*, writing from the Mayo Clinic, compared a
series of ventriculo-atrial and ventriculo-peritoneal shunts
over a 2 year time period. In the series of 37 patients
receiving the ventriculo-peritoneal shunt, there was one
revision per 13 month period per patient. Four cases of
meningitis were reported. There were 2 deaths from meningitis and one death from acute obstruction. The author concluded the ventriculo-peritoneal shunts were the procedure
of choice in infants and children.[32]

Our results with the ventriculo-peritoneal procedure

emphasize that by far our most ubiquitous and serious complications were ventriculitis and infection-related complications. Ventriculitis accounts for all of our shunt-related
mortality. 81.7% of all ventriculo-peritoneal complications
were of infectious origin. Our great fear of ventriculitis
made shunt removal and insertion of external ventricular
drainage systems our policy with only nominal evidence of
infection. This undoubtedly contributed to our very high
shunt revision rate, but on the other hand promoted our
rather low shunt-related mortality rate of 2.7%. Additionally, a large number of our shunted patients were very young
infants with newly repaired myelomeningoceles or else congenital hydrocephalus. Both groups of patients required a
relatively large number of procedures, and thus more chance
for untoward complications.

Using our very strict criterion, 31.1% of all patients
receiving ventriculo-peritoneal shunts developed ventriculitis at some time during their course of treatment. The
incidence per shunting procedure was approximately 16%.
The common flora of the skin were the chief pathogens.
Indeed, 78.1% of all cases of ventriculitis were caused by
gram positive cocci (See Table 6).

Relatively few complications could be attributed to the
peritoneal portion of the shunting procedure with only 10,
or 7.5% of ventriculo-peritoneal shunt complications being
abdominal. In almost 600 passes of the abdominal trocar,
there was no single instance of a perforated viscus. Others
have reported penetration of the intestinal lumen, vagina,
or scrotum at varying times after the period of surgery.[1,3,35,41,46,50,61] It is our impression that in many of these
cases the peritoneal cavity was opened surgically without
using the abdominal trocar. We suspect, therefore, that the

visceral surface of the peritoneum was either damaged or
penetrated surgically. Our technique consists of using the
Raimondi-Matsumoto peritoneal trocar.[44]

Five of our 10 abdominal complications were peritonitis
and were associated with infection along the course of the
shunt tract. We had one case in which the peritoneal cavity
was unable to absorb all the cerebrospinal fluid. We suspect that a preceding peritonitis had impaired cerebrospinal
fluid absorptive capacity. Several other reports of such
complications have been reported.[2,10,32,49]

We had one case of abdominal cyst, a complication which
has been reported elsewhere, especially in the absence of
silastic tubing,[16,30,34] and two cases of bowel obstruction.
We believe these were caused by adhesion formation secondary
to our shunting procedure. Such a problem has been reported
elsewhere.[5] In one instance, the abdominal tubing was lost
in the abdomen. In 6 cases shunt tubing was lost in the
ventricles.

There were 10 stitch infections, and two cases of wound
breakdown. The latter two occurred in very young patients
with congenital hydrocephalus and rather poor pre-operative
caloric intake.

In our series -- 196 patients receiving ventriculo-
peritoneal shunting procedures -- there were 5 subdural
hematomas, 4 of whom were in children whose sutures already
were closed. This rate ($<$ 2.5%) compares well with other
series reports where complication rates for this problem
average around 5%.[6,24] Concomitantly, we had one case of
"low-pressure syndrome" but no cases of craniostenosis, as
have been reported in the literature.[4,31]

There were 4 cases of unsuccessful ventricular cannulization. We defined this to mean requiring more than 3 passes

to cannulize the ventricles.   In all cases the ventricles were slit-like, as are found in a child who had previously been shunted.

Our one case of GI bleeding which required surgical intervention was of "stress" origin, and probably related to the child's other extreme medical problems rather than to his shunt surgery alone. We report one case of respiratory arrest, probably due to acute increase of intracranial pressure due to acute shunt obstruction. The child survived.

Our one case of chronic electrolyte imbalance may have been due to decreased steroid production because of the hypertensive third ventricle impinging upon the neuro-secretory axis or may have been due to inappropriate ADH secretions, or possibly large amounts of cerebrospinal fluid being sequestered in the peritoneal cavity. This patient's problem spontaneously resolved.

We report one case of brain abscess, secondary to shunt-related ventriculitis. This abscess required a craniotomy. Our one case of excessive blood loss occurred during a shunt revision. We concluded that it resulted from torn choroid plexus.

Among the different disease processes in which shunting procedures were done, the vast majority were undertaken to control congenital hydrocephalus and hydrocephalus in asso-ciation with meningomyelocele victims. In these groups, an average of 4 shunting procedures per patient were performed. The single-piece shunt, however, greatly decreased the number of such revisions and thus decreased, ultimately, patient mortality and morbidity. Moreover, the actual implantation itself was less fraught with complication than was the traditional three-piece shunting procedure. A full report of our results with the new single-piece shunt is in press.

We observed a direct correlation between the number of shunt revisions and incidence of complications. The incidence of gram negative ventriculitis was 4 times greater in the meningomyelocele group than in the non-meningomyelocele group. The complication rate found among older children with space-occupying lesions and those patients with subdural shunting procedures was lower than that found among children shunted at an earlier age for hydrocephalus. Indeed, the complication rates per procedure in these groups were only 7% and 6% respectively. There were only 3 cases of infection-related complications among 121 procedures. It has been reported that neonates, especially males, are more liable to shunt infections than are other infant groups.[11,43,48,59] Our statistics indicate that complications including infections were fairly evenly distributed among all age groups and both sexes.

CONCLUSIONS AND RECOMMENDATIONS

    1)   The ventriculo-peritoneal shunt has a lower rate of complications and mortality than the ventriculo-venous shunt.

    2)   The complication rate among infants with congenital hydrocephalus and myelomeningocele was noticeably higher than older children receiving shunting procedures for space-occupying lesions and subdural shunting procedures.

    3)   The abdominal portion of the shunting procedure caused relatively few complications.

    4)   There is a tremendous difficulty in evaluating the comparable statistics obtained from various institutions reviewing shunting complications. We suggest the need of a standardized prospective national data collection system where procedures and complications may be assembled in comparable form. Such an innovation might well start with a

commonly accepted form of reporting complications and mortality in neurosurgical center yearly reports. These reports
could be summated on a national basis. While such a policy
would not be without errors and inconveniences, it would
serve to engender a better grasp of neurosurgical data than
now exists.

  5) The single-piece shunt diminishes significantly
the morbidity, mortality and complications of shunting
procedures.

REFERENCES

1. Adeloye, A.: Spontaneous extrusion of the abdominal tube
    through the umbilicus complicating peritoneal shunt for
    hydrocephalus. *J. Neurosurg.*, *38*:758, 1973.
2. Ames, R.H.: Ventriculo-peritoneal shunts in the manage-
    ment of hydrocephalus. *J. Neurosurg.*, *27*:525, 1967.
3. Anderson, F.M.: Ventriculo-auriculostomy in treatment
    of hydrocephalus. *J. Neurosurg.*, *16*:551, 1959.
4. Anderson, H.: Craniosynostosis as a complication after
    operations for hydrocephalus. *Acta Paediat. Scand.*,
    55:192, 1966.
5. Andrews, E.G.: An improved technique in brain surgery:
    glass tubes versus gold or platinum for subdural drainage
    of the lateral ventricle in internal hydrocephalus.
    Surg. Gyn. & Obst., *13*:141, 1911.
6. Becker, D.P., Nulen, F.E.: Control of hydrocephalus by
    value regulated venous shunts: avoidance of complica-
    tions in prolonged shunt maintenance. *J. Neurosurg.*,
    28:215, 1968.
7. Bruce, A.M., Lorder, J., Shedder, W.I., et al:

Persistent bactaraemia following ventriculo-caval operation for hydrocephalus in infants. *Dev. Med. Child Neurol., 5*:461, 1963.

8. Cohen, S.J., and Callaghan, R.P.: A syndrome due to the bacterial colonization of Spitz-Holter valves: a review of five cases. *Brit. Med. J., 2*:677, 1967.

9. Davidoff, L.M.: Treatment of hydrocephalus: historical review and development of a new method. *Arch. Surg. Vol., 18*:1737, 1929.

10. Dean, F.B. and Keller, I.B.: Cerebrospinal fluid ascites: a complication of ventriculo-peritoneal shunt. *J. Neurosurg. Neurol. Psychiat., 35*:474, 1972.

11. Dossett, J.H., Williams, R.C., Quie, P.G.: Studies on interaction of bacteria, serum factors and polymorphonuclear leukocytes in mothers and newborns. *Pediatrics, 44*:49, 1969.

12. Dzenitis, A.J., Mealey, J., Jr., Waddill, J.R.: Myocardial perforation by ventriculo-atrial shunt tubing. *JAMA, 194*:1251, 1965.

13. Emergy, J.L. and Hilton, H.B.: Lung and heart complications of the treatment of hydrocephalus by ventriculo-auricolostomy. *Surgery, 50*:309, 1960.

14. Erdahagi, M., Eckstein, H.B. and Crome, L.: Pulmonary embolisation as a complication of ventriculo-atrial shunts inserted for hydrocephalus. *Dev. Med. Child Neurol. Suppl, 11*:36, 1966.

15. Ferguson, A.H.: Intraperitoneal diversion of the cerebrospinal fluid in cases of hydrocephalus. (Review) *N.Y. Medical Journal, 67*:902, 1898.

16. Fischer, E.G. and Shillito, J., Jr.: Large abdominal cysts: a complication of peritoneal shunts. Report of three cases. *J. Neurosurg., 31*:441, 1969.

17. Fokes, E.A.: Occult infections of ventriculo-atrial
     shunts. *J. Neurosurg., 33*:517, 1970.

18. Fotz, E.L. and Shurtleff, D.B.: Five years comparative
     study of hydrocephalus in children with and without
     operation (113 cases). *J. Neurosurg., 20*:1064, 1963.

19. Forrest, D.M. and Cooper, D.G.W.: Complications of
     ventriculo-atrial shunts: a review of 455 cases.
     J. Neurosurg., 29:506, 1968.

20. Freedman, S., Zita-Gogen, C. and Chatten, J.: Pulmonary
     vascular changes complicating ventriculo-vascular
     shunting for hydrocephalus. *J. Pediatrics, 64*:305, 1964.

21. Hammon, W.M.: Evaluation and use of the ventriculo-
     peritoneal shunt in hydrocephalus. *J. Neurosurg., 34*:
     792, 1971.

22. Harsh, G.R.: Peritoneal shunt for hydrocephalus
     utilizing the fimbria of the fallopian tubes for
     entrance to the peritoneal cavity. *J. Neurosurg., 11*:
     284, 1954.

23. Haynes, I.A.: Congenital intense hydrocephalus: its
     treatment by drainage of the cisternal magna into the
     cranial sinuses. *Am. Surg., 57*:449, 1913.

24. Illingworth, R.D.: Subdural hematoma after the treat-
     ment of chronic hydrocephalus by ventriculo-caval
     shunts. *J. Neurol. Neurosurg. Psychiat., 33*:95, 1970.

25. Illingworth, R.D., Logue, V., Symon, L. and Uemura, K.:
     The ventriculo-caval shunt in the treatment of adult
     hydrocephalus: results and complications in 101
     patients. *J. Neurosurg., 35*:681, 1971.

26. Ingram, F.D., Alexander, E. and Matron, D.D.:
     Polyethylene, a new synthetic plastic for use in surgery:

experimental applications in neurosurgery. *JAMA, 35*: 82, 1947.

27. Irving, M.L., Costello, P., Hail, G.E., and Richham, B.P.: Tissue reaction to pore and impregnanted silastic *J. Pediatric Surg., 5*:724, 1971.

28. Isanot, F.: Bronchovenous fistula as a late complication of a ventriculo-atriostomy: case report. *J. Neurosurg., 31*:574, 1969.

29. Jackson, I.J. and Snodgrass, S.R.: Peritoneal shunts in the treatment of hydrocephalus and increased intracranial pressure: a 4-year survey of 62 patients. *J. Neurosurg., 12*:216, 1955.

30. Keen, P.E. and Weitzner, S.: Inflammatory pseudotumor of mesentery: a complication of ventriculo-peritoneal shunt. *J. Neurosurg., 38*:371, 1973.

31. Kloss, J.L.: Craniosynostosis secondary to ventriculo-atrial shunt. *Am. J. Dis. Child., 116*:315, 1968.

32. Little, R.J., Roton, L.H., Jr. and Mallinger, F.J.: Comparison of ventriculo-peritoneal and ventriculo-atrial shunts for hydrocephalus in children. *Mayo Clinic Proc., 47*:396, 1964.

33. Long, D.M., DeWall, R.A. and French, L.A.: Unusual complication of ventriculo-auriculostomy: a report of two cases. *J. Neurosurg., 21*:233, 1964.

34. Matson, D.D.: Hydrocephalus treated by arachnoid-ureterostomy: report of 50 cases. *Pediatrics, 12*:326, 1953.

35. Mozingo, J.R. and Cauthen, J.C.: Vaginal perforation for a Raimondi peritoneal catheter in an adult. *Surg. Neurol., 2(3)*:195, 1974.

36. Murtagh, F. and Lehuan, R.: Peritoneal shunts in the management of hydrocephalus. *JAMA, 202*:1010, 1967.

37. Nosik, W.A.: Ventriculo-mastoidostomy, technique and observations. *J. Neurosurg., 7*:236, 1950.

38. Nugent, G.R., Lucas, R., Judy, M., et al: Thromboembolic complications of ventriculo-atrial shunts; angiocardiographic and pathologic correlations. *J. Neurosurg., 24*:34, 1966.

39. Nulsen, F.E., and Spitz, E.G.: Treatment of hydrocephalus by direct shunt from ventricle to jugular vein. *Surg. Forum, 2*:399, 1952.

40. Overton, M.C. and Snodgrass, S.R.: Ventriculo-venous shunt for infantile hydrocephalus: a review of five years experience with their method. *J. Neurosurg., 23*: 517, 1965.

41. Patel, C.P. and Matloub, H.: Vaginal perforation as a complication of ventriculo-peritoneal shunt. *J. Neurosurg., 38*:761, 1973.

42. Perren, J.C.S. and Lauren, R.E.: Infected ventriculo-atrial shunts: a method of treatment. *J. Neurosurg., 27*:21, 1967.

43. Provenzano, R.W., Wetterlow, B.S. and Sullivan, C.L.: Immunization and antibody response in the newborn infant. *New England J. of Med., 273*:959, 1965.

44. Pudenz, R.H., Russell, F.E., et al: Ventriculo-auriculostomy: a technique for shunting cerebrospinal fluid into the right auricle. Preliminary report. *J. Neurosurg., 14*:171, 1957.

45. Raimondi, A.J. and Matsumoto, S.A.: A simplified technique for performing the ventriculo-peritoneal shunt. *J. Neurosurg., 26*:357, 1967.

46. Ramani, P.S.: Extrusion of abdominal catheter of ventriculo-peritoneal shunt into the scrotum. Case report. *J. Neurosurg., 40(6)*:772, 1974.

47. Ransohoff, J.: Ventriculo-pleural anastomosis in the treatment of midline obstructional neoplasms. *J. Neurosurg.*, *8*:295, 1954.

48. Rosen, F.S. and Janeway, C.A.: Immunological competence of the newborn infant. *Pediatrics, 33*:159, 1964.

49. Rosenthal, J.D., Golden, G.T., Shaw, C.A. and Janes, J.A.: Intractable ascites: a complication of ventriculo-peritoneal shunting with a silastic catheter. *Amer. J. Surg., 5*:613, 1974.

50. Rubin, R.C., Shotok, N.R., Visudhipon, P.: Asymptomatic perforated vicus and gram negative ventriculitis as a complication of value regulated ventriculo-peritoneal shunts. Report of two cases. *J. Neurosurg., 37*:616, 1972.

51. Sehado, T.H., Maxwell, J.H. and Brackett, C.E.,Jr.: Intestinal volvulus secondary to a ventriculo-peritoneal shunt: case report. *J. Neurosurg., 35*:95, 1971.

52. Schinke, R.T., Block, P.H., Mark, V.H., et al: Indolent staphylococcus albus and aureus bacterimia after ventriculo-atrialostomy: role of foreign body in its initiation and perpetuation. *New England J. Med., 264*: 264, 1961.

53. Scott, M., Wyces, H.T., Myrlagh, F. and Reyes, V.: Observations on ventricular and lumbar subarachnoid-peritoneal shunts in hydrocephalus in infants. *J. Neurosurg., 12*:165, 1955.

54. Shurtleff, D.B., Christie, D. and Foltz, E.L.: Ventriculoauriculostomy - associated infection: a 12 year study. *J. Neurosurg., 35*:686, 1971.

55. Sperling, D.R., Patrick, J.R., Anderson, F.M., et al: Corpulmonale secondary to ventriculoauriculostomy.

Amer. J. Dis. Child., 107:308, 1964.

56. Strenger, L.: Complications of ventriculo-venous shunts. *J. Neurosurg., 20*:219, 1963.

57. Syamosunda, R., Molthan, M.E. and Lipow, H.W.: Corpulmonale as a complication of ventriculo-atrial shunts. Case report. *J. Neurosurg., 33*:221, 1970.

58. Teingaglou, S., Eckstein, H.B.: Pericardial tamponade by Holter ventriculo-atrial shunts. *J. Neurosurg., 35*: 695, 1971.

59. Washburn, T.C., Medearis, D.N. and Childs, B.: Sex differences in susceptibility to infections. *Pediatrics, 35*:57, 1965.

60. Weiss, S.R. and Roshina, R.: Twenty-two cases of hydrocephalus treated with a silastic ventriculo-peritoneal shunt. *Int. Surg., 51*:13, 1969.

61. Wilson, G.B. and Bertan, V.: Perforation of bowel complicating peritoneal shunt hydrocephalus: report of 2 cases. *Amer. Surg., 32*:601, 1966.

TABLE 1.

Types of Shunting Procedures 1968-1973.

Ventriculo-Peritoneal	598
External Ventricular Drainage	148
Ventriculo-Atrial	40
Subdural Peritoneal	33
Cysto-Peritoneal	16
Ventriculo-Gallbladder	9
Lumbar Subarachnoid Peritoneal	4
Ventricular-Cisternal Magna	1
TOTAL	849

TABLE 2.

Total Number of Complications (160) in 849 Procedures Performed on 231 Children

Ventriculitis	100
Stitch Infection	12
Shunt Lost in Ventricle	6
Subdural Hematoma	5
Abdominal Abscess	5
Peritonitis	5
Electrolytic Imbalance	4
Unsuccessful Attempt at Cannulizing Ventricle	4
Hemiparesis Secondary to Ventricular Cannulization	4
Accidental EVD Disconnection	3
Adhesions Causing Bowel Obstruction	2
Abdominal Cyst Formation	2
Wound Breakdown	2
Subdural Abscess	1
Shunt Lost in Gallbladder	1
Shunt Lost in Abdomen	1
Respiratory Arrest Secondary to High Intracranial Pressure	1
GI Bleeding Requiring Operative Exploration	1
Inability of Peritoneal Cavity to Absorb CSF	1
Brain Abscess	1
Excessive Blood Loss	1
Seizure Secondary to Rapid CSF Loss	1
Excessively Low CSF Pressure	1
TOTAL	160

301

TABLE 3.

Rates of Complication

Number of Patients	231
Number of Patients with Complication	91
Number of Patients with Ventriculitis (one or more episodes)	66
Complication Rate per Patient (chance of complication during total clinical course)	38.9%
Ventriculitis Rate per Patient (during total clinical course)	28.5%
Number of Procedures	849
Number of Complications	160
Average Number of Procedures per Patient	3.6
Complication Rate per Procedure (risk per individual procedure)	18.8%

TABLE 4.

Complications of Ventriculo-Peritoneal Shunting Procedures

Number of Procedures	598
Number of Patients	196
Ventriculitis	94
Stitch Infection	.10
Shunt Tubing Lost in Ventricle	6
Subdural Hematoma	5
Peritonitis	5
Unsuccessful Ventricular Cannulization	4
Wound Breakdown	2
Bowel Obstruction	2
Shunt Tubing Lost in Abdomen	1
Abdominal Cyst	1
Respiratory Arrest	1
Inability of Peritoneal Cavity to Absorb CSF	1
GI Bleeding	1
Low Pressure Syndrome	1
Electrolytic Imbalance	1
Brain Abscess	1
Excessive Blood Loss	1
TOTAL	137

TABLE 5.

Complication Rates in Ventriculo-Peritoneal Shunts

Number of Patients with Ventriculitis	61
Number of Patients with Complications other than Ventriculitis	22
TOTAL	83
Complication Rate per Patient	42.3%
Ventriculitis Rate per Patient	13.1%
Complication Rate per Procedure	22.9%
Ventriculitis Rate per Procedure	15.7%

TABLE 6.

Types of Ventriculitis

Staph Epidermidis (1 episode)	26
Staph Epidermidis (2 episodes)	8
Staph Epidermidis (3 episodes)	4
Staph Aureus (1 episode)	18
Staph Aureus (3 episodes)	5
E. Coli	8
Klebsiella (1 episode)	4
Klebsiella (4 episodes)	1
Proteus	1
Pseudomonas	1
H Flu	1
Total	94

TABLE 7.

Complication of Shunting Procedures According to
Diagnostic Categories

I. Myelomeningocele	
Number of Patients	61
Number of Procedures	247
Complication Rate per Procedure	20.5%
A. Complications	
Ventriculitis	36
Wound Infection	5
Electrolytic Imbalance	2
Shunt Lost in Ventricle	2
Unsuccessful Shunting Attempts	2
Subdural Hematoma	2
Excessive Blood Loss	1
Peritonitis	1
TOTAL	51
B. Deaths from Ventriculitis	2
C. Major Organisms in Ventriculitis	
Staph Epidermidis (1 episode)	12
E. Coli	7
Klebsiella	3
Staph Epidermidis (2 episodes)	2
H Flu	1
Pseudomonas	1
II. Congenital Hydrocephalus	
Number of Patients	85
Number of Procedures	343
Complication Rate per Procedure	21.8%
A. Complications	
Ventriculitis	43
Wound Infection	5
Shunt Lost in Ventricle	3
Hemiparesis	3
EVD Disconnected	3
Electrolytic Imbalance	2

TABLE 7. (cont.)

A. Complications (cont.)	
Wound Breakdown	2
Abdominal Cyst	2
Peritonitis	2
Bowel Obstruction	1
Generalized Seizure Activity Secondary Disconnection of EVD	1
Subdural Hematomas	1
Low Pressure Syndrome	1
EVD Disconnected	1
Shunt Lost in Gallbladder	1
TOTAL	75
B. Deaths from Ventriculitis	4
C. Ventriculitis Types	
Staph Aureus	11
Staph Epidermidis (1 episode)	9
Staph Epidermidis (2 episodes)	6
Staph Epidermidis (3 episodes)	4
E. Coli	2
Klebsiella	1
Proteus	1
III. Shunted Subdural Effusion	
Number of Patients	19
Number of Procedures	33
Complication Rate per Procedure	6%
A. Complications	
Wound Infections	1
Subdural Abscess	1
TOTAL	2
IV. Shunting Procedures Made Necessary by Space Occupying Lesion	
Number of Patients	31
Number of Procedures	78
Complication Rate per Procedure	7.6%

TABLE 7. (cont.)

A. Complications
Subdural Hematoma   2
GI Bleeding   1
Unsuccessful Cannulization   1
Peritonitis   1
Patient's Peritoneal Unable to Absorb
  all the CSF   1

TOTAL   6

V. Pseudotumor Cerebri
Number of Patients   1
Number of Procedures   1
Complication Rate per Procedure   100%

    A. Complications
    Hemiplegia   1

VI. Post Meningitic Hydrocephalus
Number of Patients   4
Number of Procedures   25
Complication Rate per Procedure   12%

    A. Complications
    Ventriculitis   2
    Bowel Adhesions   1

TOTAL   3

VII. Low Pressure Hydrocephalus
Number of Patients   12
Number of Procedures   38
Complication Rate per Procedure   18.4%

    A. Complications
    Ventriculitis   4
    Wound Infection   1
    Unsuccessful Attempts at Shunting   1
    Abdominal Portion of Shunt Lost in
      Abdomen   1

TOTAL   7

TABLE 7. (cont.)

VIII. <u>Hydrocephalus Secondary to Intracranial</u> <u>Blood</u>	
Number of Patients	4
Number of Procedures	10
Complication Rate per Procedure	10%
A. <u>Complications</u>	
Ventriculitis	1
IX. <u>Dandy-Walker and Posterior Fossa Cysts</u>	
Number of Patients	14
Number of Procedures	73
Complication Rate per Procedure	17.8%
A. <u>Complications</u>	
Ventriculitis	10
Abdominal Abscess	1
Peritonitis	1
Respiratory Arrest	1
TOTAL	13

TABLE 8.

Influence of Sex and Age on Complication Rate

Males Shunted Under the Age of One Month

Patients	25
Procedures	92
A. Complications	
Ventriculitis	11
Ventricular Tubing in Abdomen	1
TOTAL	12
Types of Ventriculitis	
Staph Aureus	5
Staph Epidermidis	3
E. Coli	3
TOTAL	11

Females Shunted Under the Age of One Month

Patients	23
Procedures	92
A. Complications	
Ventriculitis	10
Wound Infection	2
Electrolytic Imbalance	2
Unsuccessful Ventricular Cannulization	1
Bowel Obstruction	1
Peritonitis	1
Excessive Blood Loss	1
Abdominal Wall Cyst	1
TOTAL	19
Types of Ventriculitis	
Staph Epidermidis	3
Staph Aureus	3
Klebsiella	2
E. Coli	2

TABLE 8. (cont.)

Males Under the Age of One Month

Complications per Procedure	13.0%
Ventriculitis per Procedure	11.9%
Procedures per Patient	3.6

First Shunt Between the Age of One Month and One Year in Male

Patients	49
Procedures	135

A. Complications

Ventriculitis	22
Abdominal Portion of Shunt Loss	2
Wound Infection	2
Shunts Lost in Ventricles	2
Unsuccessful Pass	1
Brain Abscess	1
Bowel Obstruction	1
Electrolytic Imbalance	1
TOTAL	32

Types of Ventriculitis (cont.)

TOTAL	10

Females Under the Age of One Month

Complications per Procedure	18.2%
Ventriculitis per Procedure	9.6%
Procedures per Patient	4.7

First Shunt Between the Age of One Month and One Year in Female

Patients	47
Procedures	123

A. Complications

Ventriculitis	10
Subdural Hematoma	3
Stitch Abscess	3
Abdominal Adhesions	1
Breakdown of Wound	1
Electrolytic Imbalance	1
TOTAL	19

TABLE 8. (cont.)

Types of Ventriculitis

Staph Epidermidis (1 episode)	7
Staph Epidermidis (2 episodes)	1
Staph Aureus	6
Beta Strep	1
Klebsiella (1 episode)	1
Proteus	1
H Flu	1
TOTAL	18

Males Between the Age of One Month and One Year	
Complications Per Procedure	23.79%
Ventriculitis per Procedure	16.39%
Procedures per Patient	2.7

Types of Ventriculitis

Staph Epidermidis (1 episode)	3
Staph Epidermidis (2 episodes)	1
E. Coli	2
Klebsiella	1
TOTAL	7

Females Between the Age of One Month and One Year	
Complications per Procedure	15.4%
Ventriculitis per Procedure	8.19%
Procedures per Patient	2.6

TABLE 9.

Complication of Shunting Procedures According to Diagnostic Categories

| | 3-PIECE SHUNT | | SINGLE-PIECE SHUNT | |
	MM	Non-MM	MM	Non-MM
Number of Patients	61	135	50	111
Number of Procedures	247	351	91	206
Number of Complications	51	86	15	20
Complications Per Procedure	6%	8%	6%	2%
Infection Per Procedure	15%	17%	10%	7%
Number of Procedures Per Patient	4	2.6	1.8	1.9
Infection Per Patient	42%	26%	12%	13%
Complication Per Patient	15%	7%	12%	5%

MM = Myelomeningocele
Non-MM = Non-Myelomeningocele

AVOIDANCE OF SHUNT DEPENDENCY

Fred J. Epstein, M.D., Gerald M. Hochwald, M.D.
Alvin Wald, M.D. and Joseph Ransohoff, M.D.

Hydrocephalus is most commonly treated with a shunting procedure, the purpose of which is to reduce the volume of the ventricular system to normal and to totally restore the attenuated cortical mantle. While this procedure preserves the life of many infants and children, it is becoming increasingly clear that total shunt dependency, with all of its sequelae, is a frequent "complication" and that the long-term results have often been far from satisfactory.

On the basis of clinical investigation and laboratory research, the authors have proposed an approach to the treatment of neonatal hydrocephalus which is intended to reduce, or occasionally eliminate shunt dependency by increasing the effectiveness of remaining CSF absorptive pathways. That absorptive pathways still function may be inferred from the observation that in most cases of hydrocephalus the infant skull does not grow in proportion to the volume of CSF produced. Indeed, it has been well documented in this laboratory that it is rarely necessary to remove more than one-third of the volume of CSF produced in 24 hours to retard abnormal head growth and stabilize the disease.[1] It is, therefore, apparent that the bulk of newly formed CSF is absorbed by what remains of patent, normal pathways or by alternative pathways, and the activity of hydrocephalus is

secondary only to that relatively small volume of CSF that is
not absorbed. In order to achieve a hydrodynamic equilibrium
it is only necessary to increase the efficiency of already
functioning absorptive mechanisms and, therefore, treatment
should be directed towards that goal. This may be accomplished either by the non-invasive technique of intermittent
cranial compression,[2] or by the insertion of an "on-off"
type of shunt which is used intermittently to drain a fixed
volume of CSF.[1] The ultimate goal of both of these methods
of treatment is to bring about a state of shunt-independent
arrested hydrocephalus. If either method is not successful,
and it becomes evident that shunt dependency is unavoidable,
the shunt is nevertheless used intermittently in an effort
to maintain moderately enlarged ventricles while preserving
at least 3 cm of frontal cortical mantle. This insures that
recurrent obstructions and necessary revisions of the ventricular catheter, which are so often the basis of late morbidity
and mortality, occur less frequently. Finally, in that
group of children that are irrevocably shunt dependent, have
small ventricles and require multiple revisions of the proximal catheter, subtemporal craniectomy may break the vicious
circle.[3]

It is the overall philosophy of treatment which is
directed towards the avoidance of shunt dependency that is
the subject of this report.

METHOD

Infants with slowly progressing hydrocephalus who fulfill specific selection criteria are treated with cranial
compression. This is accomplished by the intermittent application of an elastic bandage or silastic helmet with an

lomegaly occurs.   Perhaps in both of these situations one of
the factors that contributes to progression of the disease is
that in the presence of an expansile head there is a failure
to establish an adequate pressure gradient between the
ventricle and the "Alternate" absorptive site.   Rather, the
resistance of the brain and ventricular system to expansion
is less than the resistance to CSF absorption -- therefore,
progressive ventriculomegaly results.

Additional factors may be of importance.   Although
ventriculomegaly is secondary to an interruption of spinal
fluid circulation, there is not always a total anatomic
obstruction.   What appears to be a total aqueductal occlusion
by ventriculography may in reality be a partial stenosis.
However, because of the expansile nature of the infant skull
the pressure gradient necessary to push fluid across the
compromised area does not develop and progressive ventriculomegaly results.

When cranial compression is contra-indicated or not
successful, a "volume-control shunt" is inserted.   This
apparatus has an "on-off" valve which may be regulated as
desired in order to divert only a specific amount of CSF
through the shunt.   In the immediate post-operative period,
the valve is opened for six minutes every four hours.   This
is gradually decreased, and in most infants with active
hydrocephalus, opening of the valve for two minutes every
eight hours proves sufficient.   Intrinsic to this concept of
treatment is the attempt to gradually discontinue utilization
of the shunt over a period of months or even one to two years,
and thereby bring about permanent arrest of the disease.
During this time, careful attention is directed to the size
of the ventricular system, and the thickness of the cortical
mantle.   This is documented at regular intervals by

computerized axial tomography. The criteria for successful
treatment is a 3 cm frontal cortical mantle at six months of
age. In those infants and children in which it is impossible
to arrest the hydrocephalus, the valve is nevertheless used
intermittently as an effort is made to maintain "generous"
ventricular volume while continuing to retain cortical mantle
at a minimum of 3 cm. In this way, small or "slit" ventricles
do not evolve and recurrent obstruction of the ventricular
catheter is less likely to occur. Again, ventricular volume
is monitored by regular CAT scans, and subsequent frequency
and duration of shunt utilization are regulated accordingly.

Finally, in those children who are shunt dependent and
have small ventricles with recurrent catheter obstruction
leading to episodes of coma and decerebration, subtemporal
craniectomy is performed. The purpose of this procedure is
threefold. In the first place, it vents the increased intracranial pressure and, therefore, renders the resultant
symptoms less fulminant. Secondly, it permits the palpating
finger to make a rapid gross assessment of ICP. Since shunt
dependent children frequently suffer from related as well as
unrelated headaches, this allows an immediate estimate of
whether or not the headache is secondary to shunt malfunction. Finally, and perhaps of most importance, subtemporal
craniectomy permits some dilation of the ipsilateral ventricular system if a shunt malfunction occurs. This conclusion
is based on the laboratory observation that hydrocephalic
cats subjected to hemicraniectomy develop dilation of the
ipsilateral ventricle (Fig. 3).

RESULTS

Eleven of sixteen hydrocephalic infants treated with
cranial compression have had their disease compensated. Ten

of these children have accomplished normal developmental
milestones, and one is behind. The age range of the group
is now 10 months to 4 years. Five of the original group
were treated with shunts when it became evident that cortical
mantle was not developing adequately.

In eight infants, intracranial pressure was monitored
before, during, and after cranial compression. In general,
ICP was increased from a pre-treatment baseline of 180-220
m/H$_2$O to 500 mm H$_2$O during compression. When treatment was
temporarily interrupted after a 3-4 hour period, the ICP
abruptly decreased to approximately 50% of the pre-treatment
baseline pressure, and then gradually returned to the previous level during a 2-3 hour period. It is believed that
these alterations are secondary to the displacement of CSF
from the ventricular system during cranial compression.

When both the ICP and the pressure within the inflatable
helmet were monitored simultaneously, they were initially
nearly identical at 500 mm H$_2$O. However, during the next
2-3 hours ICP dropped downward towards 350 mm H$_2$O. Again,
this probably reflects displacement of CSF secondary to
cranial compression.

Eighteen infants have been treated with intermittently
draining "volume control" shunts. Ten have been totally
weaned from the shunt, the hydrocephalus having become
compensated. Three have died, and five still require the
shunt. In the latter group, which are in fact shunt dependent, there have been few episodes of ventricular catheter
obstruction as the ventricles are moderately enlarged.
Cortical mantle in both of these groups has been maintained
at a minimum of 3 cm, and the children have normal
intelligence.

Eight children with small ventricles and recurrent catheter obstruction have been treated with subtemporal craniectomy. All of these children were between the ages of 9 months and 13 years, and had undergone multiple revisions of the ventricular catheter in the weeks immediately preceding surgery. In no case was the procedure more than transiently successful as the ventricles were small and adequate catheter placement was impossible. Four of the children have now been followed for 12 months, and four, three years, with no further malfunctioning of the proximal catheter.

In one child the peritoneal catheter became dislodged, resulting in distal obstruction. Alarming symptoms of elevated ICP which had accompanied previous episodes of shunt malfunction, did not develop as the craniectomy functioned as an adequate decompression, and elective revision was easily accomplished.

DISCUSSION

Following insertion of a conventional, continuously draining shunting system the ventricles rapidly shrink and alternate absorptive pathways cease functioning. As the ventricles are reduced to normal or subnormal volume, the ventricular catheter may become trapped between the abutting ventricular walls causing serious signs and symptoms of increased ICP. Unless revision is promptly accomplished, coma or even death may rapidly ensue (Fig. 4). It is this tragic culmination of treatment which is the most common late cause of morbidity and mortality. It has been well documented by Nulsen[8] that 3 cms of frontal cortical mantle if often sufficient for normal or superior intellectual function, and it is therefore of the greatest importance to inflatable inner lining (Fig. 1). The criteria for including infants in this treatment group are: 1) progressive hydrocephalus in the presence of normal or only slightly increased intracranial pressure; 2) cortical mantle in excess of 1.5 cm at the thinnest point; 3) good general medical condition.

Pre-treatment intracranial pressure may be evaluated by continuous epidural monitoring. If this is not possible, a lax or soft fontanelle and absence of symptoms of increased ICP is accepted as evidence for suitability for treatment.

Cranial compression is intended to bring about total arrest of hydrocephalus. This concept of therapy evolved from extensive laboratory investigation which may be summarized as follows:[4,5,6,7,9,10,11]

1) The majority of cats made hydrocephalic by intracisternal kaolin compensate despite complete obstruction of the outlet foramina of the fourth ventricle. This occurs when the ventricular volume has increased from the normal of 1 cc to 4-6 cc and is the result of alternate CSF absorptive pathways becoming function.

2) CSF absorption increases as ICP increases.

3) Cats with compensated hydrocephalus become decompensated when the head is rendered expansile by extensive craniectomy. Ventricular volume rapidly increases to 16-20 cc as a result of a marked decrease in CSF absorption (Fig.2a-c).

4) Craniectomized cats with decompensated hydrocephalus recompensate as CSF absorption is re-established following cranioplasty.

On the basis of these observations it was evident that the rigid adult skull was of importance in limiting the progression of feline hydrocephalus. In the hydrocephalic neonate, as in the craniectomized cat, progressive ventricu-

recognize that although small ventricles may be aesthetically
pleasing, they are unnecessary and, furthermore, are not
uncommonly responsible for ultimate failure of treatment.

In conclusion, it must be emphasized that the authors
do not regard this treatment sequence as a panacea for hydrocephalus. Certainly a pharmacologic agent which would permanently decrease CSF production by 25-30% would be of
greater potential value. Until this is available, however,
the method of treatment that avoids total shunt dependency
will eliminate many of the tragedies that have been inherent
in past and present techniques of treatment.

REFERENCES

1. Epstein, F., Hochwald, G., Ransohoff, J.: A Volume
    Control System for the Treatment of Hydrocephalus:
    laboratory and clinical experience. *J. Neurosurg.*, *38*:
    282, 1973.

2. Epstein, F.: Neonatal Hydrocephalus treated by Compres-
    sive Head Wrapping. *Lancet*, *1*:634, 1973.

3. Epstein, F., Fleischer, A.S., Hochwald, G.M., Ransohoff,
    J.: Subtemporal Craniectomy for Recurrent Shunt
    Obstruction Secondary to Small Ventricles. *J. of
    Neurosurg.*, *41*:29, 1974.

4. Hochwald, G.M., Sahar, A., Sadik, A.R.: Cerebrospinal
    Fluid Production and Histological Observations in Animals
    with Experimental Obstructive Hydrocephalus. *Exp.
    Neurol.*, *25*:190, 1969.

5. Hochwald, G.M., Epstein, F., Malham, C., Ransohoff, J.:
    The Role of the Skull and Dura in Experimental Feline
    Hydrocephalus. *Dev. Med. & Child Neurol.*, *14*:65,

Suppl. 27, 1972.

6. Hochwald, G.M., Lux, W.E., Jr., Sahar, A., Ransohoff,
    J.: Experimental Hydrocephalus. Changes in Cerebro-
    spinal Fluid Dynamics as a Function of Time. *Arch.
    Neurol.*, *26*:120, 1972.

7. Hochwald, G.M., Epstein, F., Malham, C., Ransohoff, J.:
    The Relationship of Compensated to Decompensated Hydro-
    cephalus in the Cat. *J. Neurosurg.*, *39*:694, 1973.

8. Nulsen, F.E.: Preservation of Intellect by Shunt Proce-
    dures - long term results. Presented at the meeting of
    the American Academy of Orthopaedic Surgeons, Hartford,
    Conn., November 1970.

9. Sahar, A., Hochwald, G.M., Ransohoff, J.: Alternative
    pathway for Cerebrospinal Fluid Absorption in Animals
    with Experimental Obstructive Hydrocephalus. *Exp.
    Neurol.*, *25*:200, 1969.

10. Hochwald, G.M., Sahar, A., Sadik, A.R., Ransohoff, J.:
    Alternative Pathway for Cerebrospinal Fluid Absorption
    in Animals with Experimental Obstructive Hydrocephalus.
    Arch. Neurol., *21*:638, 1969.

11. Sahar, A., Hochwald, G.M., Ransohoff, J.: Experimental
    Hydrocephalus: Cerebrospinal Fluid Formation and
    Ventricular Size as a Function of Intraventricular
    Pressure. *J. Neurol. Sci.*, *11*:81, 1970.

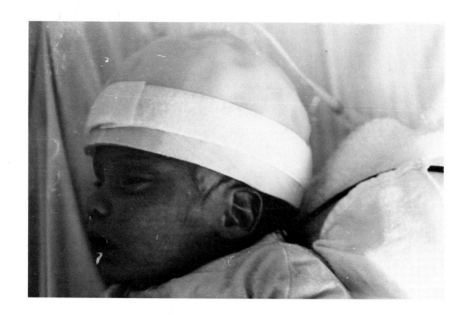

Fig. 1. Inflatable cap used in certain patients to control slowly progressive hydrocephalus.

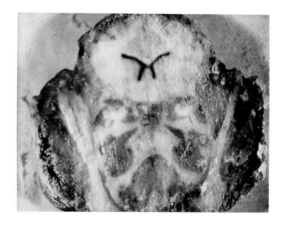

Fig. 2A. Normal feline ventricles.

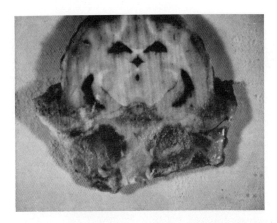

Fig. 2B.   Kaolin hydrocephalus with intact skull.

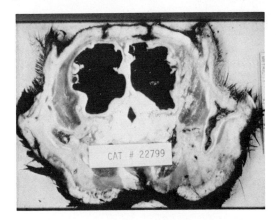

Fig. 2C.   Kaolin hydrocephalus which has
decompensated following bilateral craniectomy.

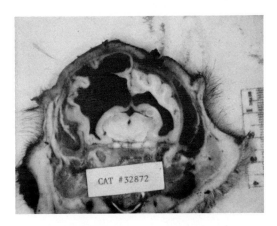

Fig. 3.   Unilateral ventriculomegaly following
ipsilateral craniectomy.

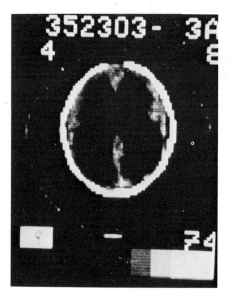

Fig. 4A. Preoperative CAT scan showing massive hydrocephalus.

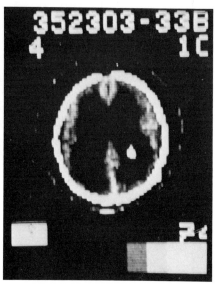

Fig. 4B. 48 hours following shunting procedure.

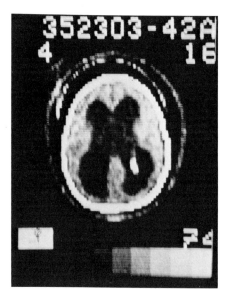

Fig. 4C. Five days following shunts.

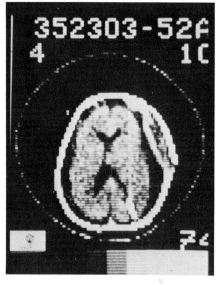

Fig. 4D. Three weeks following shunts. Note "slit"-like ventricles and subdural effusion.

MANAGEMENT OF SHUNT INFECTIONS

Robert L. McLaurin, M.D.

INTRODUCTION

The syndrome of septicemia due to colonization of Spitz-Holter valves by staphylococci was originally described in 1961.[1] Subsequent to that time several other reports appeared in the literature and in each instance the recommendation was made that shunt removal was necessary as the infection could not be eradicated as long as the foreign body was in place. In 1966 the concept was introduced[2] that shunt removal, immediate replacement, and the intraventricular and systemic antibiotics could be effective in eliminating shunt infection. Subsequent to that report, our own efforts have been toward the use of antibiotics alone without any surgical procedure. It is recognized that our results have not been duplicated by some other authors and the reason for the variation is not clear. Our experience to date, however, has led us to conclude that the majority of shunt infections can be eradicated without operative intervention if aggressive antibiotic management is employed.

CASE MATERIAL

Two forms of shunt infection can be delineated. The first is an acute sepsis occurring shortly after the insertion of a shunt system. This is usually ·associated with

inflammation at the site of insertion and evidence of
infection may spread the entire length of the shunt. The
infant usually shows systemic signs of acute infection
including fever and leukocytosis. This presentation is more
likely to be due to infection by staphylococcus aureus or by
gram negative organisms.

The second type of infection is somewhat more subtle and
although it may occur in the early post-operative period, it
can be seen months or even years after the last operative
procedure. This type of infection is usually not associated
with evidence of acute inflammation but is accompanied by an
intermittent low grade fever, anemia, a moderate leukocytosis
and the variable presence of hepatosplenomegaly. The most
common organism accounting for this type of indolent infection is staph epidermidis.

During the past 11 years, 45 patients with shunt
infection have been treated in our clinic. The emphasis from
the beginning has been on the preservation of a functioning
shunt at all times combined with the effectiveness of intraventricular and systemic antibiotic therapy. Details of the
method of treatment used in this series will be documented
later. The etiology of hydrocephalus in this series is
listed in Table I. The most significant feature of this
table is the low incidence of patients with Arnold-Chiari
deformity since this deformity accounted for approximately
50 percent of all hydrocephalic patients treated by shunting
during this same interval. It emphasizes the fact that
transient bacteremias must play a minor role in shunt
infection. Patients with myelomeningocele and Arnold-Chiari
malformations notoriously have frequent urinary tract
infections as well as transient bacteremias from decubitus
ulceration. Despite these repetitive bacteremias this group

of patients has a low incidence of shunt infections. Moreover, the organisms seen in shunt infections did not suggest
that bacteremia from urinary tract or decubitus infection has
provided the etiologic agents.

The organisms identified in the present series are
listed in Table II. As in all previous series, staph epidermidis has been the most frequent offender but is by no means
the only offending organism. In general the patients in whom
the infection has become apparent only months after the last
surgical procedure have a much higher incidence of staph
epidermidis infection. On the contrary, those patients in
whom infection has made its appearance within a few days or
a week after a surgical procedure have shown a variety of
organisms.

Prior to 1971, when ventriculo-atrial shunting was the
procedure of choice, recovery of the organism usually
occurred from the blood stream. Ventricular fluid may or
may not be contaminated under these circumstances although in
the majority of situations, the organism could be recovered.
During the past five years peritoneal shunting has been done
almost exclusively in our clinic and therefore identification
of the organisms has been entirely from ventricular fluid
analysis.

TREATMENT AND RESULTS

The essential part of the treatment of infected shunts
is the direct introduction of antibiotics into the ventricular
system. It is well known that most antibiotics do not
penetrate the blood CSF barrier to any appreciable extent
unless there is active inflammation within the CSF compartment. This is particularly true of the drugs which are most
effective against staph epidermidis. Therefore, while

adequate levels can be achieved by parenteral administration to sterilize the outside of the shunt system the inside of the system remains protected by the blood CSF barrier. The only way of achieving appropriate MIC levels is by direct installation into the ventricular cavity.

If the infection cannot be eradicated by antibiotics alone our proposal is that the shunt system can be completely replaced and antibiotics will then be more effective. By removal of the infected pumping device the reservoir and the associated lengths of tubing the clean replaced system can be effectively sterilized by the immediate institution of intraventricular therapy.

The plan of management being recommended at the present time includes accurate identification of the offending organism and establishment of its antibiotic sensitivities. When accurate identification of the organisms has been achieved, and providing the shunt system is working satis- factorily, intensive antibiotic therapy is initiated. This combines the use of intraventricular and parenteral adminis- tration of antibiotics. Intraventricular administration is done usually on a daily basis after thorough skin prepartion. We have determined that in most instances even with a patent functioning shunt, the antibiotic level exceeds MIC of the organism at the end of 24 hours. We do recommend, however, that if facilities are available for determining antibiotic levels, this is worthwhile performing early in the course of treatment.

A course of treatment has arbitrarily been set at two weeks. This includes daily injections of antibiotics and the parenteral administration is usually performed intravenously for one week and orally for the second week.

After a two week course of treatment all antibiotics are

discontinued and two days later the ventricular fluid is
cultured. Blood cultures should also be obtained if the
patient has a vascular shunt.

The above regimen has been effective in most cases, but
if it is not successful in eradicating the infection, it is
recommended that the course be repeated with a different
antibiotic to which the organism is again proven to be
sensitive.

If antibiotic therapy alone proves ineffective, it is
then necessary to consider removal of the shunt followed by
immediate replacement and immediate institution of intraventricular and systemic antibiotic therapy. While this was
our initial approach to the management of infection, it has
not been necessary to carry out this procedure within recent
years. Finally if the removal and immediate replacement are
not effective, it is then necessary to plan for removal of
the shunt without replacement. When this has been done,
parenteral antibiotics are probably effective in eliminating
the infection, although intraventricular therapy may add
some measure of assurance of sterilization of that compartment. After a course of antibiotic therapy (10-14 days) the
CSF is again cultured, prior to replacement of the shunt
system.

Results indicate that in the present series of 45
patients, 29 or approximately two-thirds of the total, have
been successfully managed by antibiotics alone (Table III).
Thirteen of the last 15 patients have been managed successfully in that manner.

Of the total 45 patients 12 have been treated successfully by removal of the shunt and immediate replacement
followed by intraventricular and system antibiotics. This
includes the 6 original patients in whom this was the only

method of treatment attempted. Therefore, of the subsequent
39 patients it has been necessary to utilize this method in
only 6 or approximately 15 percent of the instances. In only
4 patients has it been necessary to remove the shunt for a
more prolonged period of antibiotic therapy. The conclusion
reached on the basis of our own personal experience is that
the majority of shunt infections can be successfully treated
without surgery, but it is necessary to understand the
rationale for aggressive intraventricular and systemic antibiotic management.

The use of prophylactic antibiotics has been advocated
by some individuals and questioned by others. In general,
however, it appears that the trend has been toward the use of
prophylactic antibiotics. Our regimen of prophylaxis has
taken into account the possibility of infection from pre-
operative ventricular tapping and also the failure of antibiotics to enter the cerebrospinal fluid. Our present
regimen, therefore, includes the administration of parenteral
antibiotics beginning 24 hours prior to surgery. This
continued for 2 days postoperatively and then orally for
another 3 days. In addition, a single bolus of methicillin
is introduced through the reservoir into the ventricular
system at the time of replacement of the shunt. Using this
regimen, the incidence of postoperative shunt infection has
been reduced to less than 5 percent in our series and the
majority of those in which it has occurred have had CSF
leakage from the incision due to shunt malfunction. Our
conclusion at the present time, therefore, is that prophylactic antibiotics are of advantage.

REFERENCES

1. Callaghan R.P., Cohen, S.J. and Stewart, G.T.:
    Septicaemia due to colonization of Spitz-Holter valves
    by staphylococci: Five cases treated with methicillin.
    Brit. Med. J., 1:860, 1961.
2. Perrin, J.C. and McLaurin, R.L.: Infected ventriculo-
    atrial shunts: A method of treatment. *J. Neurosurg.,
    27*:21, 1967.

TABLE 1.

Etiology of Hydrocephalus

Idiopathic: communicating or non-communicating	25
Arnold-Chiari deformity	7
Dandy-Walker deformity	4
Infection; meningitis or ventriculitis	4
Subarachnoid blood	5
TOTAL	45

TABLE 2.

Organisms

Staph epidermidis		23
alone	18	
mixed	4	
strep. viridans	1	
enterobacter	1	
staph. aureus	1	
candida	1	
Staph aureus		6
E. coli		3
Meningococcus, pseudomonas, H. influenza (2), diphteroid, Gm. neg. rod (untypable) proteus mirabilis, strep. viridans, bact. antratum, Neisseria flava, Micrococcus luteus, Klebsiella, No growth		13
TOTAL		45

TABLE 3.

Treatment

Intraventricular and systemic antibiotics only	29
Removal of shunt - immediate replacement - intraventricular and systemic antibiotics	12
Removal of shunt - intraventricular and systemic antibiotics - delayed replacement of shunt	4
TOTAL	45

THE NEPHRITIS ASSOCIATED WITH CHRONICALLY INFECTED VENTRICULO-ATRIAL SHUNTS (SHUNT NEPHRITIS)

C.F. Strife, M.D., A.J. McAdams, M.D.
and C.D. West, M.D.

It has now become apparent that immune mediated renal disease may result from man's inadequate response to certain infectious agents. The association of infection and glomerulonephritis has been observed in a number of clinical situations including subacute bacterial endocarditis,[1] malaria,[2] syphilis,[3] osteomyelitis,[4] pneumococcal and staphylococcal infections,[5] certain viral infections[6] and ventriculo-atrial shunt infections.[7]

Since the first description by Black, et al of the association of nephrotic syndrome with infected ventriculo-atrial shunts in 1965,[8] more than 30 cases have been reported. It has become apparent that the renal lesion is a result of glomerular deposition of intermediate size immune complexes composed of antigen (derived from the infecting organism), antibody (IgG and IgM rheumatoid factor directed against the patient's IgG) and complement components (Clq, C4, C3).

Germuth and Rodriquez[9] have shown that rabbits injected over long periods of time with the foreign protein, Bovine serum albumin (BSA), produce three types of antibody response. They may respond with a sustained high level, an intermediate level or low level of antibody production. With

high antibody production, large immune complexes are formed
which are readily removed by the reticuloendothelial system.
Those with a low or an intermiediate level of antibody
response will form either small or moderate size complexes.
Only the small or moderate size complexes penetrate the
glomerular capillary endothelium and deposit adjacent to the
basement membrane. The result is an inflammatory response
by the kidney. As more and more complexes deposit in the
glomerular capillary wall, the inflammation increases and
the rate of complex deposition overcomes the ability of the
kidney (mesangium) to remove them. A thickened capillary
wall develops and eventually squeezes the capillary lumen
until it becomes completely closed.

Experimental chronic immune complex nephritis in the
rabbit is analogous to the nephritis seen with shunt infections. In shunt nephritis the foreign protein derives from
the infecting organism which is usually of low virulence
(*Staphlococcal epidermidis*) and is continuously released
into the blood. The response of the patient is to produce
antibody which probably varies between a high amount and an
intermediate amount. This results in the formation of immune
complexes of a size varying between large and intermediate.
The large complexes are removed by the reticuloendothelial
system thus explaining the high incidence of hepatosplenomegaly. The smaller, intermediate size complexes circulate
longer and have an opportunity to deposit in the glomerular
capillaries (Fig. 1) and, theoretically, in other small
capillaries. Only after a great amount of deposition do the
symptoms of nephritis (proteinuria, hematuria, nephrotic
syndrome) become apparent.

The evaluation of a patient who presents with clinical
findings suggestive of shunt nephritis (spiking fever, gross

hematuria, pallor and hepatosplenomegaly) should include a
urinalysis, complete blood cultures (Table 1). The presence
of significant proteinuria is the most useful sign of
nephritis. Hematuria may more readily co-exist with calculi,
infection, urethritis or irritative bleeding from ilial
bladder stomas and, therefore, is not as useful a sign for
nephritis as proteinuria. Iron resistant anemia, probably
secondary to chronic infection, has been a prominent feature.
Hypoproteinemia resulting from a combination of increased
protein loss and decreased synthesis may occasionally progress to an overt nephrotic syndrome.

Hypocomplementemia with low serum levels of Clq, C4, and
C3 parallels the course of shunt nephritis (Fig. 3). The
classical complement system is easily activated by circulating immune complexes. In addition, we have noted circulating cryoglobulins (reversible cold-precipitable globulins)
to parallel the disease course and the hypocomplementemia
in the four patients who were studied. The cryoglobulins
are thought to be the *in vitro* representation of *in vivo*
circulating immune complexes.[7]

Treatment of shunt nephritis is based on removing the
antigen or infecting organism. In five of six cases seen at
the Children's Hospital, Cincinnati, over the past seven
years, antibiotic therapy combined with removal of the entire
shunt and replacement either at one operation or at a later
time proved successful. In one patient, antibiotics alone
eradicated the infection. In three of four patients followed
for greater than two years, all symptoms of nephritis disappeared. In the one patient with the most severe renal
lesion, mild proteinuria persists. It should be mentioned
that shunt nephritis has not been reported in any patient
with a shunt other than of the ventriculo-atrial variety.

REFERENCES

1. Boulton-Jones, J.M., Sissons, J.G.P., Evans, D.J. and
   Peters, D.K.: Renal lesions of subacute infective
   endocarditis. *Br. Med. J., 2*:11, 1974.

2. Allison, A.C., Hendrickse, R.G., Edington, G.M., Honba,
   V., de Petris, S., and Adehiyi, A.: Immune complexes
   in the nephrotic syndrome of African children. *Lancet,
   1*:1232, 1969.

3. Braunstein, G.D., Lewis, E.J., Galvenek, E.G., Hamilton,
   A., and Bill, W.B.: The nephrotic syndrome associated
   with secondary syphillis: an immune deposit disease.
   Amer. J. Med., 48:843, 1970.

4. Boonshaft, B., Maher, J.F., and Schreiner, G.E.:
   Nephrotic syndrome associated with osteomyelitis without
   secondary amyloidosis. *Arch. Intern. Med., 125*:322,
   1970.

5. Michael, A.F., Westberg, N.G., Fish, A.J., and Vernier,
   R.L.: Studies on chronic membranoproliferative glomerulonephritis with hypocomplementemia. *J. Exp. Med.,
   134*:208s, 1971.

6. Smith, R.D. and Aquino, J.: Viruses and the kidney.
   Med. Clin. N. Amer., 55:89, 1971.

7. Strife, C.F., McDonald, B.M., Ruley, E.J., McAdams, A.J.,
   and West, C.D.: Shunt nephritis: The nature of the
   serum cryoglobulins and their relation to the complement
   profile. *J. Pediatr., 88*:403, 1976.

8. Black, J.A., Challacombe, D.N., and Ockenden, B.G.:
   Nephrotic syndrome associated with bacteremia after
   shunt operations for hydrocephalus. *Lancet, 2*:291, 1965.

9. Germuth, F.G. and Rodriquez, E.: Immune complex deposit
   and anti-basement membrane disease. IN Immunopathology

of the Renal Glomerulus, Boston, Little, Brown & Co., 1973, pp. 37.

10. Stauffer, U.G.: Shunt nephritis: Diffuse glomerulo-nephritis complicating ventriculo-atrial shunts. *Dev. Med. Child Neurol., Suppl. 22, 12*:161, 1970.

TABLE 1.

Clinical Findings in 13 Cases of Shunt Nephritis[7,10]

	No. Cases
General	
Spiking fever	12
Anemia	13
Hepatosplenamegaly	12
Renal	
Proteinuria	13
Edema	8
Hematuria	13
Hypertension	8
Bacteriology (pos. cultures)	
Blood	10
CSF	9

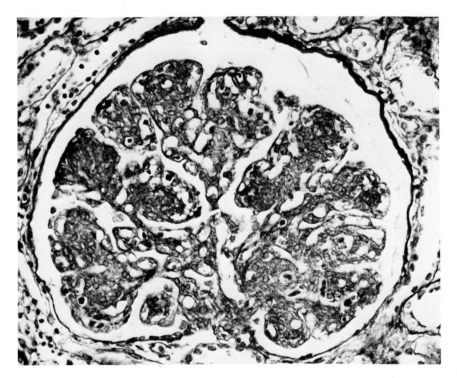

Fig. 1. Glomerulus from a patient with shunt nephritis showing enlargement and hyperlobulation. The mesangium is expanded and the widespread double-contoured appearance of the glomerular capillary walls is attributable to mesangial interposition. There is moderate reduction in the number of open capillary lumens. (Jones methenamine silver stain × 375.)

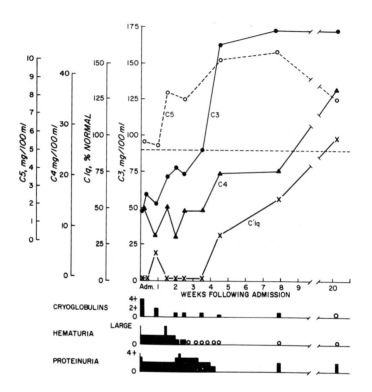

Fig. 2. Serial serum levels of the components of the classical complement pathway and cryoglobulins as they relate to urinary abnormalities and treatment. Dashed horizontal line indicates lower limit of normal range. Bacteremia with Staphylococcus epidermidis eradicated after shunt removal. Proteinuria persists two years following shunt removal.

INTRAVASCULAR MANIPULATION OF
VENTRICULOATRIAL SHUNT CATHETERS

David C. Schwartz, M.D. and
William J. McSweeney, M.D.

The disruption and subsequent migration or malposition of ventriculoatrial shunt catheters is an infrequent but nonetheless significant complication of intravascular shunt procedures for hydrocephalus. The presence of a free-floating intracardiac foreign body can result in cardiac dysrrhythmia, pulmonary embolization, sepsis or perforation.[1] Prompt removal of the dislodged catheter must be undertaken to avoid these secondary complications. Transvenous retrieval of embolized catheter fragments or manipulation of a malpositioned catheter can be safely accomplished thereby precluding thoracotomy. In the past five years, we have encountered three instances of catheter disruption or malposition necessitating intravascular repositioning or removal, Cases 1 and 2 have previously been published.[4,3] Our recent experience with Case 3 forms the basis of this communication.

CASE REPORT (YS, CHMC #253761)

This six-year-old black female was admitted to the Children's Hospital Medical Center for the first time for removal of an embolized ventriculoatrial shunt catheter.

She was originally seen at three months of age at which time diagnostic studies confirmed the presence of communica-

341

ting hydrocephalus. A right ventriculoatrial shunt was
performed and she responded satisfactorily. The shunt continued to function well until two years of age when shunt
sepsis occurred and the shunt was removed. A ventriculo-
peritoneal shunt was subsequently performed. Malfunction of
the ventriculoperitoneal shunt necessitated rehospitalization
a year later. This was satisfactorily repaired and she was
discharged from further follow-up. In December, 1972, the
ventriculoperitoneal shunt became detached and she underwent
another right ventriculoatrial shunt. In January, 1974, a
false meningocele developed over the Holter valve resulting
in separation of the atrial portion of the shunt catheter.
It was impossible to retrieve the dislodged distal segment
in the superior vena cava. A left ventriculoatrial shunt was
inserted and she was discharged from outpatient follow-up.
In the interim, the family moved and she appeared for the
first time at Children's Hospital Medical Center some twenty
months later for routine neurosurgical follow-up.

The history indicated that she had experienced palpita-
tions for several weeks. Both Holter valves were palpated
and judged to be functioning normally. Routine skull and
chest radiographs were obtained to assess the position of
the shunts. It was apparent from the AP and lateral radiographs (Figs. 1 & 2) that while the left ventriculoatrial
shunt was in good position, the right-sided shunt had
dislodged and embolized into the right heart. The distal tip
was coiled in the main pulmonary artery while the proximal
tip was lying against the lateral wall of the right atrium.
The patient was subsequently admitted for an attempt at
transvenous retrieval of the embolized catheter.

Under Ketamine anesthesia, a bi-plane angiocardiogram
was performed via the right femoral vein in order to

visualize the right heart chambers and pulmonary artery.
The angiocardiogram (Figs. 3 & 4) showed a filling defect
along the lateral wall of the right atrium but the right
ventricle and pulmonary arteries appeared normal. In view
of this, it was elected to procede with an attempt at transvenous retrieval of the dislodged shunt catheter.

A Cook catheter tip deflector system was introduced into
the common femoral vein and advanced to the right atrium.
The catheter assembly consisted of a 5F 80 cm Cook polyethylene catheter over a deflector wire. This was inserted into
an 8F 50 cm woven dacron end-hole catheter which served as a
sleeve for the movable core. The deflector tip was activated
thereby describing a gentle convexity on the wire tip. This
was utilized to hook the proximal end of the catheter. It
was apparent that the proximal end of the shunt catheter was
adherent to the lateral wall of the right atrium, however,
after gentle traction, the catheter was freed from the right
atrial wall and pulled into the inferior vena cava. The
distal end, however, remained looped in the pulmonary artery.
The deflector catheter system was withdrawn and a loop snare
device was then employed consisting of a Cook 0.025 inch
145 cm teflon wire guide which had been folded in its mid
portion and introduced into the 8F 50 cm woven dacron
catheter. The proximal end of the embolized shunt catheter
was snared in the inferior vena cava and the dacron catheter
was advanced over the wire snare pulling it tight and grasp-
ing the embolized catheter. The entrapped catheter was then
pulled down the inferior vena cava and withdrawn through the
femoral vein incision. Surprisingly, little clot was found
adherent to the catheter fragment. No arrhythmia was noted
during the withdrawal. The femoral vein was then repaired
and the wound was closed.

The patient tolerated the procedure well and was
discharged the following day without complication. She was
seen in Cardiac Clinic one week later and was found to have
no cardiac abnormalities and was totally asymptomatic.

DISCUSSION

Transvenous or non-surgical retrieval of embolized
ventriculoatrial shunts has been successfully accomplished by
several techniques.[2,5] These include endoscopic forceps, the
loop snare method and, more recently, with the use of a
deflector tip catheter system. The method of retrieval
largely depends upon the location and orientation of the
embolized catheter. With the proximal end in the right
atrium, hooking the catheter with the guide wire deflector
can be employed either to remove the catheter or reposition
it for ultimate removal by the loop snare method. Successful
retrieval from the pulmonary artery utilizing a loop snare
catheter has been reported by Picard.[5] Failure to hook or
snare an embolized fragment may be due to enclosure of the
proximal tip in thrombus. Extensive thrombus formation,
especially in the pulmonary artery, may preclude transvenous
removal since traction on the catheter could discharge clot
and result in distal embolization. It is likely that
thrombus formation is related to the duration of catheter
dislodgement. In our most recent experience, the ventriculo-
atrial shunt catheter was known to have been dislodged for
twenty-five months. In view of the duration of embolization,
a forward venous angiogram was performed to assess the degree
of thrombus formation before attempting to remove the catheter. If extensive thrombus had been visualized, particularly
in the pulmonary artery, the procedure would have been

abandoned in favor of thoracotomy and right heart exploration with cardiopulmonary bypass.

CONCLUSION

Disruption of the distal portion of a ventriculoatrial shunt with subsequent embolization into the heart necessitates prompt retrieval. Numerous reports indicate that removal can be accomplished by the transvenous method. Our experience with a guide wire deflector system indicates that this method is a simple and safe technique to reposition or remove the dislodged catheter fragment when the proximal end is residing in the right atrium.

REFERENCES

1. Bernhardt, L.C., Wegner, G.P., Mendenhall, J.T.: Intravenous catheter embolization to pulmonary artery. *Chest, 57*:329, 1970.

2. Bloomfield, D.A.: Techniques of nonsurgical retrieval of Iatrogenic foreign bodies from the heart. *Amer. J. Cardiol., 27*:538, 1971.

3. McSweeney, W.J.: Intravascular repositioning of a ventriculoatrial shunt. *J. Neurosurg., 36*:512, 1972.

4. McSweeney, W.J., Schwartz, D.C.: Retrieval of a catheter foreign body from the right heart using a guide wire deflector system. *Radiology, 100*:61, 1971.

5. Picard, L., et al: Transluminal retrieval of ventriculoatrial shunt catheters from the heart and great vessels: A new method. *Neuroradiology, 10*:159, 1975.

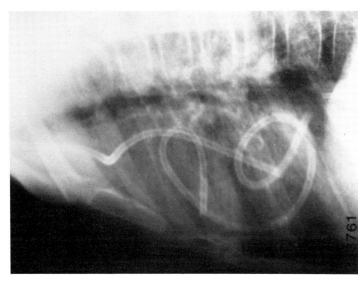

Fig. 2. Lateral chest radiograph. The dislodged shunt catheter is seen extending from the right atrium into the pulmonary artery.

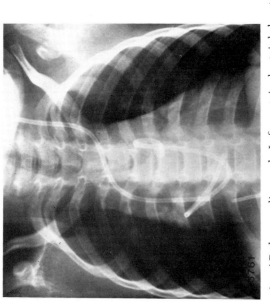

Fig. 1. AP chest radiograph. Left ventriculoatrial shunt in proper position. Embolized right ventriculoatrial shunt is coiled in the heart. The distal end is in the main pulmonary artery. The proximal end is in the right atrium.

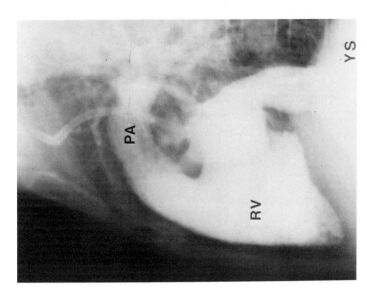

Fig. 4. Lateral view of venous angiogram. PA = main pulmonary artery; RV = right ventricle. The distal coil of the embolized catheter is seen extending to the bifurcation of the pulmonary artery.

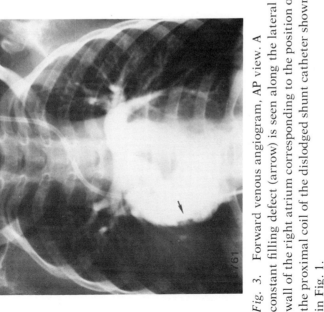

Fig. 3. Forward venous angiogram, AP view. A constant filling defect (arrow) is seen along the lateral wall of the right atrium corresponding to the position of the proximal coil of the dislodged shunt catheter shown in Fig. 1.

347

OCCULT SPINAL DYSRAPHISM

Luis Schut, M.D., Francis J. Pizzi, M.D.
and Derek A. Bruce, M.B.

Dysraphism, by definition is any lack of closure of two
structures which are normally fused. Spina bifida is a
dysraphism of osseous elements that enclose the vertebral
canal. The lack of bony closure in spina bifida may be
anterior involving the body of the vertebra, or posterior
involving the neural arches of the vertebrae (pedicles,
laminae, articular processes and spinous process). In usage,
however, the term "spina bifida" refers to a failure of
complete midline fusion of the vertebral arches. Willis, in
1958, further divided spina bifida into two categories;
spina bifida cystica and spina bifida occulta.[22] Spina
bifida cystica is the well known myelomeningocele or meningocele that protrudes from a bony defect in the vertebral
arches. Spina bifida occulta consists of a similar vertebral
defect, but there is no visable exposure of meninges or
neural tissue. Lichtenstein used the term "spinal dysraphism"
for all disorders associated with failure of fusion of vertebral or neural elements.[14]

In this paper we will restrict ourselves to occult
spinal dysraphism. The different conditions associated with
occult spinal dysraphism will be found in Table I. These
will be discussed first in general, including clinical and
radiographic similarities, then, each condition will be

discussed individually so as to elucidate unique features.

INCIDENCE AND SEX PREVALENCE

According to Record and McKeown, 60% of all congenital malformations involve the nervous system or its coverings.[19] The incidence of spina bifida ranges from 5% to 25% depending upon author and method of determining the incidence. James and Lassman found a 5% incidence of spina bifida in autopsied adults.[9] Matson, on the other hand, claimed that 25% of all children will show some minor defect of the vertebral spine or lamina on x-ray.[17] According to the review by Jones and Love, all authors agreed that spina bifida occurred at a rate of 1/1,000 live or dead births.[11] Since spina bifida occulta is frequently an incidental finding on x-ray, the true incidence could best be determined by an autopsy series using spinal column x-rays as a screening device. The 5% figure, therefore, most closely approximates the true incidence. For comparison, the incidence of spina bifida cystica is 2.5/1,000 births.

The sex ratio is slightly more than 2-1 female to male ratio in spina bifida occulta as compared to an equal sex ratio in spina bifida cystica.[9,11]

CLINICAL CHARACTERISTICS

Most commonly, defects in the vertebral arch indicating spina bifida occulta are seen at the L-5 and S-1 vertebrae. Next most common is the high cervical area followed by defects in the thoracic and upper lumbar levels.[17] As mentioned previously, the x-ray presentation of spina bifida occulta is an incidental finding associated with no symptoms or signs. There is, however, a small group of cases of spina bifida occulta that are associated with central neural axis involve-

ment. These associated neural anomalies may bind down the
spinal cord or nerve roots thus preventing them from changing
position within the vertebral column during growth of the
child. It is these cases that we must strive to diagnose
early in their course, for it has been shown that early
surgery is most beneficial for the prevention of progressive
disability.[8,9]

The central neural axis anomalies that are associated
with spina bifida occulta are not commonly evident at birth.
As the child grows, a dysraphic lesion begins to have its
effect in several different ways:

1) by preventing the spinal cord from ascending within
the canal during growth.

2) pressure from increasing size of abnormal tissue
(lipoma, dermoid tumor, etc.) within the bony spinal canal.

3) pressure from normal growth of the neural tissue
within an abnormally narrow vertebral canal. All these
mechanical distortions of the neural elements cause a progressive interference with local blood supply and neuronal
conduction manifesting clinically as neurological deficit.[9]

The presenting symptoms and signs are summarized in
Table II taken from the James and Lassman series of 100
patients with spina bifida occulta associated with intraspinal abnormalities.[9]

Signs of spina bifida occulta may be in the form of
cutaneous, neurological or orthopedic abnormalities.

CUTANEOUS

Cutaneous abnormalities indicative of an underlying
occult spinal dysraphism are situated in the midline over
the bony spinal canal or very close to the midline. A very
striking hairy patch (hypertrichosis), consisting of lengthy

silk-like hair, may be found in the upper lumbar region.
This is longest in the midline, sometimes resembling a
horse's tail, and then tapers off in density bilaterally
(Fig. 1). Frequently the patient's mother has trimmed this
hair for years prior to presentation. If the dysraphism is
located in the cervical or upper thoracic region, there is
usually a smaller patch of silky hair. The skin from which
the hair grows may be pigmented or angiomatous. There is no
association of hypertrichosis with any particular intraspinal
anomaly.[9]

Cutaneous port-wine angiomas located in the suboccipital
area are usually not significant. If the angiomata are in
the midline along the spine especially in the lumbosacral
area, there is a frequent association with underlying spina
bifida.[17]

Pigmented nevi may be found near the midline of the back
in the lumbar or lumbosacral region. These patches may be
bright red to brownish in color with mottling and can be very
large.

Atretic meningoceles may be found in the midline over
the lumbosacral spine. These are rounded 5 to 6 cm diameter
skin abnormalities consisting of a central thin white area
surrounded by a periphery of red, pink or brown. These
represent myelomeningoceles that have spontaneously closed
themselves.

Subcutaneous lipomas located at or near the midline of
the lumbosacral spine may be significant of an underlying
occult spinal dysraphism. These are subcutaneous, non-tender,
poorly circumscribed soft masses of fat. The skin over these
subcutaneous masses is either normal or hairy and dimpled
(Fig. 2). These are commonly associated with underlying
spinal dysraphism.

A dimple-like depression in the skin at or near the
midline over the spinal column may indicate occult spinal
dysraphism. There is fixation of the epithelium to the
underlying skin and subcutaneous layers (Fig. 3).

NEUROLOGICAL MANIFESTATIONS

Muscle weakness and gait disturbance is usually manifested at two years of age when the child begins to walk.
That there is motor involvement is underscored by a striking
unilateral lower extremity muscle atrophy associated sometimes with a short leg (Fig. 4). The deep tendon reflexes
may be normal, increased, hypoactive or absent.

Sensory examination is usually unreliable. However,
there may be symptomless fracture or trophic ulceration as
unequivical signs of sensory dysfunction.

Abnormalities of sphincter control may be manifested by
the mother's complaint of enuresis, inability to toilet train
or regression of bladder and bowel control after it was
learned. There may be complaints of dribbling of urine with
abdominal pressure, stress incontinence or overflow incontinence. These symptoms may be corroborated by a patulous
anus on digital examination, positive crede maneuver or a
post-voiding catheterization in search of residual urine.

ORTHOPEDIC ABNORMALITY

The most frequent orthopedic finding is a unilateral
cavovarus deformity of the foot with or without a short leg.[2]
Characteristically there is associated equinovarus deformity
or "club foot". The foot is in plantar-flexion and deviates
medially. There may be "claw toes" (Fig. 4).

The gait abnormality is due to the deformed foot and
shortened leg combined with the muscular weakness. There is

usually a complaint of pain secondary to the abnormal gait.
James and Lassman[9] described the gait as an elevation of the
first metatarsal head as though something were underneath
the foot with the great toe flexed. Sometimes there is an
associated adduction of the forefoot. If the gait abnormality persists any length of time, the cavovarus deformity
becomes evident with a high arch, adducted forefoot, with
inversion and clawing of the toes. The term "orthopedic
syndrome" has been used in reference to the combination of
gait abnormality with foot deformity.

Sharrard theorized that the limb deformities associated
with spina bifida are due to the lack of or weak innervation
of antagonistic muscles of the lower extremity,[21] that this
is due to damage of neuron groups within the affected cord
segments was proved by Lendon.[13]

RADIOLOGICAL CHARACTERISTICS

In order to make the diagnosis of spina bifida occulta,
a laminal defect on plain spine film must be seen. This
occurs between the C-7 and S-5 levels, most commonly at the
L-5 and S-1 laminae. In the majority of cases, defects
extend a distance of 3 to 4 levels.[9] Associated with the
laminal defect, there is usually an increase in the interpedicular distance over several levels (Fig. 5).

Plain spine x-rays reveal abnormalities of the vertebral
body as well as the intravertebral disc space. Hemivertebrae,
"butterfly" vertebrae, narrowing of the vertebrae in the
anteroposterior diameter or small vertebral bodies are
common. There may be fusion of bodies as well as clefts
within the body. In a small percentage of cases, there is
agenesis of the sacrum. A bony septum on anteroposterior
view, sometimes associated with a narrow disc space is

diagnostic of diastematomyelia (Fig. 5).

If clinical and plain x-ray findings are suggestive of occult spina dysraphism, the myelography is indicated. Since spina bifida occulta is associated with an intradural mass in the lumbosacral area occasionally, it is suggested that the dye be introduced by puncture of the cisterna magna rather than by lumbar puncture. It is mandatory that both A-P and lateral views be taken with the patient in the supine position (with the needle removed) as well as in the standard prone position. Occasionally, the bony spur of diastemato-myelia originates in the posterior spinal canal from the undersurface of the laminae rather than from the vertebral bodies. The intradural lipoma associated with a myelolipoma lies posteriorly as well. Both these conditions would be missed if myelography were not done in the supine position.

Abnormalities seen at myelography are a defect in the flow of the pantopaque, a space occupying lesion, a low level of the conus medullaris, or a splitting of the dye into a diamond shaped defect around the bony or cartilaginous spur of diastematomyelia. The space occupying lesion presents as a filling defect in the column of dye. There may be trans-lucencies associated with fibrous bands, nerve roots, or a wide filum terminale (Fig. 6).

Gryspeerdt, in his paper on myelography in occult spinal dysraphism, describes the technique to best define the conus medullaris attached to the filum terminale. The filum ter-minale is abnormally wide if it is greater than 3 mm,[6] and this finding is suggestive of "tethered cord syndrome".

CONDITIONS ASSOCIATED WITH SPINA BIFIDA OCCULTA

DIASTEMATOMYELIA

Diastematomyelia is defined as an abnormal cleft or

division of the spinal cord. This is to be distinguished
from diplomyelia, which is actually a reduplication of the
spinal cord. The cleft in the spinal cord in diastematomyelia may be bony, cartilaginous or fibrous. In the James and
Lassman series,[9] at the site of the septum there has always
been a completely ossified neural arch, although the spinous
process was not necessarily well formed. They noted that the
laminal defects of spina bifida are in neighboring neural
arches rather than the one over the site of the septum. The
split halves of the spinal cord are each totally invested
with a tube of dura mater. The septum lies between the two
dural tubes. There may be bands of fibrous tissue or atretic
nerve roots that pass from one or both halves of the spinal
cord to the intradural surface or pass through to attach
extradurally. The septum may be placed at the caudal point
of junction between the spinal halves. Therefore, the bands,
as well as the septum, will prevent normal cephalic migration
of the spinal cord during growth.

The purpose of surgery in these cases is prophylactic
rather than curative.[17] Surgery is indicated if on repeated
examination there is objective evidence of progression of
deficit. A laminectomy 1 to 2 segments above and below each
side of the septum is done, and the septum and both medial
walls of the dural tubes are removed. Any bands that run
from the spinal cord to the extradural areas are lysed. The
dura mater is then sewn together thus creating a single dural
tube out of two adjacent dural tubes.

CONGENITAL DERMAL SINUS

A congenital dermal sinus by definition is any depression or tract extending inward from the skin surface, which
is lined by a stratified squamous epithelium.[17] These tracts
are usually located in the lower lumbar and sacral region

and are surrounded by hairy skin.

The sinus may extend into the spinal canal and enter the subarachnoid space. This may be the nidus for recurrent bouts of meningitis. The attachment of the dermal sinus to neural tissue may distort the normal growth of that tissue and prevent its cephalic migration.

The dermal sinus, may, at any point along its tract, expand into an epidermoid cyst or a dermoid cyst. The more common is dermoid cyst, which is distinguished from epidermoid cyst by its contents. The epidermoid cyst contains epithelial debris and is lined by stratified squamous epithelium alone. The dermoid cyst contains keratin, sebacious material, hair, sebacious glands and hair follicles, namely, any of the elements of the deeper skin layers. The dermal sinus itself is much deeper than a dimple. The pilonidal sinus is sometimes confused with a dermal sinus. One must remember that a pilonidal sinus is acquired and therefore is unlikely to be found in a child. Matson and Jerva[18] stress that the final skin level of the dermal sinus at birth will be lower on the back than the point of its origin within the spinal canal. On the other hand, a cranial dermal sinus tract always passes inward in a caudal direction, extending to its neuro-endodermal equivalent level.[17]

The dermal sinus tract, when it becomes intraspinal, either goes through a bony laminal defect or through the ligamentum flavum between the laminae when there is no bony defect. If the expansion of the dermal sinus into a dermoid or epidermoid is intraspinal, it will act as a spinal cord or cauda equina tumor, causing appropriate clinical and radiologic changes.

Progressive loss of neurological function below the level of the cutaneous opening of the dermal sinus is an

indication for surgical therapy. If intraspinal extension
of a congenital dermal sinus is suspected, it is both unnecessary and unwise to probe the tract or inject any tracer
dye.[17] The intraspinal cyst may be adherent to the nerve
roots as a result of the episodes of recurrent meningitis.
The contents of the cyst should be removed, and any parts
of the capsule that are not adherent to nerve roots should be
removed as well.

NEURENTERIC CYST

Neurenteric cyst arises as a result of the transient
connection between ectodermal entodermal tissue at the region
of the posterior neuropore. If there is failure of formation
of the mesodermal layer, there is then a persistent connection between the entoderm and ectoderm. As the ectoderm
migrates, it pulls the entodermal tissues through the vertebral canal. Most commonly a neurenteric cyst arises in the
low cervical or upper thoracic region. They are less common
at the sacrococcygeal level.

Clinically, these cysts present as an intraspinal mass
lesion with concomittent neurological and orthopedic deformities. These neurenteric cysts are the counter part of the
congenital dermal sinus. Just as the epidermoid or dermoid
cyst can occur at any point along the tract of the congenital
dermal sinus, so can the neurenteric cyst occur at any point
along the tract of connection between the extodermally and
entodermally derived structures. If the cyst is located in
the neck and happens to be extraspinal, there will be a
problem with deglutition. If the cyst is extraspinal and in
the mediastinum, there may be signs of upper airway obstructions due to tracheal compression.

There may be a history of recurrent meningitis in which
no organism can be cultured. This should raise the suspicion

of an intraspinal neurenteric cyst. These cysts contain
slightly cloudy, colorless fluid, which upon leaking acts as
an irritant and causes a meningitic reaction.

Cutaneous defects such as excess hair, abnormal fat
collection, port-wine stains or dermal sinus tract openings
have never been seen in association with neurenteric cysts.[17]

There are characteristic radiological findings associated with neurenteric cysts. There may be a circular defect
in the body of the vertebra due to persistence of the tract
between the intraspinal neurenteric cyst and its place of
origin near other entodermally derived structures. There
may be a widened vertebral body due to bony proliferation in
an attempt to fill the gap which follows delayed disappear-
ance of the tract. There may be an associated hemivertebra
or fused vertebrae.

The neurenteric cyst may be extradural or intradural.
If intradural it may be within the substance of the spinal
cord (intramedullary) or outside the substance of the spinal
cord (extramedullary), yet within the dura. These neurenteric cysts present as intraspinal space occupying mass lesions.
They, therefore, should be removed at the time of diagnosis
so as to prevent further spinal cord compression and subsequent progression of neurological abnormality.

MYELOLIPOMA

Lipomas, or superficial fatty tumors, may present in the
lumbosacral region near the midline at birth. These sometimes are associated with a similar intraspinal fatty tumor
that is connected to the superficial lipoma. In this
instance the condition is called myelolipoma. There may or
may not be neurological dysfunction associated with myelolipoma (Fig. 2).

In the majority of cases in the James and Lassman

series,[12] there was a direct traceable connection from the
subcutaneous tissues to the spinal cord at or near the conus
medullaris. The site of the attachment to the cord is small.
Dubowitz and Lorber[4] found that the stalk connecting the two
masses went intradurally through the gap of the area of spina
bifida and connected to the conus medullaris or the nerve
roots of the cauda equina. They felt that the lower end of
the cord was never in a normal position, but frequently was
low in the spinal canal, sometimes as low as the first or
second sacral level. In this instance, the roots of the
cauda equina had to migrate upwards from the conus and then
angle down to exit through the appropriate foramina. In
Loeser's[15] report on myelolipoma in the adult, all patients
had spina bifida at the L-4 L-5 level. Yet the stalk between
the intraspinal and subcutaneous lipomatous mass went between
the spinous processes of L-3 and L-4, rather than through the
area of spina bifida.

It is generally agreed that early exploration with
removal of the subcutaneous and intraspinal lipomas be done
as a preventative measure even if there is no neurological
dysfunction.[4,12,15] The operation should consist of decompressive laminectomy with removal of as much of the lipomatous tissue as possible without injuring the nerve roots of
the cauda equina. The attachment of the lipoma to the conus
medullaris or spinal cord is adherent, and there is little
justification for an attempt to separate this.

HYDROMYELIA

Hydromyelia is a congenital dilatation of the central
spinal canal. It is lined by ependymal cells, and in this
way can pathologically be distinguished from syringomyelia.[1]

Gardner felt that impairment of normal cerebrospinal

fluid drainage from the fourth ventricle is the etiology of
hydromyelia.[5] This is supported by the frequent association
of the Arnold-Chiari malformation where there indeed is
impaired drainage of the fourth ventricle fluid. In this
condition, the foramina of Magendie and Luschka instead of
opening into the cisterna magna, open into the cervical
spinal canal.

Clinical presentation is as a compressive spinal cord
mass associated with bilateral radicular findings.

Unique x-ray findings are a widened cervical spinal
canal both in the A-P and lateral dimensions resembling a
funnel with the base directed cephalad.[18] There is also an
associated platybasia of the base of the skull, where the
head appears to be impaled upon the cervical spinal column.
On myelography, there is a characteristic segmentation of the
pantopaque inside the hydromyelic cavity[7,10] that resembles
the large bowel after a post-evacuation barium enema. Heinz,[7]
described the "collapsing cord sign". This was demonstrated
by performing an air myelogram after a pantopaque myelogram.
In the prone position, the cord appeared widened, while in
the sitting position, the cord appeared small due to collapse
of the hydromyelic cavity. This serves to distinguish an
infiltrating glioma of the spinal cord itself from a hydromyelic cavity. Using the above myelographic techniques,
James[10] showed an actual communication of the fourth ventricle with the hydromyelic cavity, thus further supporting the
above-mentioned theory proposed by Gardner.

Surgery should be directed at the primary abnormality,
namely impaired cerebrospinal fluid drainage from the fourth
ventricle. Therefore, posterior fossa and cervical spinal
decompression should be done as the initial procedure. If
this does not prevent progression of neurological deficit,

then a ventricular shunting procedure is recommended.

TETHERED CORD SYNDROME

The tethered cord syndrome or tight filum terminale
syndrome is caused by abnormal tissue that tethers the
intrathecal nervous tissue thus preventing its ascent in the
spinal canal during growth. The intrathecal nervous tissue
will be tethered by the maturation and contraction of fibrous
tissue connected to it.[9] Intradural nerve roots with their
site of origin on the conus medullaris may become atretic
and tether the intrathecal nervous tissue.

Jones and Love[11] described several cases of "tight
filum terminale". Anatomically the conus medullaris merges
into the filum terminale, and this then ends in the coccygeal
ligament which attaches to the lowest end of the bony spinal
canal. A thickened filum terminale would therefore tether
the conus medullaris in the bony spinal canal preventing its
ascent during growth. This would then cause an increase of
tension on the spinal cord with resultant pain and neurological dysfunction.

The symptoms are characteristically worse in the morning
due to lengthening of the spinal column during sleep. This
occurs because the supine position allows the discs between
the vertebral bodies to assume a more spherical configuration due to increased water content of the disc material and
resumption of the spherical shape of the disc due to elastic
forces. The symptoms are also worse with flexion of the
back which causes a lengthening of the vertebral canal without a concomittent lengthening of the spinal contents due to
their inferior fixation by the thickened filum terminale.

A unique myelographic finding is a widening of the
filum terminale greater than 3 mm. Also the dural sac is
displaced backwards by the thickened filum terminale and

becomes tented over it.

Lumbar laminectomy with opening of the dura and severing of the filum terminale is recommended when there is progression of neurological symptoms. Jones and Love[11] in six cases where the above regimen was followed, claimed that there was improvement of urinary symptoms, relief of low back pain and stabilization of a pre-operative unsteady gait.

REDUNDANT NERVE ROOTS

There are isolated case reports of redundant nerve roots as a cause of cauda equina compression in the absence of hypertrophic interstitial neuritis (Dejerine-Sottas disease). [3,16,20] This may be related to the condition called "meningocele manque" by James and Lassman.[9] This was felt to be a myelomeningocele that was partially developed before birth and spontaneously healed itself. Then, the nerve roots that were contained in the myelomeningocele sac therefore became redundant as they tried to resume their normal position within the spinal canal.

This condition presents as a cauda equina mass lesion with multiple radicular findings involving the lower extremities. A unique feature on myelography is a serpigenous type of defect indistinguishable from arteriovenous malformation of the spinal cord and cauda equina.

The diagnosis of redundant nerve root is made at surgery during a decompressive laminectomy. Upon opening the dura, the redundant nerve roots, enlarged and elongated, herniate themselves through the opening in the dura.[20] Just a decompressive laminectomy with opening of the dura is the recommended method of treatment. This will usually result in relief of the symptoms and neurological signs.

REFERENCES

1. Blackwood, W., McMenemey, W.H., Meyer, A., Norman, R.M., Russell, D.S.: Greenfield's Neuropathology, 2nd Ed., Great Britain, Edward Arnold Ltd., 1963.

2. Crenshaw, A.H. (Editor): Campbell's Operative Orthopedics, 5th Ed., C.V. Mosby Co., 1971.

3. Cressman, M.R., Pawl, R.P.: Serpentine myelographic defect caused by redundant nerve root. Case report. *J. Neurosurg.*, *28*:391, 1968.

4. Dubowitz, V., Lorber, J., Zachary, R.B.: Lipoma of the cauda equina. *Arch. Dis. Child.*, *40*:207, 1965.

5. Gardner, W.J.: Hydrodynamic mechanism of syringomyelia: its relationship to myelocele. *J. Neurol. Neurosurg. Psychiat.*, *28*:247, 1965.

6. Gryspeerdt, G.L.: Myelographic assessment of occult forms of spinal dysraphism. *Acta Radiol.*, *1*:702, 1963.

7. Heinz, E.R., Schlessinger, E.B., Potts, D.G.: Radiological sign of hydromyelia. *Radiology*, *86*:311, 1966.

8. Ingraham, F.D., Swan, H., Hamlin, H., Lawrey, J., Matson, D.: Spina Bifida and Cranium Bifidum. The Children's Hospital, Boston. Cambridge, Mass. Harvard Univ. Press, 1944.

9. James, C.C.M., Lassman, L.P.: Spinal dysraphism - Spina Bifida Occulta. New York, Appleton-Century-Crofts, 1972.

10. James, H.E., Schut, L., Pasquariello, P.S.: Communication of hydromyelic cavity with fourth ventricle shown by combined pantopaque and air myelography. *J. Neurosurg.*, *38*:235, 1973.

11. Jones, P.H., Love, J.G.: Tight filum terminale. *AMA Arch. Surg.*, *73*:556, 1956.

12. Lassman, L.P., James, C.C.M.: Lumbosacral lipomas: Critical survey of 26 cases submitted to laminectomy. *J. Neurol. Neurosurg. Psychiat.*, *30*:174, 1967.

13. Lendon, R.G.: Neuroanatomical and embryological studies on spina bifida cystica in man and the rat. Doctoral Thesis, 1968. Submitted to Univ. of Sheffield.

14. Lichtenstein, B.W.: Spinal dysraphism. Spina bifida and myelodipplasia. *Arch. Neurol. Psychiat.*, *44*:792, 1940.

15. Loeser, J.D., Lewin, R.J.: Lumbosacral lipoma in the adult. *J. Neurosurg.*, *29*:405, 1968.

16. Lombardi, V.: Redundant nerve root of the cauda equina. A case report. *Neurology*, *19*:1223, 1969.

17. Matson, D.D.: Neurosurgery of infancy and childhood. Charles C. Thomas, 1969.

18. Matson, D.D., Jerva, M.J.: Recurrent meningitis associated with congenital lumbosacral dermal sinus tract. *J. Neurosurg.*, *25*:288, 1966.

19. Record, R.G., McKeown, T.: Congenital malformations of the central nervous system. I: A survey of 930 cases. *Brit. J. Sociol.*, *3*:183, 1949.

20. Schut, L., Groff, R.A.: Redundant nerve roots as a cause of complete myelographic block: Case report. *J. Neurosurg.*, *28*:394, 1968.

21. Sharrard, W.T.W.: The mechanism of the paralytic deformity in spina bifida. *Cerebr. Palsy Bull.*, *4*:310, 1962.

22. Willis, R.A.: The Borderland of Embryology and Pathology. London, Butterworth, 1958.

TABLE 1.

Conditions Associated with Spina Bifida Occulta.

Diastematomyelia
Congenital dermal sinus
Neurenteric cyst
Myelolipoma
Hydromyelia
Tethered cord syndrome
Redundant nerve roots

TABLE II.

(From James and Lassman[9])

Presenting Symptoms and Signs.

59%	Gait abnormality and foot deformity (orthopedic syndrome)
25%	Cutaneous signs
10%	Bladder incontinence
5%	Scoliosis or foot deformity

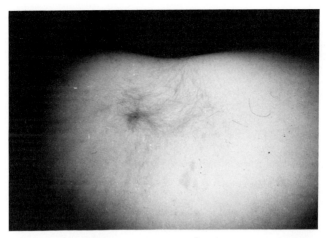

Fig. 1. Hypertrichosis.

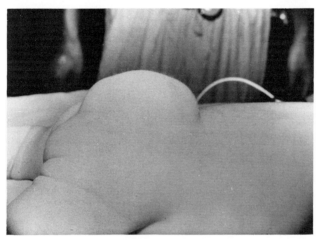

Fig. 2. Subcutaneous lipoma.

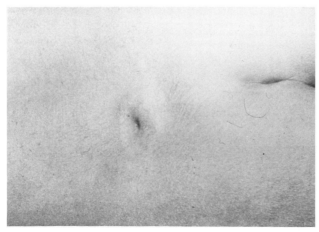

Fig. 3. Congenital dermal sinus.

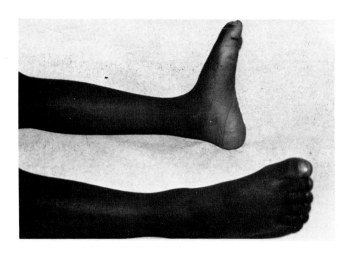

Fig. 4. Orthopedic deformity showing atrophic short leg and cavovarus deformity.

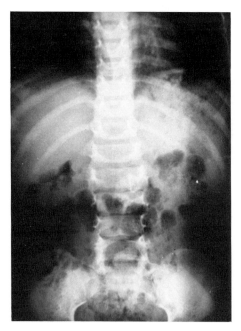

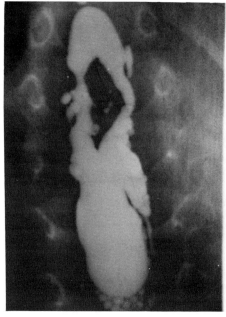

Fig. 5. AP plain spine X-ray showing: Widened interpedicular distance, spina bifida, and diastematomyelia spur.

Fig. 6. AP myelogram showing diamond-shaped filling defect of diastematomyelia.

TETHERED CORD SYNDROME

E. Bruce Hendrick, M.D., Harold J. Hoffman, M.D.
and Robin P. Humphreys, M.D.

In the present day western world with increasing degree
of social awareness, more and more attention is being paid
to the physically handicapped. While it has always been
obvious that children and infants with myelomeningocele
would develop paralytic deformities involving bladder and
lower extremities, it was only with the increasing awareness
on physical examination and with the development of better
diagnostic facilities, that the patients with diastematomyelia came to be diagnosed and treated. The neurosurgical
acquisition of these patients depended to a large extent upon
the education of the orthopedic and urologic surgeons in the
early manifestations of the problem.

In the past 5 years a new clinical problem has been
added to the scene. The so-called filum terminale syndrome
or tethered cord syndrome is now being widely discussed and
pediatricians and surgical specialties are becoming aware of
its presentation.

The work by Garceau,[1] Jones and Love[3] and others was
relatively ignored until the development of a very simple
change in myelography was publicized.[2] The Neurosurgical
Unit at the Hospital for Sick Children in Toronto paid little
attention to the existence of this syndrome until the

introducation of the technique of supine myelography. Within
the past 5 years, using this particular radiological technique, 31 children have been identified and treated for the
tethered cord syndrome. In order to eliminate any argument
or confusion in the description of this syndrome, all
patients with meningoceles, myelomeningoceles, lipomeningo-
celes, diastematomyelia and intraspinal space-occupying
dysraphic conditions such as dermoid tumours and neurenteric
cysts were excluded. We were careful to include only those
patients having a low conus medullaris and a thickened filum
terminale, which had to measure 2 mm or more in diameter.

CLINICAL PRESENTATION

     In the 31 patients in the series, there were many modes
of presentation. Fourteen of the patients exhibit the so-
called cutaneous stigmata of spina bifida occulta. In 8
cases, the defect was a hairy patch. One patient had an
angioma and a hairy patch and in one other patient there was
associated cutaneous dimple. In 2 other patients there was
an angioma alone and one patient a dimple alone and 3, the
patients had abnormal fat pads. Twelve of the patients were
under 5 years of age, 7 were between 6 and 10 years of age,
4 between 11 and 12 years of age and 8 were adolescents under
the age of 16.

PRESENTATION

     The patients typically presented with their symptoms in
periods of rapid growth and development. In 22 out of the
series, it was by the development of progressive weakness
and/or sensory loss in one or both lower limbs. This was
usually a presentation of muscle wasting, weakness and a

decrease in development of the foot on the effected side.
Pes cavus deformities were common. Absent ankle jerk and
a plantar extensor response were not infrequently present.
As one might expect, several of the patients had had previous
orthopedic surgery to their lower extremities of the progressive deformity. Several had presented with routine myelography which had failed to show in the abnormality. Some
patients have been diagnosed as Charcot Marie Tooth Syndrome,
cerebral palsy and multiple sclerosis. In only 3 patients
was the primary presentation, a disturbance of bladder and/or
bowel function alone. In 4 patients, sphincter disturbance
was accompanied by another peripheral presenting feature.
In only one patient, was bladder sphincter disturbance a
sign of disorder.

Of interest was the presence of scoliosis as the only
primary manifestation of the problem in 3 patients. There
were 5 patients, in addition in which scoliosis was a
secondary feature combined with other forms of presentation.
Characteristically, the scoliosis is usually progressive and
accompanied by weakness of one leg or by sphincter disturbance.

In 6 patients, pain was a major feature. The pain was
located usually in the lumbosacral area with frequent
radiation in one or both legs. It was typically aggravated
by movement of the back and in particular, by flexion of the
neck or assumption of the sitting position. In one patient
alone was pain the only evidence of the underlying problem.
In the remaining 5, pain was accompanied by scoliosis in 2,
progressive leg weakness in 2 and incontinence in one. Of
interest, one patient had progressive scoliosis despite a
previous spinal fusion. The pain will become so unbearable
that   she   was   unable   to   sit   up   and   had   to

attend   school   in   a   lounge   chair.

The referral pattern was interesting and might have
been predicted by the clinical presentation. Twenty-six
patients were referred by orthopedic surgeons, 2 by urologists
and 3 by pediatricians.

INVESTIGATION

Routine x-rays of the spine taken in an adequate manner
revealed a defect in the neural arch usually in the lumbosacral area in all patients. In 17 patients, both the low
conus and thick filum were seen in supine myelography (Fig. 1).
In one patient, the filum was so thickened with an intrinsic
lipoma, which is not unusual, that it could only be visualized on prone myelography in the caudal end of the dural sac.
In 3 patients a thick filum was noted but the conus could not
be visualized. In 5 patients, the low conus was noted but the
filum was not visualized. Four patients who had their spinal
cord extend to the caudal end of the dural sac were misdiag-
nosed on myelography. Two were found to have a low placed
thickened filum, one was felt to have a normal conus and
thickened filum and one patient was diagnosed as being normal.
A normal supine myelogram was also observed in one patient
with a thick filum which contained a lipoma. Two patients
with normal myelogram had a typical presentation of a tethered
spinal cord and surgery was proceeded with inspite of the lack
of radiological evidence. In 17 patients however, both the
low conus and thick filum could be seen on supine myelography.

TREATMENT

The treatment consists of laminectomy carried out on a
lumbosacral area. In 19 of the cases, there was an obvious

thickened fibrotic filum terminale. This was associated
with extradural bands in one patient. Seven patients had
small intrinsic lipomas within the thickened filum and one
patient had a small cyst, probably of arachnoid nature,
within the filum itself. In 4 patients, no filum terminale
could be visualized. The spinal cord tissue appeared to
extend to the lower end of the dural sac ending in a small
lipoma attachment of the conus to the end of the sac itself.

The filum terminale was divided between silver clips
and it was apparent in most patients that there was an upward
movement of the proximal end (Fig. 2). In those patients with
a spinal cord attachment to the lower end of the sac, the
cord was transected at the dural attachment.

In 2 patients presenting with scoliosis alone, Harrington fusions were carried out under the same anesthesia as
the laminectomy.

RESULTS

The improvement following surgical treatment depended
to some extent upon the presenting complaints. Pain was
alleviated and in most patients disappeared immediately
following release of the tethered filum. Many patients
developed increased mobility of their back and were able to
partake in athletic endeavours which have previously been
impossible. There was some decrease in motor weakness and
sensory loss in most patients. In no patients was there an
increase in neurological deficit. It was heartening to see
that in 4 patients, previously contemplated orthopedic
procedures were no longer needed.

Perhaps the most disappointing result but also the one
most to be expected was the lack of response in those
patients who had long term sphincter disturbance. One

individual was considered by the urological surgeons to be greatly improved following release of her tethered cord. This patient however, still required intermittent catheterization but did regain bladder sensation. One patient with both urinary and fecal incontinence regained urinary continence only.

DISCUSSION

While experience to date with the problem of tethered spinal cord has been limited and of short duration in terms of follow-up, the results have been most gratifying. It is hoped that the early diagnosis and awareness of the problem by all individuals dealing with children will lead to earlier treatment and hopefully, better clinical results.

Most people dealing with children are aware of the potential dangers of progressive weakness or deformity of the lower extremities or change in bladder or bowel habit. To the list of conditions previously considered offerable and responsible for the symptoms, we would like to add tethered spinal cord.

REFERENCES

1.   Garceau, G.J.: The filum terminale syndrome. *J. Bone and Jt. Surgery*, *35-A*:711, 1953.
2.   Gryspeerdt, G.L.: Myelographic assessment of occult forms of spinal dysraphism. *Acta. Radiol.* (Diagn), *1*:702, 1963.
3.   Jones, P.A. and Love, J.G.: Tight filum terminale. *Arch. Surg.*, *73*:556, 1956.

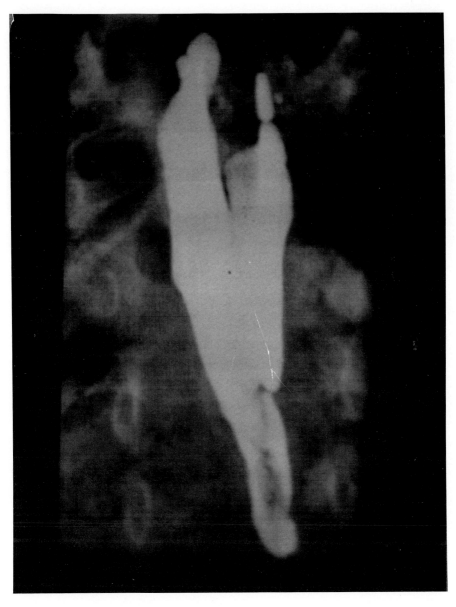

Fig. 1. Myelogram showing thickened filum and low conus.

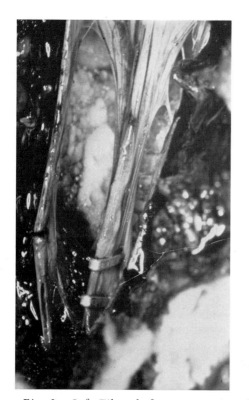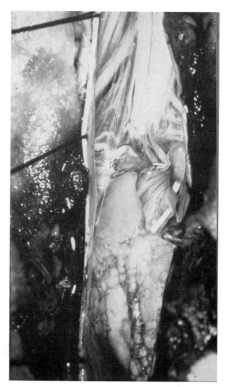

Fig. 2. Left: Filum before transection showing nerve roots pointing in a cephalad direction.*Right*: After transection showing roots pointing in a normal caudad direction.

ENDPOINT IN HYDROCEPHALUS

Martin P. Sayers, M.D.

What is the status of the treatment of hydrocephalus in 1976? Where are the trends leading us and what constitutes a satisfactory endpoint for the patient. A few patients have always survived, because hydrocephalus is sometimes a transient phenomenon and because natural events such as subsidence of inflammation, maturation and rupture of membranes as an aqueductal veil, a medullary vellum, the tela chorioidea or the lamina terminalis reestablishes satisfactory circulation and absorption.

Prior to the advent of Dr. Arn Torkildsen's ventriculocisternostomy procedure for aqueduct and third ventricle obstructions in 1936, the quality of survival was probably rarely improved much by neurosurgical procedures. Spinoureteral shunt markedly improved the outlook for a select small group between 1947 and 1956 at a time when we were having small success with ventriculomastoid, ventriculopleural and ventriculoperitoneal shunts -- actually ventriculo-every thing was tried. However, real success in all of these techniques awaited development of a good check valve like the one introduced by Mr. John Holter and Dr. Spitz in May, 1956. Dr. Nulsen and Dr. Spitz had struggled with the valve regulated ventriculovenous shunt in the late 1940's. Dr. Pudenz followed close on their heels with the Pudenz-

Heyer valve.

1956 and 1957 were the turning point, but since then we have been dusting off and reviving the old procedures because of the changed outlook for both obstructive and non-obstructive hydrocephalus. Sepsis in all of its forms was a threat related primarily to foreign body reaction in the tissues but also to operative technique, and most importantly to timing of procedures. It is gradually a smaller problem because of reduced bulk of foreign materials, a resurgence of peritoneal shunting and accumulating wisdom and experience. A series of discussions in this book have forthrightly dealt with the experience in this area.

A discussion of the selection of patients for treatment is integral because the data points increasingly to certain categories of patients who remain the least stable and have most indefinite endpoint or ultimate solution for their problem. All treatment other than ventricular shunt thus far entails a traverse through the subarachnoid space. Those cases in which this space is lost, obliterated or fails to develop prove to be our most difficult problems. Conversely the preservation and enhancement of some subarachnoid pathways is paramount.

It is probable that improved timing and technique can eventually provide a satisfactory permanent solution to the aqueduct stenosis problem through recanalization of the aqueduct, ventriculostomy or ventriculocisternostomy, providing that we do not inadvertantly lose the subarachnoid spaces.[3]

It has been my opinion that these spaces have been temporarily partially obstructed or lost in almost all advanced hydrocephalus regardless of cause, due to ventricular

distention and compression of the brain against the inner
table of the skull. The subarachnoid spaces are inadequate
in post-meningitic and post-hemorrhagic communicating hydrocephalus, but in our series the capacity to circulate and
dispose of the CSF is regained after one successful shunt in
about 80% of these cases. There is a very high spontaneous
compensation rate in hydrocephalus due to prematurity, hemorrhage or sepsis if the conditions are treated relatively
early, and if we do not encounter technical complications
which further damage the subarachnoid space, i.e., sepsis,
hygroma, new hemorrhage or excessive foreign body reaction.[2]

Preservation and enhancement of the ciliary action
within the ventricular system is probably one of the keys to
success. A large porencephalic diverticulum from the lateral
ventricle may continue to enlarge in the face of otherwise
adequate CSF pathways and arachnoidal granulations due to
lack of cilia and pulsation factors. Ventricle emptying can
often be enhanced by reducing the ventricular size to the
point that the ciliary action again becomes effective. This
has been strikingly demonstrated by Dr. Langman, anatomist,
in his work at the University of Virginia. Conversely the
poisoning, ciliary inactivating effect of biproducts of
blood breakdown in the ventricles is probably one of the
primary factors in the hydrocephalus due to the ventricular
hemorrhage and of prematurity.

Ideally, then, our ultimate treatment of hydrocephalus
may require an initial period of low pressure ventricular
shunting to encourage reopening, development, forcing,
dilation, or maturation of an adequate subarachnoid space
and ciliary activity.

In the past a fortunate few hydrocephalic children have
found compensation somewhere along the road with over-sized

heads. What is the mechanism? Probably there is more than one. Possibilities are 1) increased surface for transventricular absorption, 2) increased area for extra ventricular absorption other than pacchionian granulations, 3) perforation of membranes, and possibly 4) increased resistance to growth by thicker skull as described by Dr. Epstein. One of the biproducts may be a "forcing of the subarachnoid spaces."

It is, I think, important to be willing to accept compensation with larger than normal ventricles and possibly modestly increased pressure as one of the solutions to the problem. One of the all too common problems in my experience is categorized by a recent phone call about one of my patients treated by a single shunt for post-meningitic hydrocephalus in 1957. She is now 20 years old and has moved across the country. A high school graduate, she was gainfully employed, but experienced occasional headaches. In the course of a headache workup a C.T. scan showed just moderately enlarged ventricles. The pressure had not been measured, there was no papilledema or optic atrophy. A physician on the telephone said, "She is to be reshunted, and her family wanted you to be notified." I suggested a consultation with a neurosurgeon who wasn't far away, and who shares, I think, my conviction that early compensation most often leads to more stable and stronger compensation with advanced maturity -- not that there isn't such a thing as late decompensation. We are receiving quite a number of similar communications as CAT scans become more available. In our opinion a little increased pressure and moderately enlarged ventricles of long standing are often acceptable. One too many operations can destroy a beautiful start toward compensation and 'shunt-independence'.

Myelomeningocele constitutes in our series a cause or

the concomitant of approximately 60% of non-communicating or
50% of all hydrocephalus, i.e., 373 of 730 cases. I refer to
this as non-communicating hydrocephalus with some reserva-
tions, because the obstruction is often shown to be in the
subarachnoid space, though it is usually in the posterior
fossa, and often is very close to the foramina of Luschka
and Magendie.

All of the mechanisms of this type of hydrocephalus are
not clearly defined at present, but obstruction in the subarachnoid space is clearly one of them, as it may also be in
some forms of communicating hydrocephalus. Why is the fluid
pathway obstructed? Here we again approach the simile of the
blind men and the elephant. Is it chromosomal, chemical,
mechanical due to crowding and Arnold-Chiari malformation or
aberrant fibrous tissue as suggested by Dr. Gardner? We
really don't know. I have speculated in my own mind regarding the possibility of a reverse flow of relatively noxious
fluid from the amniotic sac through the central canal to the
4th ventricle and into the neighboring subarachnoid spaces
inducing a chemical arachnoiditis.

At any rate in our patients about 50% of the cases with
hydrocephalus and myelomeningocele have apparently developed
or found routes for communication of the CSF to adequate
absorptive areas after shunting and with maturation. This is
the major source of my jargon about "forcing the subarachnoid
space". I feel that these children are redeveloping spinal
fluid circulation in a manner parallel to the post-hemorrhagic
and post-meningitic hydrocephalic children.

In the uncompensated myelomeningocele patients, if the
subarachnoid block is largely in the posterior fossa, we
have reasoned that they may be prime candidates for third
ventriculostomy -- and they have been -- at least in many

cases. I have felt that it was wise, where possible, to
first attempt to achieve smaller ventricles and some maturation of the subarachnoid spaces then apply the ventriculostomy when and if it becomes apparent that the patient is not
one of the favorable 50% who can compensate the hydrocephalus
after a single shunt.

Not all of the ventriculostomies will function uneventfully, but it presently appears that most of them will. And
that we can improve, substantially, the success that was
attained in the period prior to satisfactory ventricular
shunting. The technique of our percutaneous anterior and
posterior third ventriculostomies is known to most of you
and is diagrammatically illustrated in Figure 1. The procedure is performed through twist drill openings, using the
McKinney leukotome to fenestrate the lamina terminalis and
the posterior floor of the 3rd ventricle between and behind
the mammillary bodies when indicated.

Our estimate of the status of our shunted patients as of
January, 1975 is depicted in Table 1. Of the 648 survivors
at that time we have relatively good evidence that 168 are
"compensated". They have either been demonstrated to be
functioning well with an obstructed shunt (shuntgram)[1] or
have functioned well for over 8 years without shunt revision.
Another 90 are probably compensated because they are
functioning well with shunts that are not working as judged
by digital testing -- but haven't yet passed the 8 year test,
and we haven't felt that we should subject them to the rigors
of a shuntgram.

It is of course probable that about 50% of the remaining
unrevised shunts are also compensated or in the process of
compensating. This figure would add about 60 more cases to
the compensated group, but that is pure speculation. 83 of

93 third ventriculostomies are judged to be functioning satisfactorily.

Assuredly over 50% of the surviving patients are presently at some type of an endpoint. This is not to say that intercurrent illness, head trauma or even the natural processes of aging will not disturb the balance. We have not addressed ourselves specifically to the quality of their survival in this paper. Almost certainly the quality can be improved with additional experience. The quality of survival is definitely better for the more recent patients than for the earlier ones in the series. Earlier mortality rates were prohibitive by today's standards.

SUMMARY

I have attempted to point up a number of salient techniques which may help to produce an earlier and more satisfactory endpoint in hydrocephalus. These include avoidance of infection, proper selection of patient, preservation and enhancement of the subarachnoid spaces and of the ependymal cilia and acceptance of large ventricle compensation.

Some form of ventriculostomy may be increasingly effective in the treatment of aqueduct stenosis, hydrocephalus with myelodysplasia and some cases of communicating hydrocephalus. We have had favorable experiences in all of these areas.

Over 50% of our 648 survivors of shunting procedures since 1957 are presently at some type of endpoint or compensation. It should be possible progressively to improve this percentage as we work to perfect new techniques.

REFERENCES

1. Dewey, R., Kosnik, E.J. and Sayers, M.P.: A simple test
    of shunt function: The shuntgram. A technical note.
    J. Neurosurg., 44:121, 1976.
2. Sayers, M.P.: Shunt complications. IN Clinical
    Neurosurgery, Vol. 23, Baltimore, Williams and Wilkins,
    1975, pp. 393.
3. Sayers, M.P. and Kosnik, E.J.: Percutaneous third
    ventriculostomy: Experience and technique. *Child's
    Brain, 2*:24, 1976.

TABLE 1.

Hydrocephalus (1957-1974)

Status January 1975 (18 years)		
Shunt survivors		648
"Compensated"*	168	
Functioning 3rd ventriculostomy	83	
"Probably compensated"**	90	
		341
Still shunt dependent		307 (47%)

*Criteria for "compensated"
1. no shunt for 8 years and/or
2. shunt demonstrated nonfunctioning[1]

**"Probably compensated"
1. 25% of survivors last 8 years

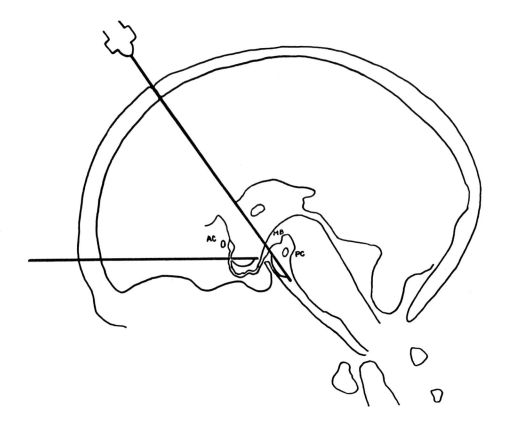

Fig. 1. Placement of the McKinney leukotome for anterior and for posterior fenestration of the third ventricle, median sagittal plane.

    A.C. (anterior commissure)

    M.B. (mammillary body)

    P.C. (posterior cerebral artery)

Part III
ORTHOPEDIC SURGERY

Participants

Norris C. Carroll, M.D., BSc, F.R.C.S. (C)
    Ontario Crippled Children's Hospital, Ontario, Canada
Robert A. Dickson, Ch.M., F.R.C.S.
    Louisville, Kentucky
Earl Feiwell, M.D.
    Rancho Los Amigos, California
Richard A. Jolson, M.D.
    Cincinnati Children's Hospital, Cincinnati, Ohio
Kenton D. Leatherman, M.D.
    Cosair Children's Hospital, Louisville, Kentucky
Richard E. Lindseth, M.D.
    Indiana University School of Medicine, Indianapolis, Indiana
John A. Odom, Jr., M.D.
    Children's Hospital, Denver, Colorado
John F. Raycroft, M.D.
    Newington Children's Hospital, Hartford, Connecticut
Michael J. Rozen, M.D.
    Cincinnati Children's Hospital, Cincinnati, Ohio
W. J. W. Sharrard, M.D., F.R.C.S.
    Children's Hospital, Sheffield, England

ASSESSMENT OF THE MYELOMENINGOCELE
CHILD

W.J.W. Sharrard, M.D., F.R.C.S.

Serial assessment of deformity and locomotor function in the spine and lower limbs is an essential part of the management of the children born with a myelomeningocele lesion. Normal lower limb function with no deformity can be expected to be present when the spinal lesion is a meningocele but when there is a myelomeningocele there is always some paralysis, partial or complete, of the lower limbs associated with deformity that may or may not be present at birth but which may develop during the course of growth.

Ideally, some assessment of paralysis and deformity in the lower limbs should be made as soon as possible after birth or, if this is not possible, within the first month of life provided that the general condition of the child makes it possible. Progressive studies can be repeated at any appropriate time interval - for instance monthly for the first six months, three-monthly for the next year and then six-monthly until growth is complete. A particularly detailed assessment should precede any prospective orthopaedic procedure or if there is any clinical suspicion of alteration in the neurological state of the lower limbs. It is useful to have some pattern of recording of assessment in the same way at each examination so that change in deformity or paralytic state can be recognised more easily.

PLAN OF ASSESSMENT

General assessment - The general state of health of the child, the presence of hydrocephalus and the condition of shunts controlling it, the overall state of renal and bladder function and the presence of any urinary infection.

General locomotor function - The general state of motor ability including sitting ability and posture, ability to crawl, kneel, stand with support, walk with bracing or aids and the general features of gait, balance and co-ordination. The general functional ability in relation to home, school and social activities.

Spine - The extent of the spinal lesion, the condition of the skin over the myelomeningocele area and the presence of any skin ulceration, the presence of kyphosis, lordosis or scoliosis and the effect of this on sitting or standing posture.

Lower limbs - A general description of the posture and overall deformity that is present at the hips, knees and feet. The general picture of spontaneous muscle activity whether it seems to be voluntary, reflex, autonomous or a mixture of types of activity.

Hip deformity - The range of passive movements of the hips with particular reference to the presence of fixed flexion, limited abduction or limited medial or lateral rotation. Clinical evidence of subluxation or dislocation.

Knee deformity - The range of passive movements in the knee with particular reference to flexion or recurvatum deformity and the presence of any valgus, varus or rotational deformity of the femur or tibia.

Ankle and foot deformity - The range of passive movements at the ankle, hindfoot, forefoot and toes with

particular reference to equinus, equinovarus, calcaneus,
calcaneo-valgus, vertical talus, pronation or supination
of the forefoot, metatarsus varus, claw toes or intrinsic
deformity of the toes.

Muscle activity - The presence of spontaneous movement
in infancy and early childhood, and of activity under
voluntary control when the child is able to respond to
instructions, charted in relation to specific muscles or
muscle groups wherever possible (Fig. 1). The presence of
reflex activity produced by stimulation of the inner side of
the thigh, the calf, or the sole of the foot. The presence
of any fine autonomous movement independent of any sensory
stimulus. The presence or absence of muscle wasting and
tone. The presence or absence of tendon reflexes, the
plantar responses and the existence of spasticity or clonus.

Sensory function - Response to pin prick and more
detailed sensory testing to pin prick and light touch in an
older child. The presence of skin colour changes and areas
of skin thickening, cornification or ulceration particularly
at the heel, underneath the metatarsal heads, upon the toes
or in the ischial, sacral or perineal regions.

Associated pathological lesions - The presence of
recent or past fractures as shown by the presence of swelling,
abnormal mobility or deformity especially in the supracondylar
region of the femur or the lower tibia. The presence of
abnormal mobility at the ankle or knee suggestive of a
Charcot joint in an older child.

Special investigations - Percutaneous stimulation
(Fig. 2) of main nerve trunks and individual muscles in the
lower limbs especially in infancy or early childhood or in
any child when operative treatment is contemplated, to
discover the presence of unrecognisable reflex or autonomous

muscle activity. Electromyography may sometimes give
additional information and, where feasible, evoked responses
to determine the presence of sensory levels in infancy and
early childhood.

Radiographs - Radiographs of the hips and spine should
be made routinely at least every 6 months and may be combined
with radiographs required for pylography. Radiographs of
the knees, ankles or feet according to the presence of
deformity or fracture.

Clinical photography - Because of the multiplicity and
complexity of the deformities that may be present, periodic
clinical photography provides an excellent record, particularly before operative correction of deformity and
immediately after removal of plaster following any operative
correction.

THE PATHOGENESIS OF PARALYSIS AND DEFORMITY

Studies of the spinal cord in myelomeningocele have
shown a bewildering variety of lesions.[5] In some instances,
the spinal cord is fully neurulated with a good nerve cell
content but there has been protrusion of nervous tissue,
some of which has degenerated or been lost due to surface
exposure. Other cords fail to neurulate or are partly
neurulated. Portions of the cord may have failed to develop
completely, particularly the distal segments or they have
suffered secondary degeneration. Even in the more proximal
parts of the spinal cord, well away from the myelomeningocele
lesion, there may be duplication or diplomyelia, diastematomyelia, hydromyelia or syringomyelia. Pressure changes may
result from the presence of lipomata or other space occupying
tumours. Superimposed on this pathological development may
be the effects of trauma or infection occurring after birth

and, in later months or years, the effects of fibrosis and
traction due to tethering of the terminal part of the spinal
cord at an abnormally low level. It is no surprise, therefore, to find that the paralysis and deformity of the lower
limbs presents a very varied picture both at birth and subsequently. This, together with the intrinsic difficulty in
making an accurate analysis of neurological function in
infancy and early childhood has made the formulation of any
distinctive patterns of paralysis extremely difficult. The
prognosis for later neurological function is also notoriously
unreliable when compared with the situation presenting at
birth in that later function may be worse, the same as, or
better than that estimated in the early days of life.[3]

Some generalisations can, however, be made.[6] Localised
and smaller lesions in the lumbosacral or sacral areas are
generally associated with much lesser degrees of paralysis,
much of it of lower motor neurone type due to involvement of
the roots of the cauda equina. Lower thoracic and upper
lumbar lesions tend to be associated with adequate lower
motor neurone innervation but with fairly severe paralysis
due to upper motor neurone defect at cord level. Lesions
affecting the whole lumbar spine give an intermediate degree
of paralysis, partly upper and partly lower motor neurone in
type. In general terms, lower limbs that show strikingly
good spontaneous movements immediately after birth are among
those that are likely to show acceptable neurological
function in later years; those that show paucity of movement
and evidence of reflex activity at birth are likely to retain
such activity permanently. Early surgical closure of the
spinal lesion is likely to preserve a better degree of
neurological function particularly in smaller and lower
lesions but in the larger and more proximal lesions, it is

doubtful whether ultimate neurological function is greatly affected whether closure is undertaken early or late. Nevertheless, there are occasionally gross exceptions in which an extensive lesion as viewed from the surface may be associated with a reasonably well neurulated spinal cord and surprisingly good lower limb function following surgical repair of the spinal lesion. The paralysis is often fairly symmetrical but not necessarily so. When there is a diastematomyelia with hemimyelocele, one lower limb may be completely normal and the other moderately or severely paralysed.[4]

In practice, it is best to assume that the level of paralysis in the lower limbs is subject to considerable variation during the first nine to twelve months of life and only after the end of the first year, can the level of paralysis be thought likely to remain stable. Even then, the possibility of a further slow deterioration in muscle function may still occur in the course of growth or as a result of fibrosis or the enlargement of tumour masses in the spinal canal. Any late deterioration in neurological function may indicate the need for further exploration of the spinal lesion. For the purposes of orthopaedic management it is but possible to take the paralytic state as one finds it and to act according to the state of neurological function and deformity that presents, whilst knowing full well that even if satisfactory correction of the deformity and muscle balance has been obtained, it is always possible that a new deformity or a different type of muscle imbalance may develop in the course of time.[10,17] As the child becomes older, the presence of a sensory level often gives a more reliable indication of the overall neurological state of the limb.

In spite of these limitations, it is useful to try to define the pattern of paralysis presenting in the limb at any one time. In some children, the paralysis presents with a very clear demarkation as to the neurological level with evidence of good voluntary activity in muscles supplied by lumbar or lumbar and sacral roots down to a specific segmental level (Fig. 3) with upper or lower motor neurone paralysis in segments distal to that level. In such an instance, the pattern of deformity that presents or which subsequently develops is reasonably closely related to the distribution of neurological loss (Fig. 4). In more than fifty percent of myelomeningoceles, the pattern of paralysis is a mixture of normal activity, mixed voluntary and reflex activity and autonomous activity arising in anterior horn cells devoid of central connections.

Deformity in the newborn[9,13] is predominantly due to partial paralysis that has been present in utero. In some limbs, the deformity is extremely rigid and associated with severe wasting and underdevelopment of the tissues generally. In such instances, it seems likely from observations of comparable abnormality in animals, that the deformity has arisen in association with paralysis at a very early stage of limb development. More commonly, the deformity, though typical of a paralytic lesion, is less rigid and to a certain extent can be corrected manually even if it tends to spring back to the deformed position. In these cases, it seems likely that the deformity has arisen in later intrauterine life and is more comparable with the type of deformity that develops post-natally. The most deceptive aspect of paralysis and deformity is that in which there is no significant deformity at birth in, for instance, a thoraco-lumbar lesion, but assessment of the paralytic state indicates that there is

probably largely reflex activity in the lower limb muscles.
In such patients, secondary deformity may develop fairly
rapidly during the first year of life in association with
that reflex activity and the development of flexion
deformities of the hips and knees and equinus deformities of
the feet (Fig. 5). Even more confusing is the situation in
which there is birth deformity, for instance with flexed
adducted hips with dislocation, recurvatum of the knee and
calcaneo-varus deformity of the foot which can clearly be
associated with active innervation down to the fourth lumbar
neurological segment and paralysis of roots distal with this
level. Subsequently, additional paralysis or the development
of reflex activity in muscles that were previously relatively
unaffected may produce, ultimately, a different pattern of
paralysis superimposed upon the deformity that was present at
birth. It is cases such as this that careful assessment of
neuromotor function by all possible means, clinical, and
electrical, is needed before decisions are made about
correction of deformity and tendon transplantation.

In addition to deformity that is probably secondary to
paralysis, an element of true congenital deformity such as
club foot (Fig. 6), vertical talus or congenital dislocation
of the hip may be present[7] and requires some elements of
treatment comparable to those which might be needed in a
normal child, as well as treatment for the paralytic lesion
that is present. Furthermore, persistent posture, especially
in a limb whose muscles are inactive, may add a further
element in the production of deformity especially if passive
movements are neglected.

Deformity of the spine is more often due to bony
abnormality than to the effects of paralysis, though, in
high lesions, asymmetrical abdominal or trunk paralysis can

produce spinal deformity[2] just as it does in poliomyelitis.
Only in kyphotic deformity does the abnormal forward displacement of trunk extensor muscles regularly result in
progressive increase in kyphosis due to abnormal flexor
action in extensor muscles displaced forwards by the bony
deformity.

Hemivertebrae, sometimes multiple, unilateral fusion of
lateral or posterior processes, congenital fusion of vertebral bodies, and other bony abnormalities such as may be seen
in congenital spine deformities independently of the presence
of a myelomeningocele may result in progressive deformity
during childhood. When the vertebral bodies are normally
formed but are in association with absent or deficient
posterior elements, there is a considerable liability for the
spine to develop lordotic or lordo-scoliotic deformity in
later childhood, particularly after the age of 10 when such
deformity may increase rapidly and become very severe,
especially in a child who spends much of the day in a sitting
posture.

[1,8,12,14,15,16]

GENERAL PRINCIPLES AND INDICATIONS FOR TREATMENT

The primary goal of orthopaedic management is to obtain
the best possible function of which the individual may be
capable. The basic limitation in any patient is the overall
degree of paralysis in the lower limbs. It is important that
all those concerned - orthopaedic surgeon, physiotherapist,
orthotist, parents and the child himself - should appreciate
what general degree of mobility and activity can be hoped
for and which features deleterious to optimum function can
be modified or aided by surgery, physical measures, bracing
and social accommodation.

In infancy and early childhood, it is reasonable to
assume that the child, however severely affected, may become
capable of walking, even if this will be limited to extent
and require bracing and other aids to achieve it. To produce
the best function requires that:

1. Deformity should be corrected and, as far as
possible, correction should be maintained.

2. A balance of muscle action should be obtained at
each joint.

3. The feet should be made plantigrade.

4. The lower limbs should be aligned to allow weight
bearing.

5. Trunk stability and balance should be maintained.

6. Appropriate bracing and aids to ambulation should
be applied.

7. Cosmesis and appearance should be respected.

8. Complications such as pressure ulceration,
pathological fractures or neuropathic joints should be kept
to a minimum.

Continued vigilance, assessment and orthopaedic action
are needed in all these respects throughout the growing
period of 16 years and, to some degree, sustained in adult
life.

CORRECTION OF DEFORMITY IN THE LOWER LIMBS

Traditionally, casting or passive stretching of the
soft tissues has been used as the primary means of correction
of deformity, especially congenital deformities. Although
passive stretching and movements retain their importance in
preventing and, sometimes, correcting deformity in the
presence of complete flaccid paralysis, casting has a much
more limited place in the management of deformity in

myelomeningocele. If applied with great care, casting can
be used to correct some birth deformities such as equinovarus
and, in older children, it may help to improve some knee and
foot deformities but if there is a paralytic cause, recurrence is inevitable[11] and surgery, at least to correct
unbalanced muscle activity will be needed at some point.
In some deformities, such as vertical talus or deformities
of the hip, only surgery can be successful in producing
correction.

Both in congenital and secondary deformity in myelomeningocele, many deformities can be corrected completely by
tendon lengthening and division of short soft tissues,
ligaments and joint capsules if performed sufficiently early.
If soft tissue surgery proves inadequate or cannot correct
deformity, for instance rotary deformities of the femur or
tibia, osteotomy may be needed primarily, in addition to soft
procedures or at a second operation.

The indications for correction of deformity[1,12] are:

1. At the hip - for more than 25 degrees of flexion
deformity, even if compensated by lumbar lordosis, or progressive limitation of abduction especially if the hip range
becomes less than 20 or 30 degrees, and for subluxation or
dislocation of the hip. Bilateral dislocation in an otherwise functionless limb may be disregarded but flexion and
adduction deformity associated with it will still need to be
corrected to allow bracing. Fixed rotation or fixed
abduction deformity also needs to be corrected to allow
braces to be applied.

2. At the knee - up to 15 degrees of fixed flexion may
be acceptable, but more than this should be treated or it
will be likely to increase rapidly because of inhibited
activity in the knee flexors, voluntary or reflex. If there

is any fixed flexion deformity at the hip, it should always
be corrected first. More than 15 degrees of varus or valgus
also needs correction, usually by osteotomy. Limited flexion
may be acceptable but, rarely, severe recurvatum may need
surgical treatment. Rotary deformity of the tibia may or
may not need correction, dependent on the alignment of the
foot in relation to the knee and hip.

3. At the ankle - limited dorsiflexion is acceptable
provided that the ankle can be dorsiflexed a few degrees
above a right angle, but fixed equinus of more than 10 degrees
and any calcaneus deformity must be corrected to avoid
pressure ulceration in later childhood.

4. At the foot, limited inversion or eversion around
the median position is acceptable but any fixed varus or
valgus of hindfoot or forefoot and most adduction of the
forefoot must be corrected. Sometimes a compromise of
deformities of the ankle, hindfoot and forefoot needs to be
accepted provided that the foot is sufficiently plantigrade
overall.

5. At the toes - deformity that might be innocent in an
otherwise normal child may be a serious problem in a child
who has sensory loss in the foot and must be corrected
before toe ulceration or vascular complications develop.

6. At the spine - deformity presents in many and varied
forms - kyphosis, lordosis, lordo-scoliosis or scoliosis.
Measures applicable in the management of scoliosis in normal
children, such as the Milwaukee brace are often difficult to
apply and very liable to cause pressure ulceration or complications of shunt tubing in the neck. If serious loss of
trunk balance, pelvic obliquity, or complications such as
ulceration over the spine develop, correction of bone is
needed at any age.

CORRECTION OF MUSCLE IMBALANCE

The correction of muscle imbalance is a complex matter, different in almost any patient, with joint deformity and often difficult to achieve. Weakening of strong muscles is produced either by lengthening of tendons, excision of tendon or muscle, partial or complete denervation or in association with tendon transplantation from a deforming position. Enhancement of weak muscle action can be produced by tendon transplantation, even, at times, when the transplant is not able to produce voluntary or functional action. It is unwise to hope that deformity will not recur if correction has been made but muscle imbalance has been left uncorrected.

Sometimes, because of difficulties in judgement of the activity of reflex muscles, a transplant may produce the opposite deformity. Such a risk must be accepted and a further procedure performed to correct the new deformity. In other instances, alteration of the paralytic pattern may be responsible for production of a new deformity.

Prolonged immobilisation beyond that necessary to allow sound healing of soft tissues (3 to 4 weeks) or bone (6 to 8 weeks) is not advisable and splinting in an exaggerated position may even create a new deformity. Prolonged splinting after operation may inhibit activity in transplanted muscles and seldom produces a better result than if the limb is allowed to move spontaneously. Night splints are not without hazard and are a common cause of pressure ulceration however carefully applied.

BRACING

The primary function of a brace is to stabilise a joint that is not under adequate muscle control. The degree of

bracing needed varies from a full set of braces from axilla
to foot level to below knee appliances. Braces need to be
carefully made and applied to avoid abnormal skin pressure
and should be as light as possible. They should not be used
just to improve the appearance when the gait is cosmetically
poor - the result may be a child who is less mobile than he
is without them. Footwear needs careful selection and
fabrication especially in an active older child and particular
care needs to be taken to produce even distribution of
pressure on the sole of the foot. At no time should braces
be used to attempt to correct deformity except when there
has been a pathological fracture, when a brace may be very
conveniently used as a method of fixation to avoid plaster
casts or traction splintage.

SENSORY LOSS AND ITS COMPLICATIONS

   Sensory loss is the one factor that differentiates
myelomeningocele from all other varieties of paralytic
problem in childhood. It dominates the requirements of
treatment and is an ever present hazard in the foot, over the
front of the knee, trochanters, ischial tuberosities and the
sacrum. The causes of ulceration (Fig. 7) are three:
prolonged pressure over a prominent bony point, friction,
persistent wetness or soiling in association with bladder and
bowel incontinence. Prevention, by avoiding the causative
factors,is much easier than cure and the parents and the child
himself must be educated in preventive measures. The treatment of a sore requires relief from pressure and friction and
it should not be forgotten that a closely applied plaster
cast may be an excellent way of preventing both causes and
producing rapid healing.

Pathological fractures or epiphysial separations (Fig.8)
are very common in myelomeningocele limbs. They are
aggravated by prolonged immobilisation in casts or in a
wheelchair. The inexperienced, seeing signs of swelling,
redness, pyrexia, raised sedimentation rate and leucocytosis
almost always diagnoses osteomyelitis, especially when the
radiological changes are minimal. Treatment should be by
the simplest possible means associated with the encouragement
of activity and non-union is rare.

Loss of proprioceptive sensation and difficulties in
balance, especially in hydrocephalics, provides additional
problems in children who already have weakness in their lower
limbs and this needs to be remembered by physiotherapists
and others concerned with education in walking.

Neurological defects in the upper limbs are not at all
uncommon and may include some degree of upper motor neurone
hemiplegia in association with hydrocephalus and its shunting,
difficulties in fine manipulation, and weakness or disas-
sociated sensory loss due to lesions in the cervical spinal
cord.

OLDER CHILDHOOD AND ADOLESCENCE

In later childhood, the presence of insuperable
difficulties such as marked hydrocephalus, mental retardation,
severe renal or cardiac insufficiency, intractable spinal
deformity, multiple and recurrent limb deformity, excessive
obesity or, occasionally, sheer lack of drive and motivation
to walk, may lead to a decision to abandon efforts to sustain
limited walking function and to accommodate to a wheelchair
life. In such patients, orthopaedic management must adjust
itself to a more limited goal and it may be acceptable to
allow flexion deformities at the hips or knees to be left

without correction. Even so, the child must be helped and instructed to obtain the maximum of independence and to appreciate the social limitations of a wheelchair life and the possible hazards of ischial or sacral ulceration, spontaneous fractures, increasing obesity, oedema of the legs and feet with vascular changes, hydronephrosis secondary to ureteric kinking and an increased liability to develop severe lordo-scoliosis.

Whatever the degree of paralysis present, some permanent deficiency in lower limb function will remain and continue into adult life. The adolescent must be taught and trained to the life that he must lead in future and, wherever possible, towards useful employment for home life. His and her problems are many and are aggravated by all the other problems of puberty and sexual awakening. With good social care and advice, most adolescents will adapt well,many will become usefully and gainfully employed and tragedies such as suicide should be anticipated and avoided.

In all children, the total management of the child must not be forgotten and the multiplicity of his medical problems - cerebral, renal, orthopaedic and social. The orthopaedic surgeon must always remember that serious lesions in the cerebral or renal field must always take precedence over orthopaedic procedures and that cerebral and renal function need to be assessed anew before any orthopaedic operation is done.

REFERENCES

1. Curtis, B.H.: Principles of orthopaedic management in myelomeningocele. IN American Academy of Orthopaedic Surgeons Symposium on Myelomeningocele. St. Louis, The C.V. Mosby Co., 1972, pp. 157.

2. Drennan, J.C.: The role of muscles in the development of human lumbar kyphosis. *Dev. Med. Child Neurol., Suppl. 22*:33, 1970.

3. Duckworth, T. and Brown, B.H.: Changes in muscle activity following early closure of myelomeningocele. *Dev. Med. Child Neurol., Suppl. 22*:39, 1970.

4. Duckworth, T., Sharrard, W.J.W., Lister, J. and Seymour, N.: Hemimyelocele. *Dev. Med Child Neurol., Suppl. 16*:69, 1968.

5. Emery, J.L.: The back lesions, lipomas, and dermoids. IN American Academy of Orthopaedic Surgeons Symposium on Myelomeningocele. St. Louis, The C.V. Mosby Co., 1972, pp. 41.

6. Emery, J.L. and Lendon, R.G.: Clinical implications of cord lesions in neurospinal dysraphism. *Dev. Med. Child Neurol., Suppl. 27*:45, 1972.

7. MacEwen, G.D.: The lower extremity in myelomeningocele. IN American Academy of Orthopaedic Surgeons Symposium on Myelomeningocele. St. Louis, The C.V. Mosby Co., 1972, pp. 166.

8. Menelaus, M.B.: The Orthopaedic Management of Spina Bifida Cystica. Edinburgh, Livingstone, 1971.

9. Sharrard, W.J.W.: The mechanism of paralytic deformity in spina bifida. *Dev. Med Child Neurol., 4*:310, 1962.

10. Sharrard, W.J.W.: The segmental innervation of the
     lower limb muscles in man. *Annals of the Royal College
     of Surgeons, 35*:106, 1964.

11. Sharrard, W.J.W.: Paralytic deformity in the lower
     limb. *J. Bone Joint Surg., 49B*:731, 1967.

12. Sharrard, W.J.W.: Paediatric Orthopaedics and fractures.
     Oxford, Blackwell Scientific Publications, 1971.

13. Sharrard, W.J.W.: Neuromotor evaluation of the newborn.
     IN American Academy of Orthopaedic Surgeons Symposium
     on Myelomeningocele. St. Louis, The C.V. Mosby Co.,
     1972, pp. 26.

14. Sharrard, W.J.W.: The orthopaedic surgery of spina
     bifida. *Clin. Orthop., 92*:195, 1973.

15. Sharrard, W.J.W.: The orthopaedic management of spina
     bifida. *Acta Orthopaedica Scandinavica, 46*:356, 1975.

16. Sharrard, W.J.W.: General orthopaedic management and
     operative treatment in spina bifida for the clinician.
     IN Clinics in Developmental Medicine, No. 57,
     G. Brocklehurst (ed.), Philadelphia, J.B. Lippincott,
     Co., 1976, pp. 84.

17. Stark, G.D. and Baker, G.C.W.: The neurological
     involvement of the lower limbs in myelomeningocele.
     Dev. Med. Child Neurol., 9:732, 1967.

Name _____

Plaque neurological level _____ Type of lesion _____

Time from birth to closure _____ hrs. ___ mins. _____

MUSCLE GROUP	BIRTH				6/12				1 YEAR				18/12			
	VOL.		FAR.		VOL.		FAR.		VOL.		FAR.		VOL.		FAR.	
	R.	L.	R.	L.	R.	L.	R.	L.	R.	L.	R.	L.	R.	L.	R.	L.
p Flexors																
Hip Adductors																
Quadricpes																
Tib. Anterior																
Tib. Posterior																
Hip Abductors																
Med. Hamstring																
Ex. Hall. Long.																
Ex. Dig. Long.																
Peronei																
Lat. Hamstring																
Glut. Maximus																
alf																
Flex. Hall. Long.																
Flex. Dig. Long.																
Toe Intrinsics																
Perineum																

Deformities   Hips   Plaque stimulation

Knees

Feet

Fig. 1. Muscle chart for recording in myelomeningocele. The muscle groups are in root innervation order.

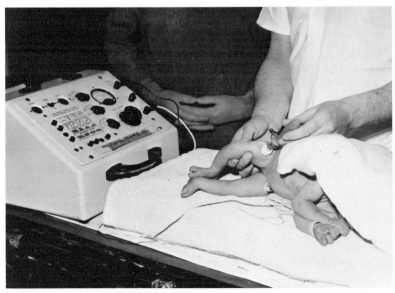

Fig. 2. Percutaneous electrical (faradic) stimulation.

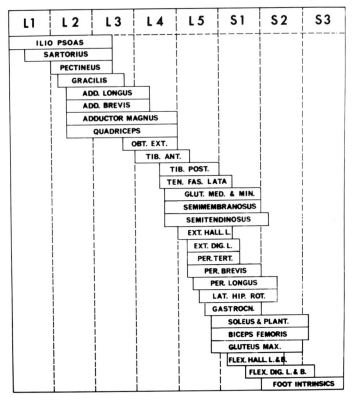

L1	L2	L3	L4	L5	S1	S2	S3

ILIO PSOAS
SARTORIUS
PECTINEUS
GRACILIS
ADD. LONGUS
ADD. BREVIS
ADDUCTOR MAGNUS
QUADRICEPS
OBT. EXT.
TIB. ANT.
TIB. POST.
TEN. FAS. LATA
GLUT. MED. & MIN.
SEMIMEMBRANOSUS
SEMITENDINOSUS
EXT. HALL. L.
EXT. DIG. L.
PER. TERT.
PER. BREVIS
PER. LONGUS
LAT. HIP. ROT.
GASTROCN.
SOLEUS & PLANT.
BICEPS FEMORIS
GLUTEUS MAX.
FLEX. HALL. L. & B.
FLEX. DIG. L. & B.
FOOT INTRINSICS

Fig. 3. Diagram of root innervation of the muscles of the lower limb.

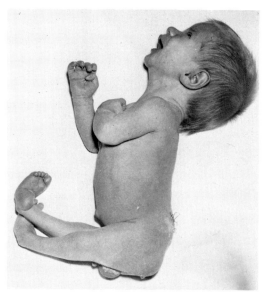

Fig. 4. Birth deformity in myelomeningocele. The hip flexors, adductors, quadriceps and tibialis anterior were all active and other muscles were paralyzed. The deformity corresponds to the paralytic pattern.

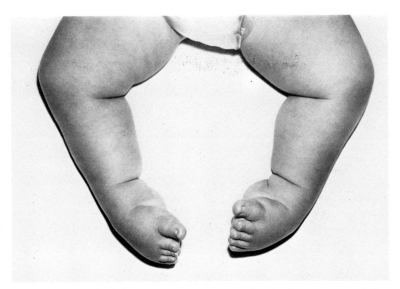

Fig. 5. Lower limb deformity at one year. At birth there was no deformity. Reflex activity in the hip, knee and ankle flexors has resulted in severe fixed deformity.

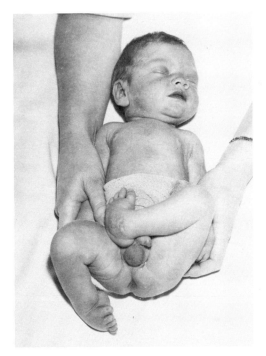

Fig. 6. Congenital talipes equino-varus at birth in a well innervated child. The deformity is a true congenital deformity, not related to the pattern of paralysis.

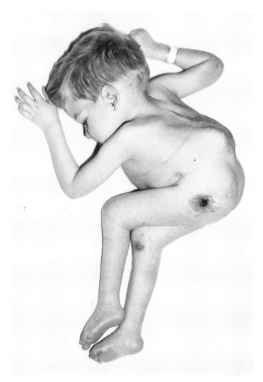

Fig. 7. Ulcers over the trochanter and knee in paraplegic myelomeningocele.

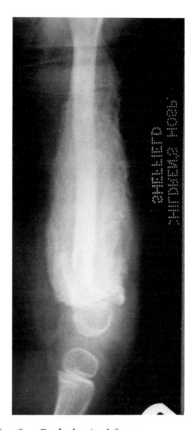

Fig. 8. Pathological fracture-separation of the lower femoral epiphysis in myelomeningocele. Extensive callus has formed within a week.

An Orthopedist's View of Bracing

N. Carroll, M.D., BSc, F.R.C.S.(C)

PRESENT STATUS - FUTURE GOALS

All spina bifida children should have functional goals
established for them; these will vary with the severity of
the motor and sensory deficit, and with the child's developmental threshold. In order to do this, it is convenient to
group them into four neurosegmental levels: thoracic, upper-
lumbar, lower-lumbar, and sacral. These children tend to be
delayed in their motor development. The major developmental
landmarks are head control, creeping, upright stance, and
upright mobility.[1]

The spina bifida child should be raised in an intellectual and physically-challenging environment. They, like all
children, benefit from a sense of achievement. Mobility is
essential in order to attain social maturation, educational,
vocational, and avocational goals.

Our recent study of 68 spina bifida children aged 12
and over found that eventual ambulatory status was primarily
dependent upon the neurosegmental level of the lesion, the
motor power within a given neurosegmental level, the extent
and degree of the orthopedic deformities, the age and stature
of the patient, the design and effectiveness of the orthosis,
intelligence, motivation, spasticity, obesity, and possibly
the sex of the child.

Goal-orientated programming requires a coordinated team effort, of which the patient is the most important member.[1]

MAJOR DEVELOPMENTAL LANDMARKS

Birth to head control. The goals are to correct deformities, to avoid contractures, to encourage development through mobility, and to protect anesthetic skin.[1]

Head control to creeping. The goals are to encourage sitting balance, prevent deformities, protect anesthetic skin, encourage the bilateral use of the hands, improve eye-hand coordination, improve upper-limb strength, expand environmental horizons, and mobility.[1]

Upright stance and mobility. Ambulation can be divided into four catagories. 1) Non-ambulators. These patients are wheelchair-bound, but can usually transfer from chair to bed. 2) Non-functional ambulators. Wheelchairs are used for transportation; however, therapy sessions of walking are done at home, in school, or in the hospital. 3) Household ambulators. These patients walk only indoors and with an apparatus; they are able to get in and out of their chair and bed with little, if any, assistance. They may use the wheelchair for some indoor activities at home and school, and for all community activities. 4) Community ambulators. These patients walk for most of their activities, and may need crutches and/or braces. A wheelchair is used for long trips only.[2]

NEUROSEGMENTAL LEVELS

Thoracic. The goals for these children are good sitting balance, ambulation at least during the first decade, ability to transfer from chair, wheelchair propulsion, self-care, social acceptability, schooling, access to environment. As an adult, the patient should learn to drive an automobile.[1]

Upper-lumbar. The goals are similar to those of the
thoracic neurosegmental level. However, it is desirable that
such a child learn to be a household ambulator.

Lower-lumbar. The aim is to make him a community
ambulator. He should be capable of standing without crutches;
practise self-care; go to a regular school; and be motivated
to be self-reliant.

Sacral. This child should be a community ambulator
with minimal bracing. The spina bifida program at the
Ontario Centre for Crippled Children comprises a preschool
parent information class, a combined spina bifida clinic, and
a spina bifida orthotic clinic. In the preschool group,
parents are shown how to avoid contractures, to encourage
development through mobility, and to protect anesthetic skin.
The combined spina bifida clinic has a neurosurgeon, an
orthopedist, and a urologist in attendance. The spina bifida
orthotic clinic is attended by an orthopaedic surgeon, an
orthotist, orthotic technicians, physiotherapists, occupational therapists, nurses, and social workers. The child is
presented at the orthotic clinic when it is felt that an
orthosis will help the child achieve the next developmental
threshold. Most of the children are 10 to 18 months old.
The child's specific functional loss is determined, goals are
established for the present and future, and decisions are
made as to the role of physiotherapy and/or surgery, and the
design of the orthoses.

ORTHOSES

A child with a thoracic or upper-lumbar lesion may have
difficulty in dragging himself from one place to another.
Therefore, we frequently prescribe a pre-bracing mobility aid

called a <u>Caster Cart</u>.[3]   The Caster Cart enables the child to move about and explore his environment; and he learns to use his hands to manipulate the wheels. His skin is protected.

When a child with a thoracic or upper-lumbar neuro-segmental level is frustrated with sitting and wants to stand, we prescribe a <u>Standing Brace</u>.[3] This is an inexpensive, pre-fabricated orthosis that allows an upright stance without delays. It is made of a tubular frame onto which parts are rivetted. The fitting can be completed in less than 2 hours, and the patient can stand and move without crutches by pivoting. Crutches can be used to achieve a swing-to or swing-through gait. As a preliminary device it enables the clinic team to assess the child in standing.

We believe that these children should stand and walk, even if later in life they will give up their orthosis for a wheelchair. When standing their lower limbs are less osteopotic and they have fewer fractures, better bladder drainage, improved bowel function, their cardiovascular system is stimulated by the increased physical activity, and upper-limb strength is increased.

Some children with an upper-lumbar neurosegmental have been fitted with a <u>Reciprocating Gait Brace</u>.[3] This device, by means of a gearbox, harnesses the power of the hip flexors on one side to produce hip extension on the opposite side. With the assistance of crutches, a reciprocal gait is possible by activating one hip flexor at a time. Swing-through gait is achieved by activating both hip flexors at the same time to keep the legs rigid. This brace is aligned so that it allows crutchless standing. It is hoped that dynamic stretching of the hip flexors will prevent progres-sive hip flexion contractures. However, we have experienced gearbox maintenance problems with this orthosis.

Children with total paraplegia (i.e., thoracic neurosegmental level) progress from the standing brace to a
Parapodium;[3] this device supports the spine while sitting
and standing. It is aligned so that the child can stand
without crutches; and with crutches the child is usually
capable of a swing-to or swing-through gait. The parapodium
is constructed from a prefabricated kit which is stable,
lightweight, adjustable for growth, easy to assemble, align,
and maintain. With the parapodium, the shoe is part of the
child, not part of the brace. Crutchless walking can be
achieved by attaching a pivot-walker or swivel-walker plat-
form to the footplate. Special-purpose attachments can be
designed and mounted easily. Crutchless standing makes it
easier for the paraplegic child to engage in activities such
as tossing a ball, dialing a telephone, reading a book while
standing, opening a bottle, or pounding a nail at a workbench.

In the last couple of years we have been making more and
more of polypropylene. Almost all our children with instability of the ankle-foot complex wear a vacuum-formed
polypropylene insert.[3] If knee stability is a problem, a
polypropylene insert can be attached with side hinges to a
polypropylene thigh support.

BRACING THE SPINE

Bracing the spine of a child with myelomeningocele is an
unresolved problem in orthotics; this results from the many
causes of the deformity. The three deformities encountered
are scoliosis, kyphosis, and lordosis; these can occur
singularly or in almost any combination. Spinal braces are
often used only as a temporary device, as surgery is
necessary to completely control the deformity.

There are many structural problems with the spine's "foundation", "super-structure", and "walls and insulation". Problems that can occur with the foundation are sacral agenesis, and pelvic obliquity which can be due to muscle imbalance, hip instability, or a leg-length inequality. Also, the size of the pelvis makes it difficult to secure a grip with a brace. Super-structure problems include deficient pedicles, laminae and dorsal spinous processes, hemi verte-brae, congenital unsegmented bars, fused ribs, muscle weakness, muscle spasticity, diastematomyelia and tethered cords. Wall and insulation problems include scarred skin, insensitive skin, and either too much or too little sub-cutaneous tissue.

Scoliosis. We have tried to control scoliosis in neonates with trough beds, and corsets that exert a three-point pressure system. However, the corset has occasionally led to hip dysplasia on the concave side of the curve. It is difficult to get a good three-point pressure system because the pelvis is small and there is often too much subcutaneous tissue overlying the ribs. Thermo-plastic jackets have been prescribed for older children.

Kyphosis. Children with kyphosis are often given a bucket insert which can be used for sitting in a chair or when riding in a Caster Cart. This device provides enough support to free the hands for actions other than maintaining balance, and protects the skin over the kyphosis. When a standing position is desirable, a back panel is constructed for use with the standing brace or parapodium.

Older children with scoliosis or lordosis who are non-walkers, often have modifications made to their wheelchairs; a sling-suspension system, which takes weight on the rib cage, is used to control the spinal position   and   relieve   buttock   pressure.

Lordosis. The commonest cause for lumbar lordosis is
severe hip-flexion deformities. When these are corrected,
better spinal alignment can be achieved with a polypropyline
jacket that grips the pelvis and rib cage posteriorly, and
has a wide band of webbing anteriorly.

A Milwaukee brace is rarely prescribed for a deformed
myelomeningocele spine.

Unfortunately, we must accept the fact that we frequently
encounter deformities caused by congenital bars, spasticity,
or severe muscle weakness; therefore, the control of these
deformities by an orthotic device is impossible.

DISCUSSION

We have listed the goals for children with varying
neurosegmental levels. How often are these goals attained?
Our recent study found that in their second and third decades,
53% of children with a sacral neurosegmental level are
community walkers; 30% with a lower-lumbar level are
community walkers; 10% with an upper-lumbar level are
community walkers; and no children with a thoracic level are
community ambulators. This is a great challenge for the
future - not to have these children ambulate during the first
decade only - but to continue to do so as an adult.

An important factor in determining ambulatory status
is the extent and degree of the orthopedic deformities in the
spina bifida child. Therefore, it is incumbent on the
orthopedic surgeon to have the spine balanced over the pelvis
and hip; the hip balanced over the knee; and the knee
balanced over the plantigrade foot. Orthotic devices must
be effective, comfortable, lightweight, low-cost, durable,
cosmetically acceptable, easy to manufacture, easy to

maintain and adjust for growth, easy to apply and remove;
they must not impede any of the activities of daily living,[3]
and they should not produce another deformity.

Through research we must develop a means of avoiding
abduction, flexion and external rotation contractures of the
hip, while still maintaining a position favoring hip
stability. We need more efficient, less cumbersome, trunk
supports. Presently, good multi-axial hip joints are not
available. We must develop a means of maintaining direc-
tional stability for limbs that are in below-knee braces.

Another important factor in determining ambulatory
status is the age and stature of the patient. We do not yet
have a good method of getting a tall, heavy paraplegic from
a sitting to standing position. We must assess the feasibility of externally-powered braces for ambulation. We need
suitable stair-climbing aids. Architectural changes are
necessary to make mobility easier within the community.

Orthotic devices used in the research and development
stage at the Ontario Centre for Crippled Children are
Plastisote shoes to protect deformed insensate feet; anterior
vacuum formed polypropylene below knee ankle-foot orthoses;
curb-climbing wheelchairs to increase mobility; a stand-up
wheelchair to enable a non-ambulator to assume and maintain
a standing position; and lightweight electric wheelchairs
that can be easily dismantled for transportation in the trunk
of an automobile; and urine collection devices.

If we are to meet orthotic challenges presented by spina
bifida children, we need total mobilization of medical,
paramedical, engineering, community, and state resources.

REFERENCES

1. National Academy of Sciences Report 1973.   The Child
    with an Orthopaedic Disability - His Orthotic Needs and
    How to Meet Them.
2. Hoffer, M.M. et al.:   Functional ambulation in patients
    with myelomeningocele.   *J. Bone Joint Surg., 55A (1)*:
    137, 1973.
3. Carroll, N.:   The orthotic management of the spina bifida
    child.   *Clinical Orthopaedics and Related Research, 102*:
    108, 1974.

CARE OF THE FLEXIBLE FOOT IN INFANTS
AND YOUNGER CHILDREN WITH
MYELODYSPLASIA

John F. Raycroft, M.D.

In myelodysplastic children with a potential for
standing, plantigrade and flexible feet are a necessity.[7] If
a child's feet are not so, great difficulty with shoe fitting
and bracing will be encountered. With growth, the feet will
deform. Repeated pressure sores, chronic infection and
progressive difficulty with balance and walking will result.
Many who have had potential for community ambulation will
become wheelchair dependent. Repeated surgical debridement
and, in a few cases amputation,[5] will be required for the
treatment of chronic osteomyelitis.[6] To forestall this
sequence, accurate diagnosis should be made, followed by
appropriate treatment and protective bracing.

DIAGNOSIS

Diagnosis is primarily a question of determining which
muscles that insert on the foot are innervated, as well as
their relative strengths. This delineation of the paralytic
pattern aids in predicting eventual deformity. The principal
diagnostic tool is physical examination. Farradic stimulation has been helpful in disclosing subclinical levels of
spasticity. Electromyography has not been of help.

In addition to identification of the paralytic pattern

it is also necessary to describe the resting position of the
foot (i.e., varus, calcaneous, etc.) and to indicate whether
spasticity is present. With this diagnostic information, it
is possible to design a logical treatment program.

TREATMENT

Again, it should be emphasized that the goal of treatment is to obtain a plantigrade, flexible foot. It is
fortunate that essentially all myelodysplastic feet are
initially flexible, that is, if motion is restricted it is
due to contracted muscles. One of the few exceptions is the
foot that is arthrogrypotic both in appearance and in
response to treatment. This latter group will be discussed
elsewhere in this symposium.

PRINCIPLES

The basic treatment principle to be followed is that
balance, both anterior to posterior and medial to lateral,
must be obtained with the foot at rest. Then balance must
be maintained by bracing against the deforming forces of
weight bearing. In a totally paralyzed, flaccid foot,
balance is obviously present so that only bracing is necessary. With muscle imbalance present, bracing alone will be
unable to control the foot. Tenotomy provides only temporary
correction and deformity will soon occur. Therefore, tendon
transfer is necessary to remove the deforming forces and to
restore balance. The tendons to be transferred will vary
with the paralytic pattern and with the preference of the
surgeon.[4,5,7]

GUIDELINES

In the past ten years, more than 200 children with foot
and ankle paralysis have been cared for in the Myelomeningocele Clinic at Newington Children's Hospital. From this

experience it has been possible to develop guidelines for
both conservative and surgical treatment of flexible feet.

1)   Tendon transfers to balance feet should be delayed
until the child is able to stand for several hours a day,
usually at about 2 years of age. Balance will never be
precise and this weight bearing is of great help in minimi-
zing error and in preventing recurrence of deformity.

2)   Plaster casting can be used to obtain a plantigrade
foot position both in the flaccid and in the partially
innervated foot. In the latter, the deformity will recur,
but a real benefit of delaying more radical treatment can be
gained. Casts must be applied with great care to avoid
pressure sores.

3)   In the performance of tendon transfer surgery:
- Medial and lateral deforming and potentially
deforming forces should be brought to the midline.
- Anterior and posterior deforming and potentially
deforming forces should be balanced as closely as
possible. Posterior strength should always be at
least slightly greater to prevent drift into the
disastrous calcaneous position.[4] If only one active
muscle is present, it should be acting posteriorly.
An important modifier of this surgical approach is that the
posterior tibial tendon should be transferred only with the
greatest caution even when it appears to be a deforming
force. Loss of this major checkrein to eversion will
frequently cause the foot to swing insidiously to a valgus
position - often uncontrollable by bracing. Lengthening of
the posterior tibial tendon is much safer in most instances.

4)   Spasticity sharply decreases the chances of
obtaining balance, and expectations should be minimal.

5)   Protective bracing is indicated to maintain
surgical gains until skeletal maturity.

Our adherence to these principles and guidelines has
resulted in increasing success in maintaining flexibility
and in obtaining plantigrade feet.   However, rarely does a
single operation achieve one's goal.   Inaccuracy in surgical
balancing and continuing growth will compromise results and
often leads to at least one subsequent procedure.

PES CONVEX VALGUS

Pes convex valgus, or paralytic vertical talus, is one
specific pattern which is markedly different.   Although the
goal of obtaining balance is the same, it cannot be treated
according to the guidelines listed above.   This foot, though
minimally involved paralytically, is dramatically deformed.
Paralysis usually is limited to the intrinsic and posterior
tibial muscles.[3]   Casting is of little value and surgery may
have to be considered early.   Several surgical procedures
used successfully have in common the restoration of normal
bony anatomy and the reinforcement of the posterior tibial
tendon.[1,8]   Bracing, including support of the arch, is again
required until skeletal maturity.

SUMMARY

The proper treatment of flexible feet in the myelomeningocele first requires accurate diagnosis and, secondly,
the proper combination of conservative and surgical techniques to gain the goal of plantigrade position and to maintain
flexibility.   Guidelines for treatment based on ten years'
experience with more than 200 feet are discussed.

REFERENCES

1. Coleman, S.S., Stelling, F.H. III and Jarrett, J.:
    Pathomechanics and treatment of congenital vertical
    talus. *Clin. Orthop., 70*:62, 1970.

2. Duckworth, T. and Smith, T.W.D.: The treatment of
    paralytic convex pes valgus. *J. Bone Joint Surg., 56B*:
    305, 1974.

3. Drennan, J.C. and Sharrard, W.J.W.: The pathological
    anatomy of convex pes valgus. *J. Bone Joint Surg., 53B*:
    455, 1971.

4. Handelsman, J.: Management of paralytic calcaneus
    deformity of the foot. *J. Bone Joint Surg., 55B*:438,
    1973.

5. Hayes, J.T., Gross, H.P. and Dow, S.: Surgery for
    paralytic defects secondary to myelomeningocele and
    myelodysplasia. *J. Bone Joint Surg., 46A*:1577, 1964.

6. Hogshead, H.P.: Management of the anesthetic, paralytic
    foot in patients with myelodysplasia. *J. Bone Joint
    Surg., 48A*:1016, 1966.

7. Sharrard, W.J.W. and Grosfield, I.: The management of
    deformity paralysis of the foot in myelomeningocele.
    J. Bone Joint Surg., 50B:456, 1968.

8. Walker, G.F. and Cheong-Leen, P.: The surgical
    management of paralytic vertical talus in myelomeningo-
    cele. *J. Bone Joint Surg.. 55B*:876, 1973.

SPLIT TRICEPS TRANSFER FOR
RECURRENT EQUINUS

Richard A. Jolson, M.D.

Perhaps the most common deformity seen in myelodysplasia
is equinus, either alone or accompanied by heel varus or
valgus. Simple heel cord lengthening, often associated with
posterior capsulotomy, usually suffices to make the foot
plantigrade. However, with continued growth, recurrence of
equinus is common. Recurrence may be secondary to inadequate
postoperative heel cord stretching, to inadequate postoperative bracing, or, as in many cases, to the failure to
recognize the spastic nature of the triceps surae muscle.
Unless spasticity is balanced, equinus usually recurs.

In the myelodysplastic foot and ankle it is imperative
to evaluate those muscle forces which cause deformity due to
their spasticity. The distorted and insensitive myelodysplastic foot cannot be braced adequately, nor can it bear
weight evenly. Since the phenomenon of spasticity causes
many types of foot deformities, certain principles must be
adhered to in order to obtain a balanced plantigrade foot.

PRINCIPLES OF SURGERY IN THE MYELODYSPLASTIC FOOT

1. Develop a balanced plantigrade foot by soft tissue
or bony release.

2. Maintain balance by tendon transfer of the active
controlled muscles.

427

3.   Neutralize spastic uncontrolled muscles by complete or split tendon transfers.

4.   Transfer tendons only after accomplishing a plantigrade foot.

5.   Maintain passive ankle motion.

6.   Maintain correction by bracing. Braces per se will not correct foot deformities.

7.   Casting either preparatory to surgery or for correction of deformity should be used with great care.

8.   Early weight bearing is important, therefore, early foot correction is necessary.

9.   The recognition of spastic muscles is of paramount importance to the eventual development of a plantigrade foot.

Foot deformities in the myelodysplastic child are seldom of positional etiology. Invariably such distortions are the product of muscle imbalance secondary to uneven neural distribution. It is not possible to equate the level of spinal paraplegia to lower extremity deformity because of the omnipresent possibility of some type of an intact reflex arc below the level of the spinal lesion leading to spasticity of certain muscle groups, often in a most irregular fashion. Thus, evaluation basically is by astute clinical examination. Treatment can not always be by rote according to the known or suspected spinal level.

SPASTIC EQUINUS

In the very young, equinus can usually be corrected surgically by simple heel cord lengthening. Often a subcutaneous approach will suffice. However, with recurrence of equinus one should suspect a spastic triceps muscle. This spasticity differs from that seen in cerebral palsy. Clonus is seldom noted. In cerebral palsy manual plantar dorsiflexion pressure will usually overcome the spasticity and allow the foot to relax into a dorsiflexed position. In the spastic equinus of myelodysplasia a rigid resistance is felt with attempts at passive stretch of the heel cord. The foot remains in fixed equinus. This spasticity is best described as a rigidity or contracture.

A typically rigid spastic equinus resists all passive attempts at dorsiflexion. The os calcis is fixed in an equinus position (Fig. 1). Often other motors innervated by the sacral segments, i.e., the long toes flexors, are similarly spastic (Fig. 2).

THE SPLIT TRICEPS TRANSFER

In order to balance the rigid triceps, the tendon and muscle is split longitudinally into equal medial and lateral halves. One half is detached from the os calcis and transferred anteriorly. The other half is split a second time and lengthened in the Z-plasty fashion. A posterior capsulotomy is necessary when passive dorsiflexion is still not possible.

TECHNIQUE

The patient is usually positioned supine if the hip and knee are supple enough to allow posterior visibility of the calf; if not, the lateral recumbent or prone position is used. A direct posterior longitudinal incision is made from the junction of the proximal and middle thirds of the calf to the os calcis (Fig. 3). The lower segment of the triceps muscle and tendo Achilles are split into equal longitudinal halves. One half is detached from the os calcis for anterior tendon transfer (Fig. 4). The remaining half is then lengthened by a long Z-plasty. A posterior ankle capsulotomy

is usually necessary. The foot is then brought into a
maximum dorsiflexed position (Fig. 5). The half to be
transferred is directed underneath the lengthened half and
brought subcutaneously to the appropriate dorsiflexor tendon
above the ankle. There is not sufficient length of tendon
in this particular transfer to permit insertion distal to the
ankle joint. Through a separate anterior incision, direct
side to side anastomosis of the transferred tendon is
performed.

Care must be taken to direct the transferred half
Achilles tendon as far distally as possible on the recipient
dorsiflexor tendon. This is accomplished by placing proximal
traction on the recipient dorsiflexor tendon, tightening the
foot into maximum dorsiflexion, and anastomosing in this taut
position.

For best results in the control of heel varus and valgus
it is important that in the transfer of the split tendo-
Achilles the correct half be directed anteriorward and in the
proper direction. If the hindfoot is in varus, the medial
half of the Achilles tendon is released, directed deep to the
lateral half, subcutaneously around the fibular side of the
ankle and into the extensor digitorum longus tendons.

Similarly if the heel is in valgus the lateral half of
the tendo Achilles is transferred around the tibial side of
the ankle into the tibialis anticus. It is important to
release the tendo Achilles from the side of the os calcis
that is pulled into either varus or valgus and then to transfer that particular half anteriorly and to the opposite side.
Thus a force contributing toward heel deformity is converted
into a corrective force quite similar to the plantarflexion -
dorsiflexion balance gained by the operation.

If the heel is in neutral position, the medial half

should be transferred directly through the interosseous membrane and sutured to all foot dorsiflexors as a unit. A long leg cast with slight knee flexion and maximum ankle dorsiflexion is applied. Some degree of knee flexion keeps the foot from slipping proximally into the cast.

From 1972 through 1975 14 transfers were performed in 10 patients. No further surgery for pure recurrent equinus has been necessary. Postoperatively, all patients have been maintained adequately by braces. X-rays reveal the preoperative equinus position (Fig. 6) and the postoperative restitution of the normal calcaneous alignment of the os calcis (Fig. 7).

Clinical results support the value of the surgery (Figs. 8 & 9). The following table illustrates a summation of our results (Fig. 10).

Mr. Sharrard has described a two-stage procedure for split triceps transfer. A routine lengthening is performed and 6 weeks later the tendon is split and transferred.

SUMMARY

The split triceps tendon transfer appears to be a worthwhile procedure for control of recurrent equinus secondary to a rigid triceps surae muscle in the myelodysplastic foot. By balancing the spastic muscles into equal plantar flexors and dorsiflexors, the foot is made plantigrade. Similarly some correction of heel varus and valgus is gained. At the time of split triceps transfer one often finds spasticity of the toe flexors. If it is present, these tendons are released proximal to the medial malleolus and transferred anteriorly with the split Achilles tendon.

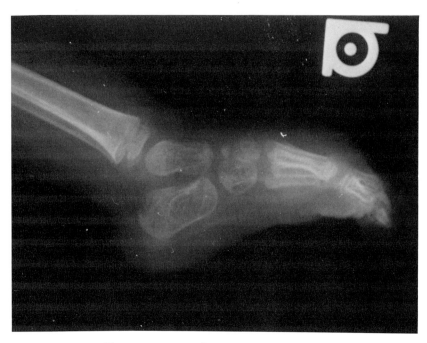

Fig. 1. X-rays of spastic equinus foot.

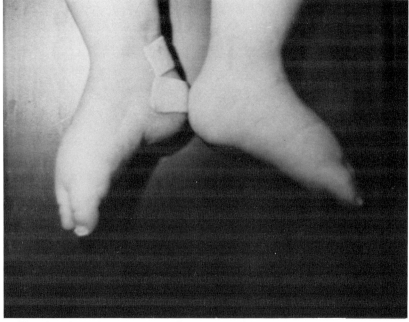

Fig. 2. Spastic equinus with associated long flexor toe spasticity.

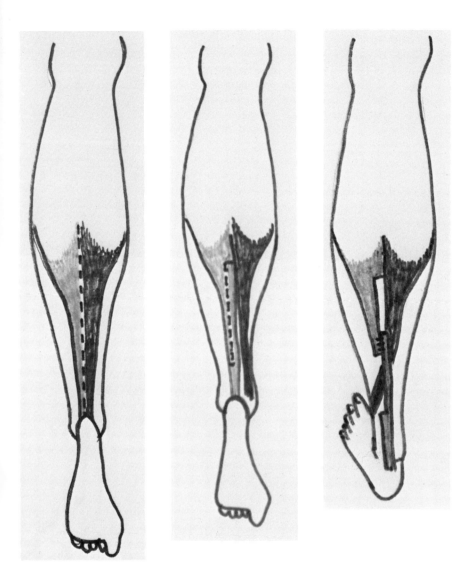

Fig. 3 (left).   Technique of split triceps transfer (STT). A longitudinal incision is made through the muscle and tendon.

Fig. 4 (middle).   Technique of STT. (cont.) One half is detached from the os calcis. The other half is lengthened by Z-plasty.

Fig. 5 (right).   Technique of STT. (cont.) Anterior transfer of one-half of the achilles tendon.

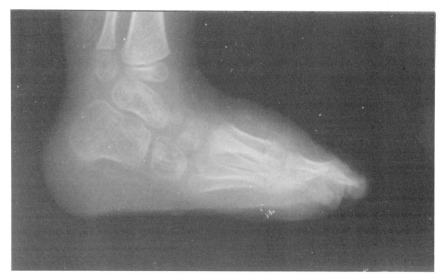

Fig. 6. Preoperative equinus, lateral view. The os calcis is in equinus.

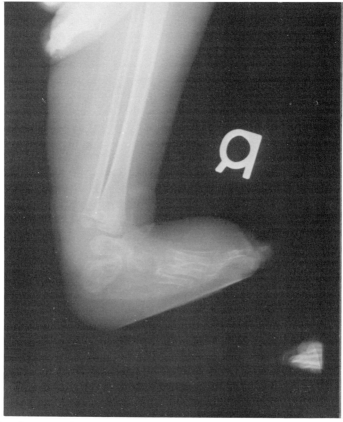

Fig. 7. Same patient as in Fig. 6—postoperative lateral view. The os calcis is now in calcaneus.

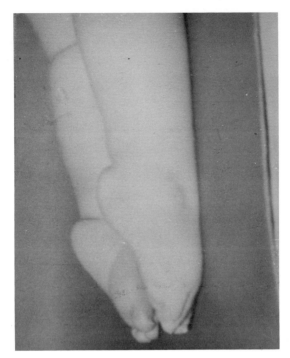

Fig. 8. Preoperative clinical picture.

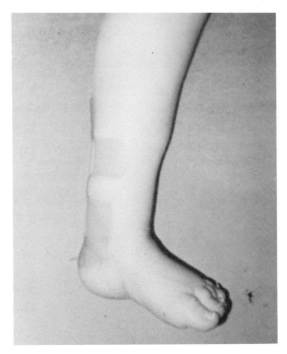

Fig. 9. Postoperative result.

Pt.	Surgery	Age	Side	TAL Prev. to STT (Months)	Follow-up (Months)	Recurrence Equinus
DW	11-17-75	2,0M	R	0	3	0
WW	04-04-72	1,0M	L	0	46	+*
	11-10-75	4,0M	R	0	3	0
SB	08-12-74	2,3M	L	+12	18	0
KC	11-25-74	8,4M	L	0	15	0
DC	06-18-72 Bilat.	3,5M	R	+15	44	0
			L	+23	44	0
TR	11-25-74	5,8M	R	+43	15	0
	03-15-73	4,1M	L	+24	35	0
SS	05-05-75	2,8M	R	0	9	0
JK	08-18-75	7,10M	R	0	6	0
CF	06-18-74 Bilat.	3,5M	R	+25	20	0
			L	+25	20	0
JR	07-15-74	5,7M	R	0	19	0

*Unrecognized spasticity of the posterior tibialis caused a later equinovarus deformity.

Fig. 10. Table of results of split triceps tendon surgery.

TALECTOMY: APPLICATION IN CHILDREN
WITH MYELODYSPLASIA

John F. Raycroft, M.D.

Excision of the talus has been advocated by several
authors in the treatment of the difficult, rigid, equinovarus
foot of the myelodysplastic child. Hogshead[2] considered it
a salvage procedure, while Sharrard and Grosfield[5] characterized it as a last resort. In contrast, Menelaus,[3] in
addition to salvage, noted broader indications. He felt that
in patients presenting late and with severe deformity, less
radical surgery was not necessarily a prerequisite.

At Newington Children's Hospital, two groups of feet
have been considered to be proper candidates for talectomy.
The first includes relapsed equinovarus feet that have been
subjected to one or more operative procedures. Previous
surgery has included medial release, posterior release, and
various tendon transfers. Relapse can be attributed to
incomplete correction, but the suspicion of low-grade,
undetected spasticity is always present. The second group
consists of the few equinovarus myelodysplastic feet so
arthrogrypotic in appearance and feel that it is possible to
predict that less radical surgery will be unsuccessful.
Rigidity, the inability to wear shoes, and persistent skin
ulceration are the common denominator of these severe
equinovarus   feet.   The   optimum   age   for   the

procedure   is   between   3   and   8   years.

TECHNIQUE

Talectomy in the myelodysplastic foot at Newington
Children's Hospital follows the technique developed here by
Dr. Burr H. Curtis. A curved incision is made along a line
extending from the lateral to the medial malleolus, crossing
the prominence of the tarsal navicular. Often it is necessary to use only the lateral two-thirds of this incision.
The extensor hallicus longus, extensor digitorus communis,
anterior tibial and peroneus tertius tendons are identified
and separated. The dorsalis pedis artery is identified and
preserved. Using the landmarks of the talonavicular joint
and the tibiotalar joint, sharp dissection around the talus
is begun. This is aided by drawing the forefoot into equinus
and adductus and subsequently by passing a large towel clip
around the neck of the talus to improve purchase. With care,
the bone can be delivered intact. Posterior remnants in some
cases have regenerated the body of the talus, resulting in
loss of good initial correction. The foot now must be
brought into plantigrade position, displaced posteriorly, and
rotated externally. The calcaneus must be in contact with
the articular surface of the tibia. This will bring the
navicula against the anterior lip of the tibia. In order to
achieve posterior displacement, the medial and lateral ankle
ligaments must be sectioned and the posterior ankle capsule
freed from the posterior tibia. If the gastro soleus tendon
is slack it does not need to be released and beneficial
stabilization results from its checkrein effect against
unlimited dorsiflexion. If tight, it must be sectioned. If
the foot will not move posteriorly with ease, the distal
tibiofibular syndesmosis should be opened. Additional space

in the ankle mortice can be obtained by reducing the inner aspects of both the medial and lateral malleoli. Occasionally it is necessary to remove a portion of the navicula to allow it to fit snugly against the anterior tibia.

With proper positioning obtained, three heavy Steinmann pins are inserted to fix the foot in the plantigrade, externally rotated position, and an above-knee cast is applied. The pins are left in place for six weeks and a weight-bearing cast is used for an additional six weeks. Following cast removal, a short leg, limited-ankle-motion brace is applied. Night splints are used and are continued until bony maturity. Residual adduction which occasionally is present can be corrected by midfoot wedge osteotomy. Carroll[1] has suggested excision of the cuboid at the time of talectomy to shorten the lateral border of the foot and resolve this problem in one step. We have had no experience with this approach.

In fifteen patients followed for more than three years, talectomy was found to be a satisfactory treatment for insensate, resistant equinovarus feet. Complications encountered included recurrent equinus and regeneration of the talus and were caused by technical errors or inadequate follow-up regarding bracing and splinting.

SUMMARY

As a salvage procedure in the repeatedly operated foot or as a primary procedure in the arthrogrypotic foot, talectomy can resolve equinovarus deformity and can provide the desired goal - a plantigrade, shoeable foot.

REFERENCES

1. Carroll, N.:   Personal communication.

2. Hogshead, H.P.:   Management of the anesthetic, paralytic
    foot in patients with myelodysplasia.   *J. Bone Joint
    Surg., 48A*:1016, 1966.

3. Menelaus, M.B.:   Talectomy for equinovarus deformity
    in arthrogryposis and spina bifida.   *J. Bone Joint Surg.,
    53B*:468, 1971.

4. Menelaus, M.B.:   The Orthopedic Management of Spina
    Bifida Cystica.   Edinburgh, E. & S. Livingstone, 1971.

5. Sharrard, W.J.W. and Grosfield, I.:   The management of
    deformity and paralysis of the foot in myelomeningocele.
    J. Bone Joint Surg., 50B:456, 1968.

HINDFOOT AND FOREFOOT VARUS

N. Carroll, M.D., BSc, F.R.C.S. (C)

Foot deformities in children with spina bifida are due to muscle weakness, muscle spasticity, and the postural effects of gravity. Weight-bearing on an unbalanced foot usually causes a progression of the deformity, and on an insensitive foot it often leads to skin breakdown. To classify forefoot and hindfoot varus, each deformity can be considered separately, and then combined. Varus or cavovarus deformities can occur in the forefoot; and varus and calcaneovarus deformities can occur in the hindfoot. A combination of forefoot and hindfoot varus is seen in neurogenic talipes equino varus.

At The Hospital for Sick Children, we initially treat these deformities by manipulations and plaster of paris casts. The skin is painted with Friar's Balsam and then carefully covered with cotton flannelette (making sure there are no wrinkles in the material). The plaster is carefully applied to maintain the position obtained by the manipulation. This procedure usually does not completely correct the deformity, but it allows easier management of the soft tissues during surgery. However, corrections have been obtained which can be maintained by a therapist.

FOREFOOT VARUS

If this persists (despite manipulations and plasters), a
medial release may be required between the ages of 6 months
and 4 years; after age 4, it is often necessary to shorten
the lateral border of the foot as well. The lateral border
can be shortened by enucleation of the cuboid, or by calcaneo-
cuboid fusion.

Cavovarus deformities are treated by release of the
plantar fascia and intrinsic muscles, progressing to a medial
release and tendon transfers. An older child with a severe
deformity may require a tarsal wedge osteotomy.

HINDFOOT VARUS

Isolated-heel varus is unusual in a child with spina
bifida. A lateral-closing-wedge osteotomy of the os calcis
is useful. If the heel is small, some correction can be
obtained by shifting the distal part of the calcaneus
laterally; thus, it is not necessary to remove as much bone.

Calcaneovarus deformities in very young children are
sometimes treated with plasters; and if a good plantigrade
position is obtained, it can be maintained with manipulations
and splints. Frequently, it will be necessary to transfer
the tibialis anterior through the interosseous membrane and
attach it to the lateral side of the os calcis where the
tendo achilis inserts. This should be delayed until the
child is 3 or 4 years old; there will then be enough contracture of the anterior capsule of the ankle so that an equinus
deformity will not occur following the muscle transfer. A
spastic muscle should never be transferred; it should be
sacrificed - it is easier to brace a flail foot than one
being deformed by a spastic muscle.

NEUROGENIC TALIPES EQUINOVARUS

This is treated initially by manipulations and plaster casts. Surgical correction is often necessary and is usually performed between age 4-6 months.

Anatomical studies of club feet have led us to conclude that, in addition to the tight tendons, capsules and ligaments the lateral malleolus is directed posteriorly, the head of the talus points laterally and the navicular is subluxed medially toward the medial malleolus. The head of the talus occupies the area that should be occupied by the front of the os calcis. The talus and os calcis are parallel; the equinus, and varus of the os calcis cannot be corrected until the talus is medially de-rotated. We have found that club feet assume a normal appearance after soft-tissue release, if the talus is rotated medially and the navicular is reduced onto the head of the talus.

OPERATIVE TECHNIQUE FOR NEUROGENIC TALIPES EQUINOVARUS

The infant is anesthetized and placed in a prone position; a tourniquet is applied to the thigh. An incision is made on the medial border of the foot, extending from the medial malleolus to the base of the first metatarsal. The abductor pollicis tendon is recessed; and, if tight, the plantar fascia is divided. The tibialis anterior tendon is identified and retracted. The flexor digitorum longus tendon is found behind the medial malleolus, and retracted to protect the neuro-vascular bundle. The tibialis posterior tendon is identified and freed from its sheath at the back of the medial malleolus; it is followed distally so that the navicular, which is completely cartilagenous in the infant under age 1, can be identified. The rather dense tissue between the navicular and the medial malleolus can then be

excised. To locate the head of the talus, dissection must
proceed in the long axis of the foot; if this is done
laterally, the joint between the navicular and the head of
the talus will be missed and the surgeon may cut into the
neck of the talus. If difficulties arise in identifying the
talo-navicular joint, the tibialis posterior tendon can be
divided in a Z fashion at the back of the leg, delivered into
the medial wound, and used to retract the navicular distally.
Once the talo-navicular joint is identified, the capsule is
divided completely, medially and superiorly. The dissection
is continued inferiorly until all the ligamentous structures
between the talus and the navicular are divided. In
addition, the tendinous slips of the tibialis posterior
running under the medial side of the tarsus are divided. It
is now obvious that the navicular is subluxated medially on
the head of the talus to lie close to the medial malleolus.

     A second incision is made along the lateral border of
the tendo achillis and dissection is carried deep. The sural
nerve is retracted laterally, and the tendo achillis is
lengthened by a Z plasty, and the medial portion is detached
distally from the os calcis. The heel is still in equinus
because the posterior capsule of the ankle joint is
contracted. The neurovascular bundle is identified and
freed; a long, thin, right-angled retractor can then be
placed in the posterior incision and out the medial incision
in such a way that the neurovascular bundle, flexor digitorum
longus tendon, and the tibialis posterior tendon lie anterior
to the retractor and are protected. After locating the
peroneal tendons on the lateral side of the ankle, the
posterior capsule of the ankle joint and the medial and
lateral ligaments of the ankle are divided. Next, the subtalar joint is opened posteriorly, medially and laterally.

The foot is dorsiflexed to a neutral position, the flexor hallucis longus, tibialis posterior, and flexor digitorum longus tendons are checked for tightness and lengthened, if necessary. It is always necessary to lengthen the flexor hallucis longus, by recession or Z plasty, and to lengthen or transpose the tibialis posterior tendon anterior to the medial malleolus.

The talus is now free to be rotated medially; this is done by placing a K-wire in the long axis of the talus from behind. After rotating the talus medially, the navicular is pushed laterally and fixed in position by advancing the K-wire through the head of the talus and across the talo-navicular joint. The foot now assumes a normal position. The bulge on the lateral side of the foot, formerly made by the head of the talus, has become an area of wrinkled skin. The foot is now at a 90 degree angle to the long axis of the leg; the forefoot no longer han s in an adducted position; and the varus of the heel is corrected.

The tendo achillis is resutured; the wounds are closed with intracutaneous Dexon sutures; the tourniquet is removed; and, if circulation is good, a bulky dressing applied. A snug plaster of paris cast is applied a week later, with the foot in the fully-corrected position.

During surgery, the significant incongruity between the talus and tibia, the talus and os calcis, and the talus and the navicular is obvious. The foot is kept in plaster for at least three months after surgery to allow for some remodelling of the cartilagenous surfaces. Later, the feet are protected by boots and splints.

The early results of this aggressive approach to a severe foot deformity have been very satisfactory.

PARALYTIC CALCANEUS IN
MYELOMENINGOCELE

Earl Feiwell, M.D.

Peabody, in 1949,[9] stated that paralytic calcaneus had
the potential for the highest grade ultimate structural
deformity of the paralytic foot, that it was the most difficult to correct by bone work, and that it was impossible to
hold by bracing.

The dropping of the heel into a more vertical position
alters the effect of the Achilles tendon attachment by dimini-
shing its leverage and thereby affecting the strength of pull.
This, however, is not a problem in the paralyzed individual
who does not have any posterior musculature and does not use
the normal push-off in gait. So why be concerned? Our concern is the structural deformity and its effect.

As is emphasized on many occasions, the plantar grade
foot is our goal in the myelomeningocele patient. With the
calcaneus deformity, the weight bearing surface is decreased
in length, thereby decreasing standing ability. The areas
of bony pressure become much more acute as the metatarsal
heads are pushed towards the surface of the forefoot. In
the insensitive foot this will lead to callosities and
ulcerations. The more vertical calcaneus also leads to a
concentration of pressure causing pressure necrosis following
prolonged weight bearing.

As Hay and Walker[3] demonstrated, ordinarily in myelomeningocele patients, greater pressures are placed on the
plantar surface of the foot than in normal children. They
assumed that this increased pressure was due to the smaller
feet in the myelomeningocele child thereby increasing the
pressure per unit of surface. Additionally, they demonstrated greater pressure on the hindfoot. If the calcaneus
is more vertical then the plantar surface will be even
smaller and greater pressure per square inch on the prominent
heel.

Other considerations adding increased pressure may be
the lack of motion in the knee and ankle which normally
reduce impact on foot strike and stance phase in ambulation.
This increase in weight bearing is more likely to lead to
ulcerations over prominent hard rigid areas of the foot as
the child grows older and thereby larger and heavier.

The foot deformity itself becomes a major problem in
fitting shoes. There is no posterior heel to help keep the
shoe on and when cavus is present, the dorsal prominence of
the mid-foot is difficult to accommodate. Additionally, if
cavus is present, clawing of the toes creates ulcerations
due to rubbing the shoe. Wearing of shoes is important, even
in the nonambulatory patient. The young lady who is confined
to a wheelchair is very proud to have a nice pair of shoes
protruding, her legs usually being covered by pants or long
dresses. On the more practical side, wearing of shoes in a
cold climate becomes a necessity. In regard to the functional
aspects, the lack of stability of the forefoot due to
increased incline of the foot and the lack of posterior
stability in gait cause knee flexion, leading to decreased
knee stability.

The cause of calcaneus is the imbalance of forces in the foot. The absence of the gastrocsoleus pull with the presence of dorsal musculature creates the deformity (Fig.1). The tibialis anterior is the prime deforming factor. The central portion of the foot is pulled upward and the os calcis downward. The metatarsal heads come closer to the calcaneus. The plantar fascia tightens. When short plantar muscles are active, either through voluntary or involuntary contractions, marked cavus results. Any other active force in the foot creates additional deformity, such as calcaneus valgus when the extensor digitorum longus is active, peroneus tertius or peroneus longus and brevis; calcaneal varus occurs when posterior tibial or toe flexors are also active.[8]

The L4 and L5 level lesions classically produce this problem in that the anterior tibialis is functioning, being the highest level of muscle innervation going to the foot, and no gastrocsoleus innervation is present.

Treatment consists of removing the deforming forces. Rather than discard a functioning tendon it is transferred to the heel to provide posterior stability to the ankle, as well as help correct the existing deformity.

The technique consists of removal of the anterior tibialis attachment from the dorsum of the foot and passing it posteriorly through the interosseous membrane to the calcaneus. Peabody describes this procedure and his results in the 1949 Academy of Orthopaedic Surgeons instructural course lectures for paralytic deformities.[9]

Westin, in his lecture in the 1965 series, accurately describes the principles of surgery of tendon transfer and his results in poliomyelitis patients.[15]

Campbell's Operative Orthopaedics gives an excellent detailed description of the procedure itself. The tendon is

released at its most distal insertion obtaining the most
maximum length possible through a medial longitudinal incision at the first cuneiform. The tendon is then brought up
through an incision in the anterior compartment at the
middle third of the leg. Dissection is carried out over the
interosseous membrane. An adequate window or flap is cut,
the muscle is passed through the opening and down bluntly
to an incision at the heel. Care is taken with the interosseous membrane to avoid a tight opening or free margins from
squeezing the muscle belly. The tendon should be distal to
the foramen. The tendon is reattached through a drill hole
in the posterior calcaneus and is tied over a well-padded
button on the medial plantar surface of the heel. Different
techniques, however, have been used by surgeons, including
splitting the Achilles tendon and actually suturing the
anterior tibialis tendon to the bone itself. This avoids
the problem of pressure ulcers which can occur beneath the
button despite all precautions of padding. Drill holes
through the apophysis have not been found to be a problem in
regard to future growth or development of the heel.[15]

Post operatively, the ankle is placed in 20 degrees of
equinus. If the anterior tibial tendon has been considerably
shortened by the dorsiflexed position of the foot and it
cannot reach to the calcaneus itself, then the tendon is
sutured to the Achilles tendon. Excessive equinus is avoided.

Immobilization is carried out for six weeks in a cast,
preferably the first two weeks in a long leg cast (which we
splint anterolaterally), then a short leg cast is substi-
tuted. Bracing is then carried out in 15 degrees to 20
degrees of equinus with gradual stretching to neutral over
the next six months. A light rocker bottom sole is used to
spread the pressure over the plantar surface of the foot and

allow for better walking. It is important that the equinus
position not persist and that the foot is stretched about
5 degrees past the neutral position. The equinus position
of the ankle can lead to excessive pressures on the metatarsal heads and knee recurvatum and force hip flexion during
stance. Slight equinus or even neutral position will
significantly affect the gait.

Perry points out in her excellent article on kinesiology
of the lower extremity bracing that plantar flexion of 15
degrees will push the center of gravity backward as the knee
is pushed into extension.[10] The patient who ambulates without crutches must have added impetus to come forward over
the end of the flat rigid sole and will tend to vault over
the foot, consequently increasing the tendency to trip and
fall. Forward flexion of the hips and trunk must be utilized
just to maintain the center of gravity over the weight bearing area.

The child who compensates for hip flexion contractures
by slight flexion of the knee has a greater difficulty with
balancing as the trunk is flexed and the center of gravity
is far forward. Crutches are required to maintain balance.
The ankle, fixed in neutral, will have a definite effect
on the gait of the child with hip flexion contracture who
depends on slight knee flexion and ankle dorsiflexion for
maintenance of balance. It is extremely important that a
permanent equinus position be avoided and that some dorsiflexion motion be obtained ultimately.

The surgical result may be compromised to achieve this
end. That is, insertion of the tendon under less tension
than one would desire in order to have maximum strength of
transferred muscle.

Crutches may be consistently required in the child who previously went without crutches in the house. This should be explained to the parent preoperatively so that discouragement of the program does not occur. People love to see good results by seeing their child walk better after surgery, but in surgical corrections in which we are carrying out procedures to prevent future deformities, there is frequently some setback in their previous physical program. It is for this reason that we must be sure that the procedure we are doing has a good likelihood of success.

The maximum that we can anticipate from this surgical procedure is good strength to manual testing,[15] but poor for rising on his toes. Most of our patients do not have normal strength of the anterior tibialis preoperatively and even good strength to manual testing is not achieved.

Our primary goal in the myelomeningocele is to attain correction of the calcaneus position. This operation is successful in preventing deformity and ataining correction in the younger child. Menalaus, in his report on 51 cases, felt that the calcaneus was corrected, but additional procedures were not indicated to correct valgus or varus deformities.[8] Seventeen feet became valgus when weight bearing and required subtalar arthrodesis. Five feet required transfer of the peronei to the heel or division of the peronei. Sharrard's 62 cases reported, had a 20 percent failure rate in providing a plantar grade foot; this apparently also being due to the occurrence of valgus or varus after anterior tibial transfer.[13]

Calcaneovalgus is present when muscles are present about the dorsal and lateral aspects of the foot. The long toe extensors and peroneus tertius are a frequent source in the L5 level patient. If present, these should be transferred through the interosseous membrane to the heel along with the tibialis anticus. Attempting to balance the foot by transferring these tendons to the mid-dorsum of the foot may be performed; however, failure is encountered if spasticity is present or if the tibialis anticus transfer has lost considerable strength, whereas the dorsal musculature has maintained greater strength. If the dorsolateral muscles are weak, a simple sectioning can be done at the time of the Peabody procedure.[8]

Calcaneovarus can be associated with an active posterior tibial muscle or functioning long toe flexors. These may be voluntary or involuntary. These tendons should be transferred to the heel.[8]

At times, no functioning muscle is found and it is assumed that intrauterine position has caused the varus position. A plantar medial release is indicated, along with the anterior tibial transfer.[13]

If all structures are weak but causing deformity, simple sectioning can be carried out. Transferring weak muscles to the heel and performing an Achilles tenodesis has been effective[5-8] in correcting the deformity.

Surgery is preferably performed before significant fixed bony deformity occurs. We prefer carrying this out between the ages one to two years as the structures are large enough and adequate observation of muscles has been performed. Faradic stimulation to determine muscle function as recommended by Sharrard is being performed.[13] In using faradic stimulation we can determine which muscles are voluntary or involuntary; however, this is not important in that either causes deformity and requires removal. Similarly, both will cause a stabilizing effect on the heel. A determination of relative strength can also be made by stimulation.

A good follow-up program is necessary in these children.
Placing the child in too much equinus postoperatively and not
following through with an adequate stretching program or
simply performing the procedure on a child who is nonweight
bearing and not obtaining the adequate follow-up can lead to
significant problems. In addition, unrecognized active
musculature can result in future deformity and require
additional surgical treatment.[8]

A two-year-old child had a transfer of the tibialis
anticus and peronei at seven months of age for calcaneus
feet, fitted in braces for protection, and was subsequently
lost to follow-up. She was then seen in our clinic at just
under two years of age with severe equinovarus deformities
of both feet. Complete posterior medial and plantar releases
were necessary, along with lengthening of the posterior
tendons. The deformity was so great on the right that it
was necessary to swing a dorsal flap to close the posteromedial portion of the incision due to the marked bony correction postoperatively preventing closure of the wound.

A tight calcaneus deformity at an early age can be
casted gently in a well padded cast to obtain some correction
before transfer. Gradually taking up the slack and holding
the foot in the position in which it can be readily placed
has been successful without complications. Changing the
cast every two weeks is necessary.

If the skin is excessively tight and the foot cannot
be placed in equinus at the time of transfer, a Z-plasty or
lengthening with a Z-Y repair as performed by Sharrard may
be performed.[12] The latter leaves a more transverse scar
which we prefer to avoid. Vertical incisions are used on
these feet wherever possible in order to avoid occurrences
of circumferential scarring. These children frequently

require multiple procedures throughout their childhood
beginning with medial transverse incisions for medial released and ending with lateral incisions for subtalar fusion
or triple arthrodeses. Stasis ulcerations can result in the
adult.

In situations in which calcaneus deformity is occurring
but the anterior tibialis is weak and is balanced by both
posterior tibialis and peronei, an Achilles tenodesis can
be performed with the transfer.[5-8] This procedure was
described by Gallie and his subsequent results in poliomyelitis were reported in 1916.[2] Jacobs reported his results
in 1966 in poliomyelitis patients.[4] His procedure had been
used on many patients with poliomyelitis in our institution
with satisfactory success. We attempted to use this in four
myelomeningocele patients to counter balance the dorsiflexor
of the foot. However, these were doomed to failure and
required revisions, since an active tendon force will tend
to stretch the opposing tenodesis. Success is achieved in
a patient who has weak dorsiflexors, by transfers to the
heels in conjunction with an Achilles tenodesis.

The procedure is performed by a posteromedial incision
approximately 2 inches in length beginning at the musculo-
tendinous junction of the Achilles tendon and extending
distalward. The tendon may be split and drill holes made
suturing the tendon through on itself as described by Jacobs,
or sutured to the bone. Westin has tenodesed the Achilles
tendon to the fibula through a posterolateral incision
providing stimulation for growth of the distal fibula as
well as providing a tenodesis effect on the heel.[5] This
procedure should be carried out only in the immature foot,
preferably between ages four and ten.

Plantar fasciotomies should be performed subsequent to this procedure in approximately three to six months. Any other procedures for correction of cavus foot should also be performed at that time.[5] This then allows for an effective force holding the heel while the mid-foot is dorsiflexed. Cast pressure, however, is not utilized to maintain the corrected position, for even with a plantar fascial and ligamentous release for cavus correction, or with wedge osteotomy, postoperative pinning is used to avoid the need for cast pressure. Casting is then used as only a protective device.

In the older child with an immature foot and a marked calcaneal deformity, calcaneal osteotomy as described by Samilson, along with plantar fasciotomy and tendon transfer can be selected.[11] In this procedure the osteotomy is made through a 1½ inch posterolateral incision at the calcaneus and a crescent-shaped osteotomy posterior to the subtalar joint. Plantar fasciotomy is carried out and the posterior portion of the calcaneus is moved superiorly and either stapled or pinned. The crescent osteotomy allows for repositioning of the tuber of the calcaneus, lengthens the heel and still provides for ready healing postoperatively.

Open wedge osteotomies as described by Lipscomb are less likely to be satisfactory in insensitive feet.[6]

Weight bearing postoperatively should be avoided until the calcaneus is united and the pin removed. Six weeks is a satisfactory period of time.

Stabilization of the foot is frequently indicated due to uncontrolled varus or valgus. Subtalar arthrodesis has not been a satisfactory procedure in our hands in correcting valgus deformity. Even with a well-stabilized subtalar joint, the valgus persists and appears to be due to deformity within

the ankle joint. Some improvement, however, from stabilization is seen, and at a later date, a distal tibial osteotomy
may be performed to provide the additional improvement of
position.[14]

Triple arthrodesis is performed when the foot is
sufficiently matured at age 12 to 14. Feet in myelomeningocele are generally smaller than normal and therefore, an
early triple arthrodesis is utilized. Weight bearing is
avoided until union is achieved since these insensitive feet
fuse more slowly and a nonunion is more likely to occur if
weight bearing is begun at the same time one normally would
allow it in a foot with sensibility. Delayed and nonunions
are much more frequent in the insensitive foot, and when
allowed to persist can lead to Charcot joints.

Prior to the performance of a triple arthrodesis, one
should determine the presence of a normal ankle joint. The
few Charcot ankle joints I have seen occurred in those ankles
with flattened tali that had been present prior to the triple
arthrodesis. If the ankle joint is poor, it would seem that
a talectomy would be the procedure of choice.

Talectomy is a satisfactory procedure for correcting
marked calcaneal varus deformities,[7-13-16] particularly when
accompanied by appropriate soft tissue releases about the
medial and plantar aspect of the foot. Postoperatively, the
calcaneus is pinned in the desired position.

In summary, it can be said that paralytic calcaneus
foot deformity is due to absence of the gastrocsoleus and
the presence of functioning dorsiflexors. The primary
deforming tendon in the L4 and L5 level patient is the
tibialis anticus. The primary treatment, therefore, is
transfer of the tibialis anticus to the heel. In the
presence of other extensor tendons which may cause

progressive valgus position, these are also transferred to
the calcaneus. In the presence of weak extensor tendons,
a simple sectioning may be performed or they may be transferred to the heel along with an Achilles tenodesis to the
fibula.

Calcaneal osteotomy with soft tissue releases may be
utilized in the older immature foot with deformity along
with tendon transfer, or may be associated with a triple
arthrodesis. The latter is used only in the mature foot.
Talectomy is used for severe deformities.

REFERENCES

1. Crenshaw, A.H.: Campbell's Operative Orthopedics.
    St. Louis, C.V. Mosby Co., 1971.
2. Gallie, W.E.: Tendon fixation in infantile paralysis:
    A review of 150 operations. *Am. J. Orthop. Surg., 14*:
    18, 1916.
3. Hay M. and Walker, G.: Plantar pressures in healthy
    children and in children with myelomeningocele. *J. Bone
    Joint Surg., 55B*:838, 1973.
4. Jacobs, J.: Achilles tenodesis for paralytic calcaneo
    cavus foot. *Clin. Orthop., 47*:143, 1966.
5. Lesin, B.E.: Tendo-achilles tenodesis in the treatment
    of paralytic calcaneo-cavus deformity in the immature
    foot. Resident research project, given at Shriners
    Hospital, Los Angeles, 1974.
6. Lipscomb, P.R.: Osteotomy of calcaneus, triple arthro-
    desis and tendon transfer for severe paralytic calcaneo-
    cavus deformity. *J. Bone Joint Surg., 51A*:548, 1969.

7. Menelaus, M.B.: Talectomy for equinovarus deformity in arthrogryposis and spina bifida. *J. Bone Joint Surg.*, *53B*:468, 1971.

8. Menelaus, M.B.: The Orthopedic Management of Spina Bifida Cystica. Edinburgh E & S, Livingstone, 1971.

9. Peabody, C.W.: Tendon transplantation in lower extremities. IN The American Academy of Orthopedic Surgeons Instructional Course Lectures, VI, 1949, pp. 178.

10. Perry, J.: Kinesiology of lower extremity bracing. *Clin. Orthop.*, *102*:18, 1974.

11. Samilson, R.L.: Crescentic Osteotomy of the Os Calcis for Calcaneo-Cavus Feet. Proceedings of the Foot Society. To be published.

12. Sharrard, W.J.W.: Paralytic deformity in the lower limb. *J. Bone Joint Surg.*, *49B*:731, 1967.

13. Sharrard, W.J.W. and Grossfield, I.: The management of deformity and paralysis of the foot in myelomeningocele. *J. Bone Joint Surg.*, *50B*:456, 1968.

14. Sharrard, W.J.W.: Supra malleolar wedge osteotomy of the tibia in children with myelomeningocele. *J. Bone Joint Surg.*, *56B*:458, 1974.

15. Westin, G.W.: Tendon transfers about the foot, ankle and hip in the paralyzed lower extremity. American Academy of Orthopedic Surgeons Instructional Course Lectures. *J. Bone Joint Surg.*, *47A*:1430, 1965.

16. Whitman, R.: Further observations on the operative treatment of paralytic talipes of the calcaneus type. *Am. J. Orthop. Surg.*, *8*:138, 1910.

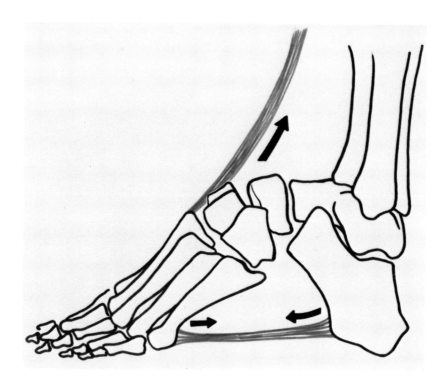

Fig. 1.

PARALYTIC CONVEX PES VALGUS
(PARALYTIC VERTICAL TALUS)

W.J.W. Sharrard, M.D., F.R.C.S.

Paralytic convex pes valgus is an uncommon congenital
foot deformity which presents in ten percent of children born
with myelomeningocele (Fig. 1). Even less often it may
present as a secondary paralytic deformity in early childhood. The external appearance and clinical features in
paralytic and non-paralytic types of convex pes valgus are
the same.[2] The sole of the foot is convex with the head of
the talus prominent in the sole of the foot. The hindfoot is
plantarflexed and in valgus and the forefoot is in calcaneus,
valgus and abduction at the mid tarsal joint with dislocation
of the talo-navicular joint. The deformity is a rigid one
and cannot be corrected manually.

PATHOLOGY

Two types of feet in myelomeningocele present with this
deformity. In the majority of patients, studies of motor
innervation indicate an intact innervation down to the
muscles supplied by the first sacral segment with paralysis
of muscles supplied by the second and third sacral segments.
[3,4] A second group of patients, less often seen because they
are severely affected before birth, show complete paralysis
of all muscles but in this group of patients, there is
evidence, from a study of the posture in the newborn, that

461

the lower limbs have been compressed one against the other
with the production of a convex pes valgus foot on one side
and a talipes equinovarus on the other side, the two feet
fitting together side by side.[3]   Studies of the pathological
anatomy[1,6] suggest that the deformity arises as a result of
strong activity in the dorsiflexors of the forefoot in the
absence of activity in intrinsic and long toe flexor muscles
resulting in a dislocation of the talo-navicular joint. As
a secondary consequence of this, the tibialis posterior
becomes splayed out and ineffective so that the evertors pre-
dominate over the invertors to produce valgus deformity of
the forefoot and to a lesser extent of the hindfoot. Plantarflexion by the triceps surae, though weak, is unopposed
because of the dislocation of the mid foot so that the hindfoot is in an equinus position, a situation that is not
obvious in the clinical appearance but is well shown on
lateral radiographs in which the talus and calcaneus are in
marked plantarflexion relative to the line of the tibia
(Fig. 2). Antero-posterior radiographs demonstrate the
abducted position of the forefoot (Fig. 3).

TREATMENT

       The deformity is so rigid that attempts at conservative
management by passive stretching or plaster casts is almost
invariably ineffective. Operative treatment by release of
tight soft tissues combined with tendon transplantation is
indicated.[2,4,5] A study of the results of various combinations of soft tissue release and tendon transfer have shown
that the best results are obtained when release procedures
are combined with transfer of the peroneus brevis to the
tibialis posterior and of the tibialis anterior to the neck
of the talus.

OPERATIVE TECHNIQUE

The operation is performed under tourniquet; provided
that it is done expeditiously, correction of all elements
of the deformity can be performed within the tourniquet time
of 1 to 1¼ hours.

The operation is performed through three incisions. The
first incision passes from the dorsum of the foot to the
lateral aspect of the subtalar region exposing the tight toe
extensor tendons and peroneus tertius which are lengthened
by alternate division of toe tendons. It is not wise to
leave the tendons unsutured because of the possibility of the
development of secondary flexion deformity of the toes in
later childhood. The peroneus longus is elongated by a Z
incision and the peroneus brevis is detached from its insertion. The subtalar joint is opened from the lateral side and
the interosseous talo-calcaneal ligament divided.

Through a second medial incision, extending from below
the medial malleolus to the talo-navicular joint, the joint
and the tibialis tendons are exposed. The tibialis anterior
is detached from its insertion to the navicular. When this
has been done, the talo-navicular joint can usually be
reduced quite easily bringing the forefoot into its truly
corrected position of plantarflexion. The talo-navicular
joint is held in the corrected position by means of a
Kirschner wire. At this point, it will usually be found that
the whole foot is now in a position of equinus. Through a
third incision anterior to the lateral border of the tendo-
calcaneus, the tendon is exposed and elongated by a Z
technique. The peroneus brevis tendon is pulled through from
the foot and transplanted across the posterior aspect of the
ankle joint deep to the neurovascular bundle and threaded
down the sheath of the tibialis posterior to be attached to

the navicular bone. The subtalar joint, which has now been
reduced from its everted position is held in position by a
Kirschner wire passed up through the heel. Finally, the
tibialis anterior tendon is sutured to the neck of the talus.
The wounds are closed and a below knee plaster applied with
the foot in the slightly over corrected position. Radiographs should show a correction of the vertical position of
the talus (Fig. 4).

In cases in which there is paralysis of all the muscles
below the knee associated with a convex pes valgus, simple
division of all the tendons combined with reduction of the
joint deformities alone is appropriate.[7]

RESULTS

In two out of three patients, the deformity remains
corrected and the foot is a satisfactory plantigrade foot.
In a few patients, instability at the subtalar joint in later
childhood may indicate the need for a Grice extra-articular
subtaloid arthrodesis. In other patients, overbalanced
action of invertors may result in an equinovarus foot, for
which secondary elongation of the transplanted tibialis
posterior and a further elongation of the tendo-calcaneus
may be needed. Below knee bracing is likely to be needed in
the majority of patients until early adolescence when a
triple arthrodesis allows them to be discarded.

Inadequate correction of the deformity or failure to
correct it surgically in early life has severe penalties in
later childhood. Because most of these children have good
lower limb innervation generally, they are active and can
usually attend normal school and partake of sporting activities. If the sole of the foot remains convex, pressure
ulceration inevitably occurs under the head of the talus with

serious secondary consequences. For an uncorrected foot seen before such events have occurred, it is still appropriate to attempt a measure of correction by excision of the navicular, wedge correction of the mid tarsal joint and subtalar joints and tendon transfer as may be appropriate.

REFERENCES

1. Drennan, J.C. and Sharrard, W.J.W.: The pathological anatomy of convex pes valgus. *J. Bone Joint Surg.,* *53B*:455, 1971.

2. Duckworth, T. and Smith, T.W.D.: The treatment of paralytic convex pes valgus. *J. Bone Joint Surg.,* *56B*:305, 1974.

3. Ralis, Z. and Duckworth, T.: The pathology of the congenital vertical talus deformity associated with spina bifida. Proceedings of Heidelberg symposium on cerebral palsy, May, 1972. Zeitschrift fur Orthopadie und ihre Grenzgebiete, 1974.

4. Sharrard, W.J.W.: Paediatric Orthopaedics and Fractures. Oxford and Edinburgh, Blackwell Scientific Publications, 1971, pp. 673.

5. Sharrard, W.J.W. and Grosfield, I.: The management of deformity and paralysis of the foot in myelomeningocele. *J. Bone Joint Surg.,* *50B*:456, 1968.

6. Specht, E.E.: Congenital paralytic vertical talus. An anatomical study. *J. Bone Joint Surg.,* *57A*:842, 1975.

7. Walker, G.F. and Cheong-Leen,P.: The surgical management of paralytic vertical talus in myelomeningocele. In proceedings of the British Orthopaedic Association. *J. Bone Joint Surg.,* *55B*:876, 1973.

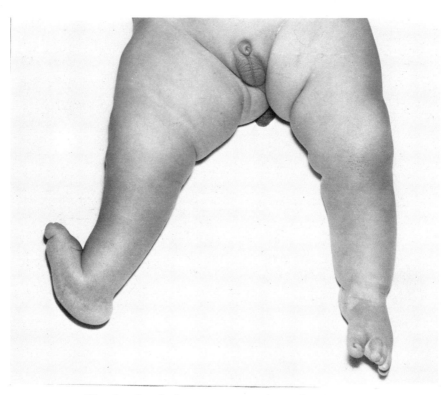

Fig. 1. Paralytic convex pes valgus of right foot.

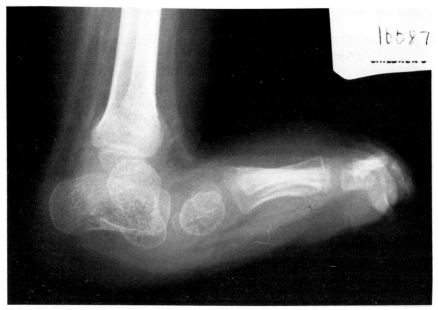

Fig. 2. Radiograph of paralytic convex pes valgus. Lateral view showing vertical talus with hindfoot equinus and forefoot calcaneus.

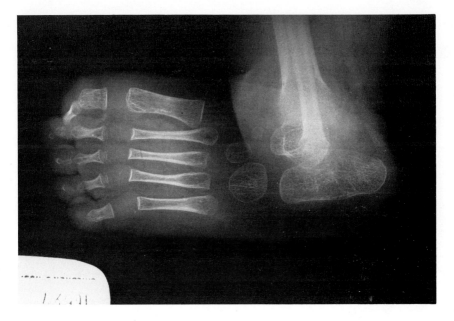

Fig. 3. Radiograph of paralytic convex pes valgus. Anteroposterior view showing abduction deformity of forefoot.

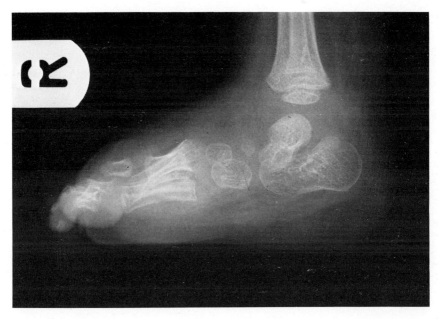

Fig. 4. Radiograph of paralytic convex pes valgus after operative correction.

PARALYTIC PES CAVUS AND CLAW TOES

W.J.W. Sharrard, M.D., F.R.C.S.

Cavus deformity or cavus associated with varus deformity of the forefoot relative to the hindfoot with clawing of the toes is associated with paresis or paralysis of the intrinsic muscles of the sole of the foot.[1,2] Sometimes the deformity is present at birth or it may not become obvious until the second or third year of life (Fig. 1). Although the deformity appears to be an innocent one, it is potentially dangerous because of loss of sensibility in the tips of the toes and underneath the metatarsal heads. At first the deformity is mobile but later becomes a fixed deformity. Children with this level of innervation are usually active and pressure ulceration on the dorsum of the toes, on the tips of the toes or underneath the metatarsal heads is very likely to develop in later life.

TREATMENT

While the toes still retain mobility and cavus deformity is not too marked, correction of the clawing deformity of the toes and tendon transplantation alone is sufficient. It is best performed in a child between the second and fourth years.

Through a medial incision at the junction of the plantar and medial surfaces of the heel, the plantar fascia is exposed and any tight plantar fascia released on the medial

and plantar aspects of the calcaneus. Particular attention
is paid to the mobilisation of fascia and tendons on the
medial side of the foot to obtain correction of the plantarflexed first metatarsal.

Clawing of the lesser toes is corrected by transplantation of the long toe flexor to the dorsum of the toes in each
lesser toe.[3] An incision is made just lateral to the proximal phalanx of each lesser toe. The extensor expansion and
the lateral side of the proximal phalanx are exposed. The
osseotendinous tunnel for the long flexor tendons is opened
on the lateral side to expose the long toe flexor tendons.
The flexor digitorum longus tendon is identified, divided
as distally as possible and mobilised to be attached to the
extensor expansion, the toe being held in plantarflexion at
the metatarso-phalangeal joint and in extension at the interphalangeal joints.

Clawing of the great toe must be treated differently.[2]
Through an incision along the medial side of the whole extent
of the great toe, the extensor hallucis longus tendon is
exposed and, if it is tight, is elongated together with
dorsal capsulotomy of the first metatarso-phalangeal joint.
The osseotendinous tunnel of the flexor hallucis longus is
opened from the medial side in the region of the proximal
phalanx. With the toe held in the corrected position,
vertical drill holes are made in the proximal phalanx from
dorsal to plantar surface, through which a wire suture is
passed attaching the tendon as a tenodesis to the proximal
phalanx. The plantar surface of the proximal phalanx is
rawed to provide a surface for attachment of the tendon.
If the flexor hallucis longus tendon proves to be excessively
short, the incision can be prolonged along the medial side
of the first metatarsal to allow elongation of the flexor

hallucis longus in the sole of the foot. The corrected
position of the great toe is held by a Kirschner wire passed
through the phalanges of the great toe into the first metatarsal. All the incisions are closed and the position held
by a plaster below the knee extending down to the tips of
the toes. Fixation is required only for three weeks.

In an older child in which the deformity has become
more fixed, the first metatarsal may be considerably depressed (Fig. 2) with valgus deformity of the forefoot
relative to the hindfoot. This deformity is a deceptive one,
because, when the patient stands, the heel is forced into
varus, giving the impression of a varus deformity of the
hindfoot. The temptation to perform an osteotomy of the
calcaneus to produce valgus of the hindfoot must be resisted.
Operative corrections needs to be made in two stages. The
plantarfascia is released as described above. The forefoot
and hindfoot are placed in as much inversion as possible.
If the first metatarsal proves to have a fixed plantarflexion
deformity, additional correction may be obtained by an
osteotomy of the base of the first metatarsal and, at the
same time, the flexor hallucis longus tendon can be elongated.
The inverted position of the foot is maintained in a below
knee plaster for one month. A second operation is then
performed to transplant tendons in the toes with correction
of any claw deformity as described above. In a child over
the age of twelve, fixed deformity at the interphalangeal
joint may require, in addition, arthrodesis of the interphalangeal joints.

REFERENCES

1. Sharrard, W.J.W.: Paediatric Orthopaedics and Fractures.
    London, Blackwell Scientific Publications Ltd., 1971,
    pp. 675.

2. Sharrard, W.J.W. and Smith, T.W.D.: Flexor hallucis
    longus tenodesis in the management of paralytic clawing
    of the hallux in childhood. *J. Bone Joint Surg., 58B:*
    in press.

3. Taylor, R.G.: The treatment of claw toes by multiple
    transfers of flexor into extensor tendons. *J. Bone Joint
    Surg., 33B:*539, 1951.

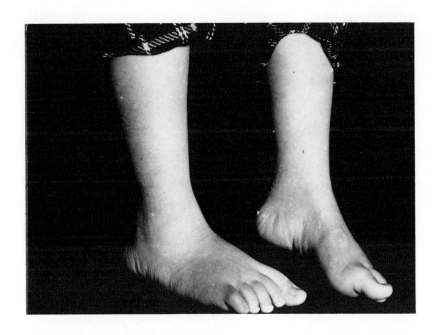

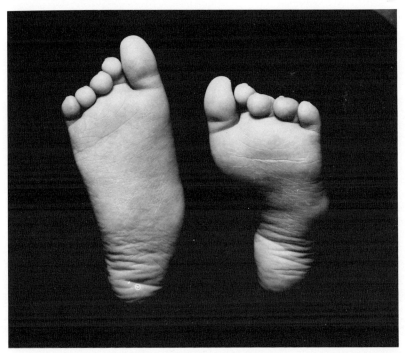

Fig. 1. Paralytic pes cavus and claw toes, left foot.

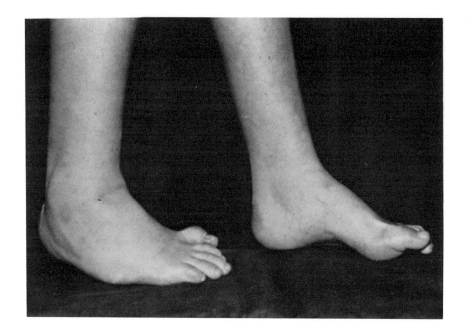

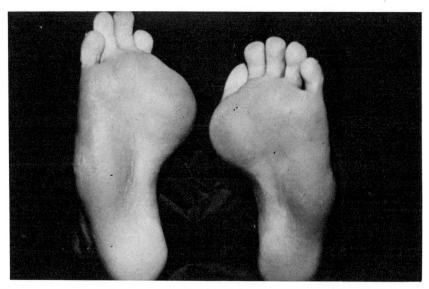

Fig. 2. Uncorrected pes cavus and claw toes. The first metatarsal head is depressed and the forefoot is in valgus relative to the hindfoot. Weight is being taken on the first metatarsal head and the cuboid and there is imminent danger of ulceration.

VALGUS AND ROTATIONAL DEFORMITIES OF
THE KNEE, ANKLE AND FOOT IN
MYELOMENINGOCELE

Richard E. Lindseth, M.D.

Structural deformities of the lower extremity occur
commonly in children paralyzed by myelomeningocele.[6] Some
of these are major structural deformities such as flexion
contractures of the hips, knees, and severe club foot
deformity of the feet which interfere with function of all
the children regardless of the level of paralysis. Other
deformities of the legs are less crippling for many of these
children and interfere with function only in the ambulatory
patient. These deformities include rotational deformities
of the lower extremity and valgus deformity of the knee,
ankle and foot. For example, valgus deformity of the knee
and ankle is of little consequence to a child confined to a
wheelchair, but becomes a problem to a child who is trying to
balance on insensitive feet and achieve some degree of
ambulatory independence. The children who are particularly
handicapped by valgus and rotational deformities have a level
of paralysis that allows extension of the knee and weak
flexion of the knee but no hip abduction nor plantar flexion
and inversion. Approximately twenty-five percent of the
children with myelomeningocele in our clinic have this level
of paralysis. Children with lower levels of paralysis,
primarily those with the sacral innervation, walk despite

valgus deformity and those of higher levels of paralysis
seldom walk.

Rotational and valgus deformities of the legs cause
many problems to these ambulatory children. The axis of the
knee and ankle joints do not line up and brace fit becomes
almost impossible. Even when a brace can be manufactured to
fit the deformed extremity, pressure sores are common,
commonly over the medial malleolus and the braces wear out
rapidly and occasionally break. Shoe wear is very rapid and
repair is frequently needed, often on a weekly basis. Gait
is also severely effected. When there is a valgus deformity
of either the foot and ankle or knee, the floor reaction
force falls lateral to the ankle joint and the knee joint
(Fig. 1). This increased the valgus deformity with further
growth and adversely affects the gait by requiring the center
of gravity to shift further to the outside than usual so that
it can be over the contact point of the foot on the floor.
This will cause a marked exaggeration of the Trendelenburg
gait. If the knee is flexed due to contracture during mid-
stance this lateral shift of the center of gravity will also
cause the tibia and foot to externally rotate producing
rotational deformity. Internal rotational deformities,
usually caused by muscle imbalance, may also cause tripping
and inability of the legs to pass one another during the
swing phase and require a wider based gait. Finally, the
cosmetic appearance of these children is also adversely
effected.

If proper treatment is to be given to these deformities
it is necessary to understand what causes them. In each
child one or all of the factors may be functioning and the
correction of only one factor will only lead to frustration
and failure. The causes for these deformities can be divided

into two groups; the first group contains factors present at birth and includes muscle imbalance and the second group contains factors developing after birth and includes the forces of standing and walking on partially innervated extremities.

Valgus deformity of the foot is usually caused by unopposed contraction of the peroneal muscles. This contraction may be either voluntary or reflex and causes progressive deformity, which eventually becomes fixed by adaptive changes in the distal tibia (Fig. 2). In some children the valgus deformity may be caused by over zealous treatment of a club foot deformity, especially if surgery is performed and the posterior tibial tendon is released. A spastic or contracted posterior tibial tendon may completely mask weak function of the peroneal muscles and following a posterior tibial tendon release the loss of the pull of the posterior tibial tendon will allow the foot to swing into increasing valgus. Procedures that shorten the lateral column of the foot, such as the Evans procedure, may likewise produce valgus deformity. Even conservative treatment of the club foot by manipulation and casting, if the metatarsus adductus and mild foot deformity is not corrected first, may result in hindfoot valgus and external rotation of the tibia[8] (Fig. 3).

Once the child begins to walk the forces of ambulation may also contribute to the formation of valgus deformity. Because most of these children do not have gluteus medius function and walk with a Trendelenburg gait, the center of gravity moves laterally over the foot and the hip adductors pull the knee medially which causes the floor reaction to pass lateral to the knee and to the mid-portion of the ankle joint forcing the ankle into valgus (Fig. 4). As growth occurs the distal tibia joint surface also tilts into valgus

and the ankle deformity becomes fixed (Fig. 5). Many of the
children in our clinic had normal alignment of the leg when
they were walking at age two to four years only to develop
severe valgus deformity of the ankle as they approached
adolescence.

Another cause of ankle valgus is abnormal gait mechanics
due to other lower extremity deformities. If there is an
external rotation of the tibia, knee flexion during the
stance phase will place the floor reaction force lateral to
the ankle forcing the foot into valgus. Also a fixed equinus
deformity of the ankle that will not allow the foot to dorsiflex above neutral position is detrimental to gait mechanics.
When this situation occurs the child is unable to come past
the mid-stance phase of his gait without raising his center
of gravity. Since his muscle paralysis prevents him from
raising his center of gravity, he will externally rotate
the leg and roll over the medial side of his foot as his
forward motion progresses past mid-stance. Eventually this
will produce an external rotation deformity of the tibia and
valgus deformity of the foot and ankle.

The causes of knee deformity are closely related to
those of the foot and ankle and in many children they are
interrelated so that deformities of the foot cause deformities
of the ankle and vise versa. Muscle imbalance caused by the
sartorius, adductor, and medial hamstring muscles can cause
a variety of deformities of the knee, particularly valgus
deformity associated with either internal or external
rotation of the tibia depending on which force appears to be
the most dominant. It is often surprising how much rotational
instability of the knee may be present in these children,
particularly those children with unopposed pull of the
sartorius and medial hamstrings. Contractures of the

iliotibial band cause valgus deformities of the knee and may contribute to flexion contractures as well.[1]

When the child walks, the same abnormality of gait that causes valgus of the ankle may cause valgus deformities of the knee. The adductor lurch causes the center of gravity to move lateral to the knee joint. Likewise a valgus deformity of the foot will cause the floor reaction force to move outside of the knee. If the foot is externally rotated to accommodate an equinus deformity then this force is also transmitted to the knee. It should be noted that in these children a ninety degree stop on a brace does not produce an extension movement at the knee helping to overcome a knee flexion contracture but rather causes the child to externally rotate the foot and ankle, producing an external valgus deformity to the foot as mentioned earlier. Another cause for deformity around the knee is mal-united fractures. These children have frequent fractures during the early childhood period. Many of these fractures due to m cle imbalance will heal in a valgus and external rotation deformity.

Rotational deformities of the leg and foot are relatively common and are rarely symmetrical. Many of these children have an internal rotation deformity of one side and an external rotation deformity on the other side, and yet no discernable difference in the level of motor paralysis can be found. Perhaps in some children the deformity is due to persistance of fetal position which does not change due to the presence of motor paralysis. In other children minor differences in muscle contractures not under conscious control may also be a factor. Nevertheless in most children muscle imbalance around the hip appears to be the major cause for the deformity. The most common muscles which appear to be involved are the iliopsoas, sartorius and short external

rotators.[4] Occasionally the tensor fascia lata will also be
a contributing factor.[1] Fractures around the hip joint often
lead to deformity since they are difficult to hold without
internal fixation of the hip (Fig. 6). Pelvic obliquity and
severe lumbar lordosis also contribute to the deformities of
the hip.

TREATMENT

The treatment of these deformities is often frustrating
and unrewarding. Seldom will one surgical procedure correct
all of the deformities. It is important to consider all of
the etiological factors that may produce the deformity and
correct each of them. Failing to do so will only permit
recurrence of the deformity while exposing the child to the
complications of surgery.

Conservative non-operative treatment is rarely of
benefit for the rotation and valgus deformities of the leg.
Although braces may be used to support the undeformed leg,
thereby equalizing the forces of ambulation and preventing
the appearance of deformity, once the deformity has occurred
braces will only produce pressure sores and interfere with
gait. Rotation deformities of the hip can sometimes be
controlled by torsion braces, however care must be used since
they may also produce external rotation and valgus deformities
of the foot and ankle. A brace across the ankle joint must
allow ten degrees of dorsiflexion if it is a movable ankle
joint or be set in ten degrees of dorsiflexion if it is a
fixed ankle joint in order to allow the child to get beyond
mid-stance (Fig.7). Otherwise the brace may produce the
deformity that we are trying to prevent by forcing the child
to externally rotate his leg and roll off the medial side of

his foot. Obviously more work and understanding must go into the design of our orthotics system so that they will not only prevent these deformities but also improve the child's gait.[3]

The treatment for deformities already present is surgical. When performing the surgical correction of these deformities it is important to treat the force imbalance caused by contracted or overactive muscles before the bone deformity is corrected. Otherwise the deformity will only recur. Multiple procedures are often needed but must be carefully timed to prevent common complications which include joint stiffness and fractures.

Rotational deformities around the hip are often common and difficult to treat effectively. Muscle transfer is the most common procedure used although the final result of the surgery is difficult to anticipate. Transfer of the iliopsoas tendon posterior laterally can often help control external rotational abnormalities.[5] At the time of the transfer it is often necessary to release contracted external rotators of the hip, primarily the piriformis, quadratus and gemellus.[4] Posterior transfer of the tensor fascia muscle origin can also be performed to help correct internal rotational deformities. Despite the muscle transfers, femoral torsion often persists and requires a rotational osteotomy.

At the knee, release of the iliotibial band will correct the valgus deformity of the knee in the young child. In the older child the deformity is in the distal femur and it is also necessary to perform a distal femoral osteotomy in order to bring the weight bearing line underneath the femoral condyles. Transfer of the sartorius muscle laterally is helpful in correcting the medial rotational instability often found in these children.

The valgus deformity of the foot in the young child

usually responds to muscle balancing procedures. However,
before performing muscle transfers consideration needs to be
made of the all of the muscles acting across the foot and
then an attempt made to balance the forces on the medial
side of the foot equal to those on the outside of the foot.
The muscles that are usually suitable for transfer are the
tibialis anterior, the extensor hallicus longus, the extensor
digitorum communis and the peroneals. Many different combinations of transfers have been proposed for these feet but
the one that should be chosen will depend upon the relative
strength of each muscle.[7] In most of these children the
peroneal muscles are strong and one or both of the peroneal
tendons are transferred posteriorly either into the os calcis
or to the Achilles tendon, although occasionally the peroneus
longus is transferred to the medial side of the foot to act
as an invertor. One must remember that equinus deformities
should be avoided since it will not help extend the knee
but will only cause the foot to go into external rotation
as the child progresses forward past mid-stance and will
eventually produce valgus deformity. Procedures to correct
fixed deformity include a distal tibial osteotomy if the
ankle mortise itself is in valgus and a calcaneal osteotomy
if the child is young and the hindfoot is deformed.[2] For
severe deformities a triple arthrodesis may be necessary,
although this will take away some of the mobility of the foot
and may lead to severe degenerative changes of the ankle
joint.

CONCLUSION

     Our treatment for children with myelomeningocele has
progressed rapidly over the last twenty years. No longer are
we worried only about survival, nor are we concerned

primarily about whether the lower lumbar paraplegic will be able to walk. We have progressed to the point that we are concerned about the quality of gait and how it can approach normality. It is for these children who have the ability to approach a normal gait pattern that the problem of rotational instability and valgus deformity of the foot, ankle and knee becomes a problem. For these children it is not a question of whether they will walk, but how they will walk. To correct these deformities extensive bracing and multiple surgical procedures are necessary. It is important for the treating physician to weigh the benefits of surgical treatment against the possible complications. For many children the answer will be to the affirmative and an attempt should be made to correct these deformities in order to help the child walk better. However, in others it may be better to accept the deformity, particularly if it is mild, and spare the child multiple surgical procedures, repeated hospitalizations and possible multiple complications.

REFERENCES

1. Irwin, G.E.: Iliotibial band, it's role in producing deformity in poliomyelitis. *J. Bone Joint Surg., 31A*: 141, 1949.
2. Dwyer, F.C.: Osteotomy of the calcaneum for pes cavus. *J. Bone Joint Surg., 41B*:80, 1959.
3. Lindseth, R.E. and Glancy, J.: Polypropylene lower-extremity braces for paraplegia due to myelomeningocele. *J. Bone Joint Surg., 56A*:556, 1974.

4. Menelaus, M.B.: Dislocation and deformity of the hip in
    children with spina bifida cystica. *J. Bone Joint Surg.*,
    51B:238, 1969.

5. Sharrard, W.J.W.: Posterior iliopsoas transplantation
    in the treatment of paralytic dislocation of the hip.
    J. Bone Joint Surg., *46B*:426, 1964.

6. Sharrard, W.J.W.: Paralytic deformity in the lower limb.
    J. Bone Joint Surg., *49B*:731, 1967.

7. Sharrard, W.J.W. and Grosfield, I.: The management of
    deformity and paralysis of the foot in myelomeningocele.
    J. Bone Joint Surg., *50B*:456, 1968.

8. Swann, M., Lloyd-Roberts, G.C. and Catterall, A.: The
    anatomy of uncorrected club feet. *J. Bone Joint Surg.*,
    51B:268, 1969.

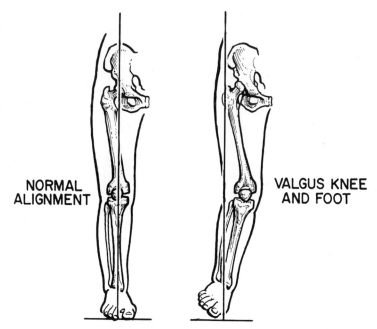

Fig. 1. The floor reaction force normally passes through the heel, mid-ankle and mid-knee to the hip. When there is valgus deformity of the ankle or knee, the floor reaction force passes to the outside of the ankle and knee joints causing increasing valgus deformity of the leg.

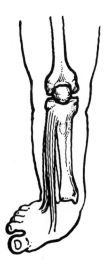

Fig. 2. Valgus deformity of the foot in lower lumbar paraplegics is usually caused by unopposed pull of the peroneal muscles.

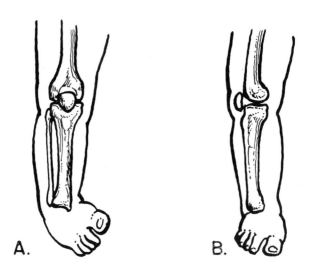

Fig. 3.   When the uncorrected club foot (A) is placed in a brace with the foot pointing ahead, the remainder of the leg will be forced into external rotation (B).

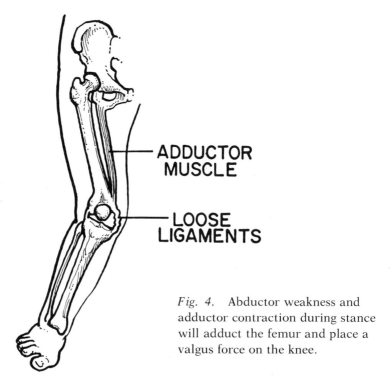

ADDUCTOR
MUSCLE

LOOSE
LIGAMENTS

Fig. 4.   Abductor weakness and adductor contraction during stance will adduct the femur and place a valgus force on the knee.

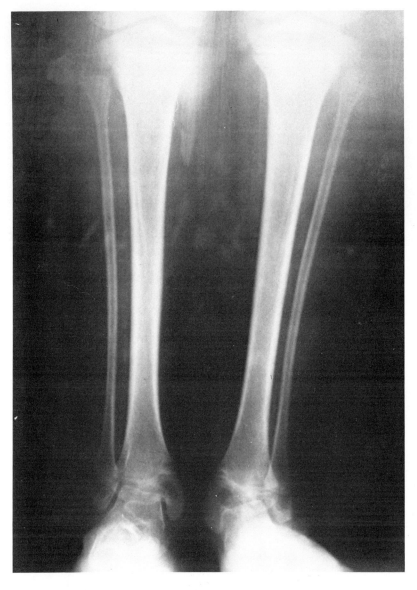

Fig. 5. Persistent valgus deformity of the foot will produce a valgus tilt of the distal tibia and the deformity becomes fixed.

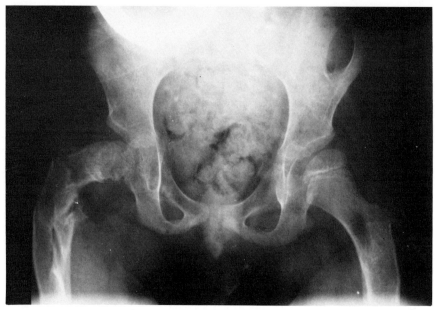

Fig. 6. Fractures are frequent in these children and often heal in deformity.

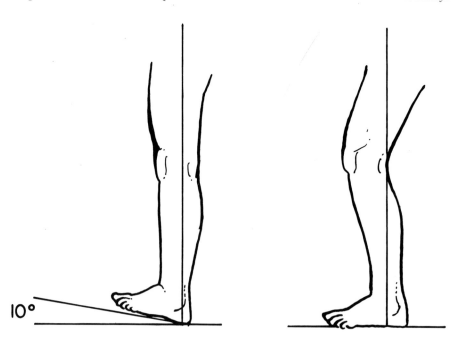

10°

Fig. 7. The ankle must be allowed to dorsiflex ten degrees if the leg is to move post mid-stance and the gait cycle completed.

THE KNEE

Richard A. Jolson, M.D.

In a review of the literature related to the orthopaedic
aspects of myelomeningocele, one notices that little
attention is given to the knee. Because the knee joint is
often stabilized with long leg braces, interest is concen-
trated upon more complicated and perhaps more intriguing hip
and foot pathology. No where else in our field is the knee
joint given such a minor role. A re-evaluation may be in
order.

MECHANICAL ASPECTS OF THE KNEE JOINT

The knee is not a true hinge joint (Fig. 1). In
extension the tibia glides forward under the femoral condyles.
This forward gliding can be mechanically restricted by
hamstring spasticity, contracture of the anterior cruciate
or posterior capsule, or a combination of these (Fig. 2).
Iliotibial band and sartorius contractures can also
contribute to flexion deformity.

Similarly, backward tibial glide is prevented by
quadriceps contracture and spasticity, contracture of the
anterior capsule or posterior cruciate ligament, or a
combination of these.

Joint contractures in myelodysplasia are usually the
result of muscular rigidity, secondary to spasticity about

489

those joints. In the knee joint such spasticity will involve either the quadriceps mechanism or the hamstring muscle group. Major contractures will occur in either extension or flexion, although the latter is much more common. However, varus, valgus, and rotational deformities also appear frequently. For proper management it is mandatory to evaluate specifically all motors crossing the knee joint and to determine whether each muscle is (a) normally functional; (b) normally functional and weak; (c) uncontrolled and flaccid; or (d) uncontrolled and spastically rigid. Spasticity in myelodysplasia occurs basically as a rigidity secondary to some continuity of the reflex arc below the level of the spinal lesion. Resultant contractures become fixed, unyielding, and resistant to manual stretching forces.

Flexion contractures are invariably associated with posterior subluxation of the tibia on the femur, because of the inhibition of forward tibial glide when knee extention is attempted.

Hyperextension contractures, the result of quadriceps spasticity, can be as much as 90 degrees but are usually in the 15 to 30 degree range. Valgus contractures may be secondary to iliotibial band contracture or to biceps femoris spasticity. However, one may find no obvious etiologic agent. Varus deformity is more unusual and seldom seen.

A cross section of muscles at the knee joint (Fig. 3) is particularly helpful in the analysis of deforming forces. Knee flexion motors are primarily innervated from L5, S1, S2 segments with some higher levels contributing through the sartorius (L2-3) and the gracilis (L3-4).

Medial rotators of the tibia include those muscles comprising the pes anserinus, which illustrate a wide range of spinal innervation. Any spasticity of this group will tend to exaggerate the internally rotated posture of the tibia on the flexed knee. With an associated knee flexion contracture, internal tibial torsion may be greatly exaggerated.

External tibial torsion may be secondary to spasticity of the biceps femoris muscle inserting at the fibular head; iliotibial band contracture may also contribute. Equal medial and lateral hamstring spasticity will present clinically as a pure flexion contracture without a torsional component.

Growth (Fig. 4) is another factor to be considered in the mechanical aspects of knee contractures. As the limb increases in length, knee contractures will place the foot farther from its most ideal position for weight bearing, i.e., directly beneath the knee joint.

Gross flexion, extension, varus, valgus or rotational contractures are unacceptable. Surgical management should be directed toward proper realignment of the tibia beneath the femur.

TREATMENT

Care of the myelomeningocele knee is dependent upon the integrity and relative strength of the quadriceps mechanism. If quadriceps strength remains normal or near normal and no significant contracture exists, bracing below the knee is permissible.

It is mandatory to balance the flexion-extension spasticity about the knee joint. Ideally a range of motion from full extension to 90 degrees flexion is desirable. Often this amount of motion cannot be achieved because of spasticity involving either the flexors or extensors. The

importance of full knee extension, either active or passive,
cannot be overemphasized. Bracing is more stable with the
knee in full extension. If extension can be maintained,
increasing contractures with further growth are less likely
to occur.

The Flail Knee with No Contractures

When the knee is flail without contractures (or even if
there is a balanced flexion-extension spasticity at 180
degrees), simple long leg bracing is all that is necessary.

The Weak Knee Without Contracture

In the weak knee without contracture some quadriceps
power exists, but is insufficient to fully extend the knee.
The weak knee without flexion contracture requires long leg
bracing but an outrigger spring assist (Fig. 5) may be added
anteriorly to increase the extension force. Surgical
advancement (Fig. 6) of the quadriceps mechanism may effectively shorten the origin-insertion distance and strengthen
a weakened quadriceps. Such advancement may be accomplished
by either plication of the patellar tendon if a patella alta
exists or by a suprapatellar quadriceps advancement.
Approximately one inch of the quadriceps mechanism is over-
lapped; particular care is taken to advance the medialis
portion of the quadriceps.

The Knee with Flexion Contracture 20 degrees or Less

When there exists a knee flexion contracture of 20 degrees or less, passive stretching should be considered.
Serial or wedging casts (Fig. 7) well padded and performed
slowly and carefully, may correct the deformity. A simple
method of cast wedging allows the tibia to glide forward as
knee extension increases (Fig. 8). X-rays demonstrate this
anterior tibial shift as the cast is widened posteriorward.

Surgical measures should be designed to correct deforming forces and reinforce weak structures. Simple release of
the iliotibial band, if tight, may be sufficient to correct
a flexion deformity. X-rays taken for tibial glide, lateral
views at 90 degrees flexion (Fig. 9) and in maximum extension,
(Fig. 10) usually will demonstrate a hinge effect between
the tibia and the femur rather than the normal forward glide
effect. Release of the anterior cruciate ligament (Fig. 11)
through an anterior incision frequently will allow the tibia
to shift forward. If full correction still is not gained,
then simple wedging casts will usually accomplish the desired
result. Lengthening of the hamstring tendons alone is seldom
adequate, as these muscles are usually spastic, and a rapid
recurrence of the flexion contracture then occurs. A more
effective measure is to recess the spastic hamstrings to the
femoral condyles and convert a deforming knee-flexion force
into a possible extension mechanism. On the other hand,
selective hamstring muscle transfer into the patella will
maintain knee balance. This tendon transfer is more
effective, however, when combined with complete surgical
release of the knee flexion contracture.

The Knee with Flexion Contracture Greater than 20 degrees

With a knee flexion contracture greater than 20 degrees,
one should not consider any form of wedging cast correction,
since the heel will not tolerate the skin pressure forces
necessary for correction. The common complication of heel
decubitus can be disastrous. A complete posterior release is
usually necessary, including the release of the posterior
capsule, the anterior cruciate ligament from behind, the
hamstring tendons, and the gastrocnemius origins. The
hamstrings (usually the gracilis and biceps femoris) may be

selectively transferred anteriorly, even if spastic, in order
to reinforce extension power. To avoid an extension
deformity, care must be taken to leave some posterior
musculature intact, even if it be by simple hamstring
lengthening. Correlated pre- and postoperative (Fig. 12,13,
14,15) photographs and x-rays illustrate the degree of
correction obtainable in a previously untreated 11 year old
girl.

Femoral supracondylar extension osteotomies should be
done only in special cases (Fig. 16). With severe knee
flexion contractures osteotomy realigns femur and tibia by
creating an opposite severe extension deformity. Whereas
the general alignment may be acceptable, a badly deformed
distal femur results with the knee joint still contracted
in flexion.

The Knee with Extension Contracture

If the knee can be passively flexed 10 degrees, then
simple treatment with a long leg brace is all that is
necessary. If the quadriceps is spastic and the knee cannot
be flexed to a neutral position, a split quadriceps tendon
transfer will create balance (Fig. 17). The rectus femoris
and intermedius are lengthened in a Z-plasty fashion while
the vastus medialis is transferred to the medial hamstrings
and the vastus lateralis transferred to the biceps femoris.
Following this procedure, the knee is occasionally stable
and balanced well enough to permit the conversion of a long
leg brace into a below knee type.

Supracondylar flexion osteotomy may be of value but
extension contracture often recurs because of the continuing
quadriceps spasticity. If the quadriceps is active and
controlled but the knee hyperextends excessively, osteotomy
may be considered. Also the quadriceps may be lengthened by

patellar tendon Z-plasty.   There is a limit to the amount of
permissible lengthening but usually 15 to 20 degrees more of
knee flexion may be gained.

Varus and Valgus Deformity

Varus and valgus deformities may be easily corrected by
supracondylar or proximal tibial closing-wedge osteotomies.
Proper knee alignment offers stability and lessens later
problems.   Any obvious deforming forces, i.e., contracted
iliotibial band, should be released.

SUMMARY

The knee joint should be given the same careful consideration as normally accorded the hip, foot and ankle.
Gaining proper alignment through surgery is feasible.
Balancing spastic motors is mandatory.   Development of full
extension with proper bracing is important for optimum
functional ambulation.

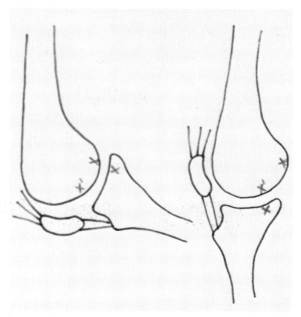

Fig. 1. The tibia glides forward from X to X' with knee extension.

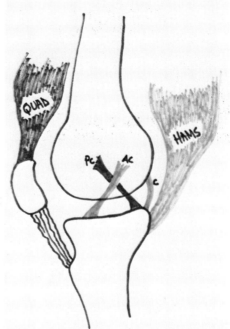

Fig. 2. Those structures inhibiting knee extension:

AC-anterior cruciate ligament; C-capsule.

HAMS-hamstring musculature. Those structures inhibiting knee flexion:

PC-posterior cruciate ligament.

QUAD-quadriceps femoris muscle.

496

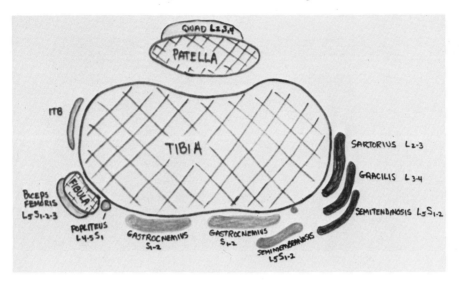

Fig. 3. Cross section muscles at the knee joint with their innervation.
Muscles of the pes anserinus, contributing to flexion, internal rotation contractures.
Pure knee flexors—gastrocnemius, semimembranosis.
Pure knee extensors—quadriceps.
Muscles contributing to flexion, valgus external rotation contractures—ITB, biceps.

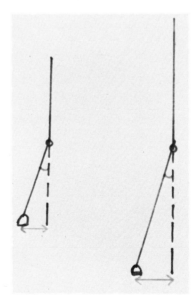

Fig. 4. The effect of longitudinal growth with a fixed angle of deformity at the knee. The foot becomes displaced further from the midline of the tibia.

497

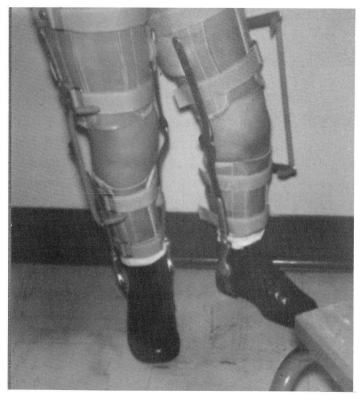

Fig. 5. Anterior spring assists to reinforce extension. (Compliment of Mr. Albert Feldman.)

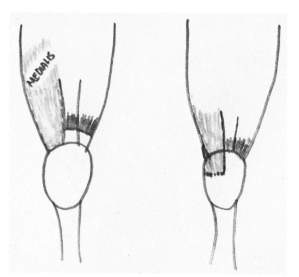

Fig. 6. Method of surgically advancing the quadriceps mechanism.

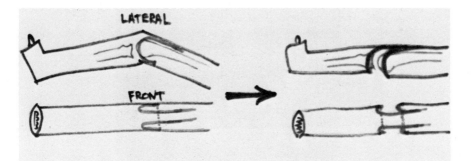

Fig. 7. A method of cast wedging allowing forward glide of the tibia on the femur with increased knee extension.

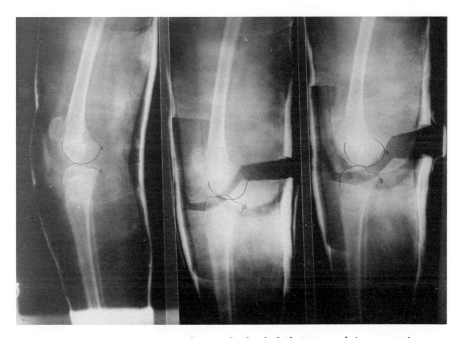

Fig. 8. X-rays demonstrating forward tibial shift in a wedging cast. As extension increases, point B (tibia) is seen to shift forward to point A (femur).

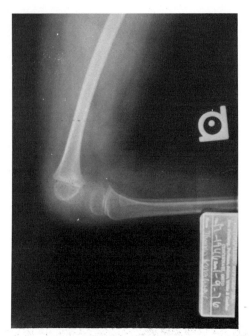

Fig. 9.   Lateral knee at 90 degrees flexion.

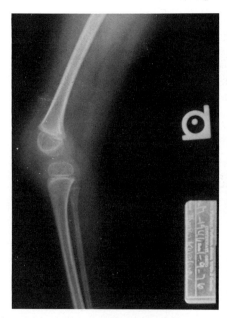

Fig. 10.   Lateral knee in maximum extension. Note the posterior sub-luxation of the tibia.

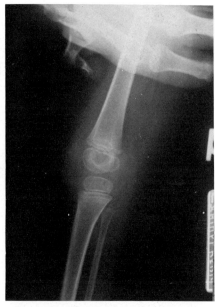

Fig. 11.   Maximum knee extension after simple release of the anterior cruciate ligament anteriorly.

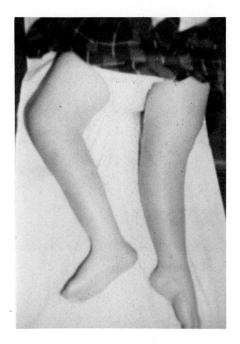

Fig. 12. Maximum extension right knee in untreated 11-year old patient.

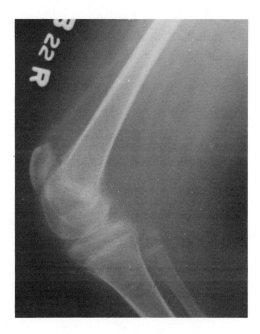

Fig. 13. X-ray of Fig. 12.

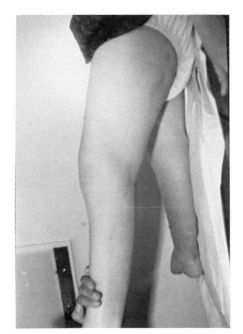

Fig. 14. Postop maximum extension right knee.

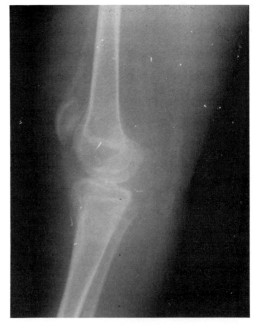

Fig. 15. X-ray of Fig. 14.

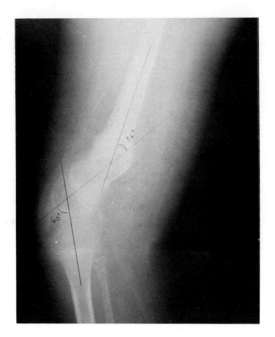

Fig. 16. Postop supracondylar osteotomy for gross knee flexion contracture.

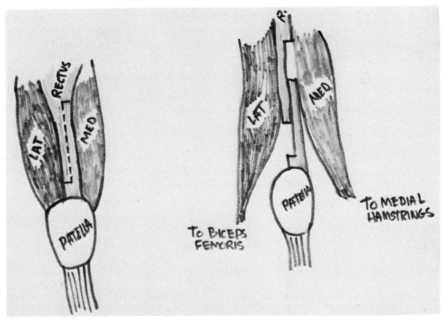

Fig. 17. Diagrammatic representation of split quadriceps transfer for spastic hyperextension of the knee.

CARE OF THE HIP IN INFANTS AND
YOUNGER CHILDREN WITH MYELODYSPLASIA

John F. Raycroft, M.D.

Dislocation of the hip in a child with myelodysplasia is a particularly disasterous event. It produces functional leg length inequality, pelvic obliquity, and often decreased motion. The beginning of paralytic lumbar scoliosis can be attributed to the dislocation and if a curve is present its progress is speeded.[5] Bracing becomes more difficult and, with that, ambulation progress is slowed. Children who have been ambulatory often become sitters. Even when sitting, unequal weight distribution secondary to skeletal deformity can produce severe skin breakdown.

Dislocation occurs most often in the group of patients with paralysis at the midlumbar level.[6] Unfortunately, this is by far the largest group of survivors, increasing the magnitude of the problem. Also of concern is the fact that this group has an excellent potential for community ambulation[3,9] if hips are located and general care is good.

Recognition of this disasterous sequence has led to the development of treatment methods designed to prevent or remedy the problem. Posterior iliopsoas transfer as described by Sharrard[6] and modified by others[2] has been a most effective method of controlling an unstable hip and by far the most common technique utilized. Its greatest success has been obtained in children over 18 months of age, as

originally recommended. However, it has been recognized
increasingly that many hips dislocate in the first year and
a half of life and that some are dislocated at birth. Moreover, adaptive changes of the acetabulum secondary to the
absence of a properly seated femoral head occur rapidly
during this time, resulting in an incompetent acetabulum.
In most cases with persistent unstable hips identified in
Sharrard's long-term review, the instability was traced to
an incompetent acetabulum.[8]

The emerging problem of the unstable hip in the infant
and younger child has been managed in various ways. Old
solutions were tried first. Splinting in the frogleg
position was unsuccessful. Fixed deformities of flexion
and abduction developed secondary to shortening of the
unopposed psoas and iliacus. Repeated adductor tenotomies
were only partially and temporarily successful, and psoas
tenotomies were rarely done. Posterior iliopsoas transfers
were performed at an earlier and earlier age with the lower
limit eventually being set at age 4 months.[7] This produced
a new set of problems. First, as the technical difficulties
of the surgery in infants increased, the complications likewise increased. Secondly, the child under 2 years of age
could in no way cooperate in a postoperative physical therapy
program, and that important aspect of the over-all program
was lost. Thirdly, as pointed out by McKibbin,[4] the eventual
potential for habilitation in younger patients often is not
clear; therefore, those with poor habilitation potential
often were operated on. He thought that extensive hip
surgery should be delayed until its usefulness could be
demonstrated clearly. To that end, abduction, internal
rotation, and splinting following reduction of the unstable
hip were utilized.

As a solution to these problems, the treatment program
developed by McKibbin is excellent. It would seem, however,
that the presence of hip instability or acetabular changes
indicate that adaptive changes already were well established
and progressive. Acknowledging that myelodysplastic children
have no intrinsic abnormalities of bony development of the
hip, it then follows that all bony changes must be secondary
to the abnormal forces generated by muscle imbalance. As
these forces develop in the fetal period and therefore are
present at birth, the earliest possible institution of
treatment is indicated. Our program to be described, then,
is essentially an extension of McKibbin's concept.

The goal of treatment emphatically should be to allow
and encourage normal acetabular development. If some degree
of instability exists, the stabilizing of the hip becomes an
important second goal. The somewhat prophylactic nature of
this approach is justified by the fact that without a good
acetabulum true hip stability can never be achieved.

In our clinic all children under age 18 months are
included in the program if the muscle pattern across the hips
is capable of producing dislocation. This excludes the
minimally involved child with no more loss than foot intrinsics. It also excludes the thoracic paraplegic with no
active musculature crossing the hip. We have been very
cautious in labeling these "thoracic paraplegic," for in
many children a minimally innervated iliopsoas is present
which, in time, is capable of producing dislocation. The
selected patients are examined, muscle power is recorded,
and hip range of motion and stability are determined. Prerequisites to splinting are a concentric reduction, 45
degrees of abduction, full extension, and slight internal
rotation of the hip. If these conditions are met, splinting

is applied. If not, the cause of the persistent deformity is
thought to be some combination of shortened psoas and adductor tendons. Arthrography is used to rule out the possibility of a physical block to reduction, such as an inverted
limbus. If none is found, surgical release of the offending
tendons is performed. Through a medial approach as described
by Ferguson[1] the adductors are examined and selectively
sectioned if tight. Dissection is then carried down to the
psoas insertion on the lesser trochanter. Release of the
psoas usually allows an unrestricted range of motion.
Occasionally, the medial hip capsule has appeared to be
contracted, maintaining a lateral position of the hip.
Longitudinal sectioning of the capsule as described by
Ferguson[1] has resolved this. Originally, the sectioned psoas
was allowed to retract, but on several occasions subsequent
posterior iliopsoas transfers were complicated by the gross
muscular nature of the distal end of the tendon. Feeling
that a tendon of better quality would result if some tension
was maintained, the released psoas was attached to the
anterior hip capsule and tagged with a metal suture to aid
in future identification. This may result in a secondary
benefit - preservation of some flexor power of the psoas
from an insertion less likely to produce dislocation. Satisfactory positioning is then demonstrated by x-ray and the
child is placed in a cast for 3 weeks. Following this,
splinting is applied. For splinting we have utilized a
posterior Vitrathene shell extending from toes to axillae.
We have found it necessary to abduct the splint to at least
50 degrees to achieve true 45 degress of femoral-pelvic
abduction. Full hip extension, and slight internal rotation
completes the prescription. With growth, brace modifications
such as detachable shoes, hip hinges, and standing capability

are added. Use of the splint is restricted to the time that the child is unattended by a parent. This allows for a full quota of physical contact and general activity while still providing adequate positioning time. In addition to active exercise, the parents are instructed in a program of passive range of motion exercise performed daily, designed to maintain flexibility and to prevent hip, knee, and ankle contractures. We have tried to continue use of the splint for 2 years, feeling that there is potential for acetabular molding up to that time. Some children with less severe paralysis demonstrate a desire to walk before that time are fitted with the necessary bracing and encouraged to do so. In these cases, abduction splinting is continued at night. At the conclusion of the splinting program, children are fitted for conventional bracing appropriate to their level of innervation, and habilitation training is intensified.

Following abduction splinting, occasionally there is some tightness of the iliotibial band, presumably caused by lack of tension on this structure in the abducted position. In all but a few cases, this condition has responded to stretching over a period of several weeks. A simple Yount fasciotomy has resolved the remaining problems.

The quality of results has varied with the age at institution of treatment but generally has been very satisfactory. The goal of normal acetabular development has been achieved in all hips in which treatment was started prior to evidence of adaptive changes. When adaptive changes have been present they have not increased, and normal development has been noted in all cases. Initial concentric reduction of all hips was obtained either by positioning or through the surgical procedures described. Reduction has not been lost in any hip under treatment. Loss of reduction after

completion of treatment should not be considered a failure
but, instead, an indication that in the presence of continuing muscle imbalance, tendon transfer is indicated.

Long-term effects will have to await later evaluation.
Early major hip surgery almost certainly can be delayed,
but whether a significant number of subsequent tendon transfers can be avoided remains to be seen. The fervent hope is
that, through early attention to acetabular development, the
need for pelvic osteotomy and acetabular reconstruction which
produce so many stiff hips and such a high incidence of re-
dislocation can be eliminated.

REFERENCES

1. Ferguson, A.B., Jr.: Primary open reduction of congenital
    dislocation of the hip using a median adductor approach.
    J. Bone Joint Surg., *55A*:671, 1973.

2. Freehafer, A.A., Vessely, J.C. and Mack, R.P.: Iliopsoas
    muscle transfer in the treatment of myelomeningocele
    patients with paralytic hip deformities. *J. Bone Joint
    Surg.*, *54A*:1715, 1972.

3. Hoffer, M.M., Feiwell, E., Perry, R., Perry, J. and
    Bonnett, C.: Functional ambulation in patients with
    myelomeningocele. *J. Bone Joint Surg.*, *55A*:137, 1973.

4. McKibbin, B.: The use of splintage in the management of
    paralytic dislocation of the hip in spina bifida cystica.
    J. Bone Joint Surg., *55B*:163, 1973.

5. Raycroft, J.F. and Curtis, B.H.: Spinal curvature in
    myelomeningocele: natural history and etiology. Part V.
    Orthopaedic and developmental problems. American Academy
    of Orthopaedic Surgeons, Symposium on Myelomeningocele,

Hartford, Connecticut, 1970. St. Louis, C.V. Mosby,
1972, pp. 186.

6. Sharrard, W.J.W.: Posterior iliopsoas transplantation
in the treatment of paralytic dislocation of the hip.
J. Bone Joint Surg., 46B:426, 1964.

7. Sharrard, W.J.W.: Paediatric Orthopaedics and Fractures.
Oxford and Edinburgh, Blackwell Scientific Publications,
1971.

8. Sharrard, W.J.W. and Carroll, N.: Long-term follow-up
of posterior iliopsoas transplant for paralytic dislocation of the hip. In Proceedings. J. Bone Joint Surg.,
52B:779, 1970.

9. Spengler, K.C.: Analysis of ambulatory function in
older myelomeningocele patients. Presented to the
Fourteenth Annual Orthopaedic Clinical Meeting and
Alumni Reunion, Newington Children's Hospital, Newington,
Connecticut, 1976.

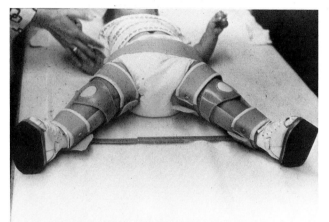

Fig. 1. Splint of Vitrathene in 45 degrees of abduction bilaterally with neutral rotation.

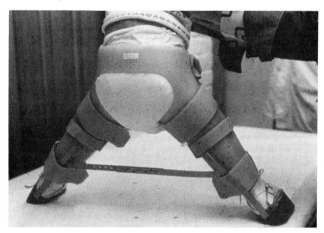

Fig. 2. Posterior view, standing.

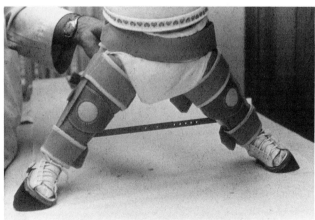

Fig. 3. Anterior view, standing.

CONSERVATIVE TREATMENT OF HIP
DISLOCATION IN THE MYELOMENINGOCELE

Earl Feiwell, M.D.

McKibbon presented a group of 11 patients treated to
the age of two years in abduction splints with controlled
neutral to slightly internal rotation and provided extension
of the hips through positioning and the weight of the splint.[5]

His initial concept was to prevent deterioration of the
hip during the early years while evaluation of the patient as
to survival and future function was carried out.

The splints allowed concentric reduction and thereby
development of the acetabulum and avoidance of iliopsoas
contracture by extension of the hip and avoidance of the
externally rotated position.

The results showed no deterioration in reducible hips
and improvement of the acetabulum in six children with
flexors and adductors. The five flail hips did not show
bony improvement. It was anticipated that surgery would
follow removal of the splints at age two. But progression
of subluxation had not occurred up to the longest period of
follow-up at one year. One patient, however, did require
iliopsoas tenotomy. Flail hips did not appear to benefit
from treatment.

Our experience with paralytic subluxations indicates
that progression will occur during childhood if a sufficient
imbalance of forces is present[6-10] (see etiology). If

513

displacement is to be treated, it must be done surgically.
There is no conservative treatment for paralytic hip dislocation. There is only conservative treatment of the patient.
The hips are treated in the most conservative surgical manner
indicated.

Our initial treatment involved surgery utilizing the
principles of balancing the forces about the hip,[8] adductor
muscles were transferred to the ischium to reduce adductor
strength past the mid-line. Iliopsoas transfers were performed; first anteriorly as described by Mustard,[7] then
laterally through a hole in the ilium as described by Garceau[2]
in 1949 article, and finally more posterolateral in the
position advocated by Sharrard. Femoral osteotomies and
acetabular procedures were performed.[10] These worked adequately on our polio patients, but as more myelomeningocele
patients entered the series, greater problems arose and
results were less optimum. We felt that greater selectivity
of patients was indicated and a study in 1970 was carried out
to determine which patients would ambulate and what were the
factors that prevented ambulation.[4]

Our conclusions were that thoracic level patients, that
is those who do not have sensation past the hips or muscles
crossing the hips, would not be adult ambulators. Ambulation
can be subdivided into community and household and exercise
levels. The community ambulator is that patient who goes out
into the community and walks with or without braces or
crutches, and who uses a wheelchair only for extreme ambulatory conditions or for great speed such as in crossing
college campuses. The household ambulator is that patient
who ambulates within the house for short distances but is
unable to reasonably ambulate any distance. Exercise
ambulators are those patients who walk as an exercise but are

unable to initiate ambulation from a sitting position or
to engage in any practical walking.

The primary goal, then, in the thoracic patient is to
provide a level pelvis and loose hips for good sitting, as
this will be their primary activity as a wheelchair patient.
A hip that does not flex to at least 90 degrees and cannot be
placed in neutral ab- or adduction position will have unequal
weight distribution on the pelvis in sitting and cause the
most disabling adult condition; the decubitus ulcer.

Surgical treatment of the hip should be limited to the
appropriate releases of soft tissues.

The lumbar patients were classified into two functional
groups for convenience of evaluation. Those with upper
lumbar lesions have flexors or adductors of the hip and/or
knee extension. The lower lumbar patient has functional
knee flexors and/or ankle extensors at their lowest level.
Sensation is variable in these groups. Knee control, that
is the functional flexors and extensors, are the primary
dividing area. Therefore, Sharrard's group three, or the
L3-4 division falls into both categories for at the L4 level
some patients have medial hamstrings. The older children and
adults with lumbar level lesions have an equal number of
ambulators and nonambulators. The primary factors were
scoliosis, mental retardation, and spasticity; these last two
factors were closely associated in effects as well as their
occurrence with hydrocephalus.

If the patient in the upper lumbar category did ambulate,
it was with long leg braces and crutches whereas many of the
lower lumbar ambulatory patients performed with short leg
braces. Some did not use crutches for household or other
short distance ambulation.

The sacral level patient is defined as the patient who has a level low enough to have hip extensors and/or ankle plantar flexors. These patients all ambulated. Hip dysplasia was not a problem. In Sharrard's series[10] there were four subluxed hips and one dislocated hip in his group of 53 in the S1 or S2 level. Appropriate adductor releases or possible varus osteotomies may be indicated in the occasional sacral patient whose spasticity gives the overall effect of a spastic subluxing or dislocating hip.

With this experience, surgical programs were directed toward those patients who were felt to be within the ambulatory levels of paralysis. A number of these patients were above the age of five.

Reduction of hips in nonambulatory patients did not result in improvement of their ambulatory status. Multiple surgical procedures were performed with little change in the functional results with the exception that some patients stopped walking with stiffness of their hips or fractures of their extremities. Subsequent spinal fusions in the teenage patients caused further decompensation of abilities for sitting, in patients with limited hip motion. Failure to achieve reduction of hips was frequently associated with pelvic obliquity.

In our rehabilitation center many children are transferred from other institutions at an older age. However, in those patients who were seen as infants or very young children, we attempted prophylactic iliopsoas transfer when the appropriate imbalance of forces appeared to be present. In some of these, late subluxations occurred, particularly when femoral osteotomies were not performed.

Attempts at treating high dislocations resulted in an increase in poor results, particularly in bilateral cases in which one might readily reduce whereas the opposite hip did not.

Questions related to our surgical abilities entered our minds. However, subsequent articles began appearing, such as that of Carroll and Sharrard, demonstrating the high incidence of late failures of surgery, particularly in high dislocations, as well as the high complication rate of stiffness.[1] In their article, 17 out of 58 hips were unable to flex to 90 degrees, 25 percent had avascular necrosis, and and frequent fractures occurred. The overall success of treatment at that time demonstrated 34 patients had stable hips, 23 were unstable and one stable hip was fused.

Parker and Walker reported in their series and demonstrated that 24 patients had good results and 19 were poor; a total of 72 hips being operated on. This resulted in 22 fractures; nine had sepsis and eight had avascular necrosis.[9]

These are formidable odds to the performance of any surgical procedure. The rate of failure has been high and complications which may make sitting extremely difficult are not infrequent. For example, the inability to flex the hip to 90 degrees or bring the hip to a neutral ab-adduction position will lead to marked pelvic obliquity in sitting. Sitting balance is then askew creating the increased chance of decubitus ulcers because of localized pressure on one ischium. Further inability to balance without depending on his arms while sitting places a tremendous burden on the patient who otherwise could function well from a society of wheelchairs.

Is it worth gambling against these great odds to produce a stable hip? Will the patient ambulate that much better to compensate for the possible complications? Are the gains reasonable to account for his losses, or are we treating the x-ray and not the functional abilities of the patient?

In our group of patients, it was found that no patient
failed to ambulate because of hip dislocation. Hips do not
continue to displace superiorly, but actually stabilize in
the displaced position. The fear of an unstable hip piston-
ing up into the axilla (Fig. 1) is not warranted. Ambulation
in the displaced position does not result in a gait that is
dissimilar from the patient who has a paralyzed or very weak
abductor. Cruse and Turner did not find, in their series
that a functioning iliopsoas transplant eliminated a Trendelenburg gait and our experience has been the same, no
matter which method of iliopsoas transplant was carried out.[12]
Even in the polio patient in whom most other musculature was
present about the hip despite a successful transfer, the
Trendelenburg gait continued.

The lower lumbar patient who may ambulate with short leg
braces and who can be a good community ambulator has some
adductor power, but walks with a Trendelenburg or gluteus
medius limp, throwing his body over his hip joint in order to
maintain balance. Many of these patients will not use
crutches about the house. The gaits of these individuals who
have reduced hips demonstrate the marked gluteus medius limp.
Patients with bilateral dislocations demonstrate a similar
gait.

It is questionable as to whether lower extremity
stability is improved by reduction of the hip.

Certainly, in our upper lumbar patients, all of whom in
our series ambulate with long leg braces and crutches, there
has been no difference in appearance or ability with the
swing-through gait, if the hips are dislocated or reduced.

No patient in our series complained of pain in or about
the hip. Complaints of pain in younger adults are rare, even
on a congenital hip dislocation that has never been treated.

Unilateral dislocation caused difficulties because of
the short lower extremity and will, unquestionably, require
some type of crutch aide. It is unlikely, however, that it
will prevent ambulation. At present, I believe that unilateral subluxation in potential ambulator should have
treatment if a limited procedure can be performed and the
pelvis is level. It is questionable as to whether lateral
iliopsoas transfer should be done unilaterally.

Bilateral subluxations should be treated by subtrochan-
teric osteotomy and iliopsoas release or anterolateral transfers in potential ambulators, but one should avoid doing any
significant open reduction or extensive bony surgery in order
to avoid limiting range of motion.

Tendon releases of the iliopsoas and sartorius, and
possibly extension osteotomies of the femur, are done for
hip flexion contractures in potential ambulators, avoiding
significant scarring over the hip joint. Ridding the hip
flexion contracture allows the patient to stand better,
reduces the presence of lumbar lordosis and knee flexion
contractures.

Conservative treatment is functional treatment. Treatment is based on the functional needs of the patient and not
on the x-rays. The nonambulating patient should be given
what he needs, namely, loose hips, a straight back and a
level pelvis. The potential ambulator requires the need to
be contracture-free and have plantargrade feet. These
patients require a great deal of bracing, multiple surgical
procedures and much work from various members of the health
team. They do not need surgical procedures on their hips
to provide better x-rays if the functional results are
questionable and the complications great. Any surgical
procedure   should   be   simple,   sure   and

definitely   provide   functional   improvement.

REFERENCES

1. Carroll, N. and Sharrard, W.J.W.: Long-term follow-up of
    posterior iliopsoas transplantation for paralytic dis-
    location of the hip. *J. Bone Joint Surg., 54A*:551, 1972.
2. Cruess, R. and Turner, N.: Paralysis of hip abductor
    muscles in spina bifida. *J. Bone Joint Surg., 52A*:1364,
    1970.
3. Garceau, G.J. and Kinzel, J.W.: Transplantation of the
    iliacus muscle for loss of hip abductor power. *Quarterly
    Bulletin, Indiana Univ. Med. Center, 13*:27, 1951.
4. Hoffer, M., Feiwell, E., Perry, R., Perry, J. and Bonnett,
    C.: Functional myelomeningocele. *J. Bone Joint Surg.,
    55A*:137, 1973.
5. McKibbon, B.: The use of splintage in the management of
    paralytic dislocations of the hip in spina bifida cystica.
    J. Bone Joint Surg., 55B:163, 1973.
6. Menelaus, M.B.: Dislocation and deformity of the hip in
    children with spina bifida cystica. *J. Bone Joint Surg.,
    51B*:238, 1969.
7. Mustard, W.T.: Iliopsoas transfer for weakness of hip
    abduction. *J. Bone Joint Surg., 34A*:647, 1952.
8. Nickel, V., Perry, J., Garrett, A. and Feiwell, E.:
    Paralytic dislocation of the hip. *Proceedings of the
    American Academy of Orthopedic Surgeons, 48A*:1021, 1966.
9. Parker, B. and Walker, G.: Posterior psoas transfer and
    hip instability in lumbar myelomeningocele. *J. Bone
    Joint Surg., 57B*:53, 1975.

10.   Sharrard, W.J.W.:   Posterior iliopsoas transplantation
      in the treatment of paralytic dislocation of the hip.
      J. Bone Joint Surg., *46B*:426, 1964.

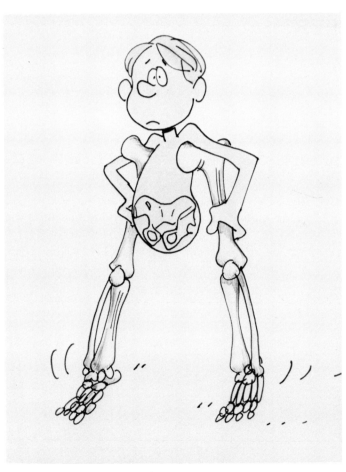

Fig. 1.

TABLE 1.

Summarized from Tables of Functional Ambulation
in Patients with Myelomeningocele.[4]

Lumbar level patients	Community ambulators (14)	Non-ambulators (19)
Retarded	0	11
60 degree scoliosis	2	9
Hydrocephalus	3	9
30 degree hip and/or 20 degree knee flexion contracture	0	19

MUSCLE BALANCING PROCEDURES IN HIP
DEFORMITY IN MYELOMENINGOCELE

W.J.W. Sharrard, M.D., F.R.C.S.

There are four main varieties of deformity that may
develop at the hip in myelomeningocele. In order of
frequency they are:

1. Flexion-adduction deformity with subluxation or
dislocation (at birth or later).

2. Flexion-lateral rotation deformity.

3. Pure flexion deformity.

4. Abduction extension deformity.

Each requires a different approach in its management to
attempt to gain muscle balance, satisfactory hip development
and prevention of recurrent deformity.

ADDUCTION-FLEXION DEFORMITY

Adduction-flexion deformity is characteristic of paralysis in which there is predominance of activity in the lumbar
roots with paresis or paralysis in the sacral segments. In
its most severe form (Fig. 1) it presents with fixed deformity
at birth with a congenital dislocation[7] which has almost
certainly been present since the first trimester of pregnancy.
This variety is uncommon but presents specific problems in
management greater than the more common situation in which
there is a lesser degree of flexion and adduction deformity
at birth possibly with subluxation or a dislocatable hip

523

comparable to that in non-paralytic dislocation and extremely
liable to progress to irreducible dislocation during the
early months of life. When there is some activity in the
gluteus medius, a much slower development of subluxation may
occur but even this may ultimately lead to dislocation in
late childhood or even early adolescence.

Muscle balancing procedures are required either to
prevent recurrence of deformity and dislocation once it has
been corrected or to halt the progress of progressive deformity. The key to the situation lies in the diminution of
excessive power in the hip flexors and adductor muscles and
the enhancement of action in the abductors and extensors by
release of the adductors possibly with posterior transfer of
their origin and postero-lateral or lateral transplantation
of the iliopsoas. The choice of procedure depends on the
extent of imbalance and the condition of the hip.

The timing of the operation depends on the severity of
the problem. Fixed flexion and adduction deformity with
congenital dislocation or rapidly progressive subluxation
requires operation in the early months of life, preferably
between the fourth and ninth months. Less rapid subluxation
can await progress in the development of gluteal function
but, if gluteal abduction power does not reach more than
grade 3, muscle balancing procedures are required before the
child reaches the ages of two or three.

ADDUCTOR RELEASE AND TRANSPOSITION

Dislocation of the hip or progression towards dislocation is always associated with limitation of abduction and
must always be corrected.[4,7] When the hip is dislocated at
birth, the adductors are always extremely tight and all of
them are affected. Through an incision in the groin,

parallel and 2.5 cm distal to it, the adductors are exposed, the fascia over them being incised along the line of the thigh. Adductor longus, gracilis, brevis and magnus all need to be divided from their attachment to the pelvis and, very frequently, the tendon of origin of the medial hamstring muscles also needs to be divided. The dislocated hip can be reduced (Fig. 2) in more than 75 percent of patients even those with severe deformity provided that sufficient abduction is obtained and the hip is allowed to flex and laterally rotate to relax the iliopsoas, which, at this stage, is normally left untouched.

In the presence of less severe deformity without dislocation, adductor longus and gracilis division and stretching of the adductor brevis and magnus is often sufficient to obtain a full range of abduction. Procedures additional to adductor release will depend on the state of muscle balance. If a very complete adductor release has been performed, it is not usually appropriate to divide the anterior branch of the obturator nerve and only occasionally does the strength of the adductors in relation to the glutei require this to be done. Posterior transplantation of the adductor longus, gracilis and brevis to the ischial tuberosity have been recommended recently[4] as a means of obtaining additional power of extension so that a lateral transfer of the iliopsoas rather than a postero-lateral transfer may achieve muscle balance. The author has no personal experience of this approach but it would appear to have much to recommend it.

If the hip is subluxated or has relatively recently dislocated, the iliopsoas transfer can be undertaken immediately following adductor release and relocation of the hip. In severe birth dislocations, however, it is probably

advisable to defer iliopsoas transplantation until one or
two weeks later to avoid excessive disturbance of the blood
supply to the femoral head associated with sudden and extreme
alteration in the position of the hip.

POSTERO-LATERAL ILIOPSOAS TRANSFER[1,6,7]

     This operation (Fig. 3) has its strongest indication in
children with congenital paralytic dislocation of the hip
associated with complete paralysis of all gluteal muscles,
or when progressive subluxation has led to dislocation in an
older child. The approach is made through an incision
passing along the anterior two-thirds of the iliac crest and
then obliquely down the anterior aspect of the thigh along
the medial side of the sartorius to a point half way between
the anterior superior spine and the knee. The incision in
the gluteal region is deepened to expose the outer side of
the iliac crest, the abdominal muscles, which often overhang
the iliac crest being mobilised upwards. The thin gluteal
fascia and the posterior part of the origin of the tensor
fascia latae are incised to expose the gluteal muscles which
are often degenerate or almost absent. The fibres of the
gluteus medius and minimus are mobilised from the outer side
of the ilium by extra-periosteal stripping. Unless there is
severe fixed flexion deformity, the anterior part of the
origin of the tensor fascia latae, the origin of the sartorius
and the origin of the rectus femoris should be left undis-
turbed since they will act as the flexors of the hip in
future. It should be possible to work beneath these muscles
to expose the hip joint and to perform capsular reefing.

     The thigh incision is deepened to expose the sartorius
and the inguinal ligament. The femoral nerve is identified
beneath a thin layer of fascia just below the inguinal

ligament and its branches carefully preserved. The object of
the next part of the dissection is to expose the lesser
trochanter. The choice lies between exposing the trochanter
between the femoral nerve and femoral vessels, which involves
the need to perform a careful and sometimes slightly difficult dissection to expose, ligate and divide the lateral
femoral circumflex vessels at their origin from the femoral
vessels or to approach on the outer side of the femoral
nerve, dividing the branches of the lateral femoral circumflex
and working beneath the femoral nerve and vessels. The
author's preference is for the first approach which allows
better mobilisation of the iliopsoas from the anterior and
medial aspects of the hip joint. The iliopsoas tendon is
then defined right down to its insertion into the lesser
trochanter. The tip of the lesser trochanter is divided with
an end-cutting knife to allow the iliopsoas tendon to be
mobilised proximally. There is often a deeper layer of the
tendon closely applied to the front of the hip which must be
identified and divided so that the sub psoas bursa can be
entered.

In the third stage of the operation, the inguinal
ligament is defined from its underlying structures and the
abdominal muscles mobilised proximally by incising the
cartilage of the iliac crest along its anterior two-thirds.
There will then be exposed in the false pelvis, the iliacus,
psoas and femoral nerves. The iliopsoas tendon with its
attached piece of lesser trochanter is passed beneath the
femoral nerve and mobilised proximally, the iliacus being
separated from the inner side of the ilium along its whole
extent to the level of the posterior superior iliac spine.
At this point, the anterior aspect of the sacro-iliac joint
can be seen. There is no requirement to proceed more

medially than this and attempts to do so may damage the ilio-
lumbar vessels or the ureter. An oval foramen is made in
the ilium just lateral to the sacro-iliac joint, with the aid
of a curved osteotome. The whole of the iliopsoas tendon
and the iliacus are passed through the foramen to the gluteal
region, the nerve supply of the iliacus arising from the
femoral nerve in the pelvis being preserved.

At this point, the hip joint can now be visualised on
the whole of its anterior, medial and lateral aspects. If
the hip has been completely dislocated before operation, the
hip capsule should be opened even if the hip has been able to
be reduced at the first operation of adductor release. An
incision is made parallel to the acetabulum and extended well
laterally and medially to allow good visualisation of the
acetabular cavity. It is not usually difficult to seat the
femoral head deeply in the pelvis and it is seldom necessary
to remove a limbus or ligament teres. Capsular reefing is
performed with removal of a V shaped portion of capsule
anteriorly and mobilisation of the redundant superior capsule
towards the anterior and medial aspect of the hip joint.
Closure of the capsule is not performed until the iliopsoas
tendon has been transplanted through the greater trochanter.

In the fourth part of the operation, the antero-lateral
aspect of the upper part of the femur is exposed by incising
the tensor fascia latae. The front of the greater trochanter
is identified and a hole made in the trochanter passing
posteriorly 20 degrees upwards and 20 degrees medially using
a Paton's burr or a drill. A tendon cannula is passed
through the foramen so that its tip emerges in the gluteal
region. The iliopsoas tendon must be trimmed adequately to
such a size as will allow its easy passage through the hole
in the trochanter. Using a suture passed through the tendon

cannula, the cannula is used to pull the iliopsoas tendon
through the tunnel in the trochanter so that the tip of the
lesser trochanter emerges through the front of the greater
trochanter.   If the lesser trochanter does not appear at the
front of the greater trochanter, a check must be made to
ensure that the tendon is not stuck posteriorly at the
entrance of the foramen; in all but a very few patients,
tendon length is sufficient to be able to bring it out
anteriorly.   If the capsule has been opened, it is now
sutured and the tip of the trochanter and the iliopsoas
tendon are sutured to the cartilage of the greater trochanter
with the hip held abducted and extended as much as possible
and with slight medial rotation.

The iliac crest is sutured back with strong sutures.
The lateral part of the inguinal ligament is sutured to the
pectineal line to close the gap produced by the removal of
the iliopsoas tendon, the suture passing between the lateral
cutaneous nerve of the thigh and the femoral nerve.   The
remainder of the wound is closed and a plaster spica applied.
Fixation in the abducted and extended position is needed for
a maximum of four weeks in a child below the age of two years
and five or five and a half weeks in a child older than this.
The hip is then allowed to mobilise so it may be appropriate
to sustain the range of abduction by means of a simple carefully padded night splint for two or three months.

Lateral transfer of the iliopsoas[2,3,4] can be used in
some cases in association with posterior transfer of the
adductor muscles.   The approach to the iliopsoas tendon and
to the pelvis is similar to that described above.   The
iliopsoas tendon is transferred beneath the femoral nerve to
the lateral or slightly postero-lateral aspect of the greater
trochanter where it is attached to the bone through a bony

tunnel. A notch is cut in the ilium to allow the tendon to lie comfortably. Treatment after operation is as described for postero-lateral iliopsoas transplantation.

RESULTS

If an adequate operation has been performed and the hip well reduced before the age of two years, there is seldom need to perform osteotomy either of the upper end of the femur or of the innominate bone. The acetabular socket will become adequately established as in non-paralytic dislocation of the hip and valgus and anteversion of the neck of the femur will correct spontaneously[1,6] as a result of the action of the iliopsoas transplant (Fig. 4). Only in patients in whom spontaneous mobilisation of the hip after operation from the abducted position fails to occur, or if the hip threatens to re-dislocate, is varus osteotomy of the upper end of the femur indicated. Although, in earlier transplants, only half the hips gained satisfactory quality of hip joint, more experience in the operation and better technique has led to much more satisfactory results with more than 80 percent of hips showing long term congruity and adequacy.[5] Recurrence of subluxation has usually been due to inadequate adductor release and, should it develop, a further release of the adductors with division of the anterior branch of the obturator nerve will suffice to restore the situation.

Avascular necrosis of the femoral head is an ever present possibility, especially if the adductors have been inadequately released but it should not occur in more than 5 to 10 percent of cases and, in most of these, spontaneous restoration of vascular supply occurs in early childhood without necessarily producing deformity of the femoral head.

In older children or in neglected cases, the soft tissue
operations and transfers described above are still indicated
but there is much more likelihood that additional bony procedures such as innominate osteotomy or upper femoral osteotomy
may be required to obtain satisfactory stability of the hip
joint. Obliquity of the pelvis is also a complicating factor
in association with subluxation or dislocation of the hip and
should, if possible, be corrected before iliopsoas transfer
is performed.

FLEXION-LATERAL ROTATION DEFORMITY

Flexion-lateral rotation deformity (Fig. 5) develops
when there is isolated action in the upper one or two lumbar
segments with activity in the iliopsoas and sartorius muscle
and paresis or paralysis in other hip musculature. The hip
falls into flexion, abduction and lateral rotation but, in
contrast to patients with fixed abduction-extension deformity,
the hip can be adducted to the neutral position when it will
be apparent that there is a marked flexion deformity present.

FLEXOR RELEASE AND ANTERO-LATERAL ILIOPSOAS TRANSFER

The iliopsoas acts as a strong lateral rotator as well
as a flexor of the hip. Elongation of the iliopsoas leaving
it attached to the lesser trochanter invites the strong
possibility of recurrent flexion and lateral rotation deformity. Flexor release should therefore be combined with transplantation of the iliopsoas to the anterior aspect of the
greater trochanter (Fig. 6). The flexor region is approached
through an oblique incision similar to that described for the
thigh portion of the dissection for postero-lateral iliopsoas
transplantation. If the flexion deformity is 40 degrees or

less, the iliopsoas should be exposed as described above,
detached from the lesser trochanter and mobilised beneath
the femoral nerve to be attached to the anterior aspect of
the greater trochanter. This alone may succeed in correcting
all flexion deformity but if flexion deformity is greater
than 40 degrees, it is usually necessary to release the
sartorius, rectus femoris and anterior part of the tensor
fascia latae from the ilium and, sometimes, to divide the
ilio-femoral ligament, though it is unwise to open the hip
capsule or the head of the femur may dislocate anteriorly.
The incision is closed and the hip spica applied with the
hip extended and medially rotated. Plaster fixation should
be maintained for not longer than four weeks.

If incomplete correction of flexion deformity to less
than 20 degrees has not been achieved by soft tissue release
alone, an extension osteotomy of the upper end of the femur
may be needed in addition, either at the same procedure or on
a second occasion one month later.

PURE FLEXION DEFORMITY

Pure flexion deformity is usually seen only in children
with innervation of all hip flexors and abductors but some
weakness of the extensors especially the gluteus maximus.
Flexion deformity develops slowly, usually in later childhood.
If it becomes greater than 30 degrees a progressive crouch
gait may develop and walking ability diminishes steadily.

Provided that deformity has not become too great,
correction can be obtained by elongation of the iliopsoas
combined, if necessary, with some lengthening of the other
hip flexors. There is no indication to transplant the
iliopsoas muscle.

ABDUCTION-EXTENSION DEFORMITY OF THE HIP

This deformity is a rare deformity but extremely difficult to manage. It develops when there is complete paralysis
of the lumbar neural segments associated with reflex activity
in the sacral segments. The hip goes into abduction, (Fig.7)
extension and lateral rotation with development of fixed
deformity so that the child is unable to sit or be accommo-
dated in a chair. Correction by release of the gluteal
muscles from the ilium and mobilisation downwards has not
proved to be a satisfactory method of correction and recurrence is likely to develop extremely rapidly. Correction is
better achieved by separation of all the gluteal muscles
from their attachments to the greater trochanter and the
upper part of the femur combined with a radical adduction-
medial rotation upper femoral osteotomy. If recurrent
deformity threatens, denervation of the glutei by division
of the superior and inferior gluteal nerves may be needed.
It has not been possible to devise any transplant to regain
adduction and flexion to combat the power of reflexly
innervated gluteal musculature.

REFERENCES

1. Carroll, N.C. and Sharrard, W.J.W.: Long-term follow-up
    of posterior iliopsoas transplantation for paralytic
    dislocation of the hip. *J. Bone Joint Surg.*, *54A*:551,
    1972.
2. Cruess, R.L. and Turner, M.S.: Paralysis of hip abductor
    muscles in spina bifida. Results of treatment by the
    Mustard procedure. *J. Bone Joint Surg.*, *52A*:1364, 1970.

3. Freehafer, A.A., Vessely, J.C. and Mack, R.P.: Ilio psoas muscle transfer in the treatment of myelomeningocele patients with paralytic hip deformities. *J. Bone Joint Surg., 54A*:1715, 1972.

4. London, J.T. and Nichols, O.: Paralytic dislocation of the hip in myelodysplasia. The role of the adductor transfer. *J. Bone Joint Surg., 57A*:501, 1975.

5. Parker, B. and Walker, G.: Posterior psoas transfer and hip instability in lumbar myelomeningocele. *J. Bone Joint Surg., 57B*:53, 1975.

6. Rueda, J. and Carroll, N.C.: Hip instability in patients with myelomeningocele. *J. Bone Joint Surg., 54B*:422, 1972.

7. Sharrard, W.J.W.: Posterior ilio psoas transplantation in the treatment of paralytic dislocation of the hip. *J. Bone Joint Surg., 46B*:426, 1964.

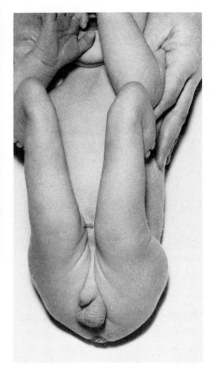

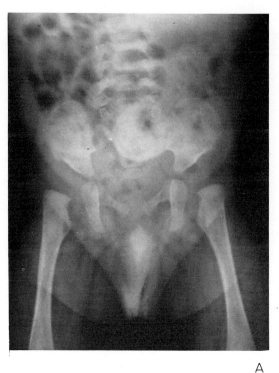

A

Fig. 1. Flexion-adduction deformity of the hips at birth. There is strong action in lumbar innervated muscles and paralysis of sacrally innervated muscles. The hips are dislocated.

Fig. 2. Radiographs of dislocated hips in myelomeningocele. A) Before operation. B) After bilateral radical adductor release.

B

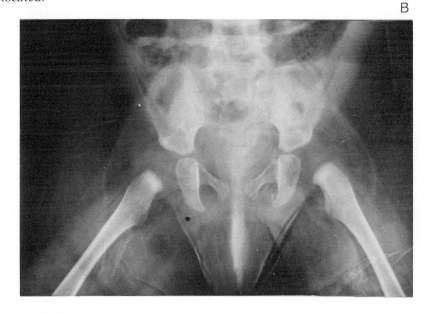

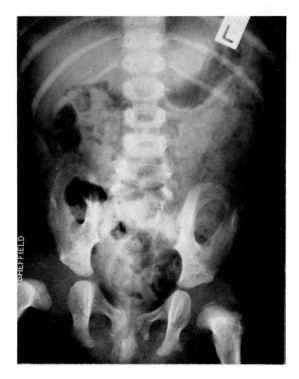

Fig. 3.   Radiograph of hips after bilateral postero-lateral iliopsoas transfer.

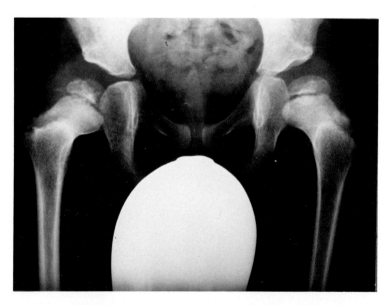

Fig. 4.   Radiograph of spontaneous correction of valgus and anteversion after iliopsoas transfer. The hips are stable and the acetabula adequate.

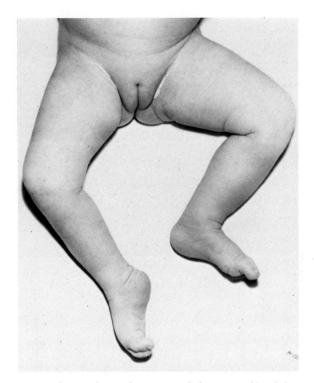

Fig. 5. Flexion-lateral rotation deformity of both hips.

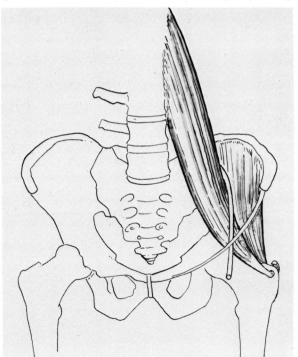

Fig. 6. Diagram of antero-lateral iliopsoas transfer.

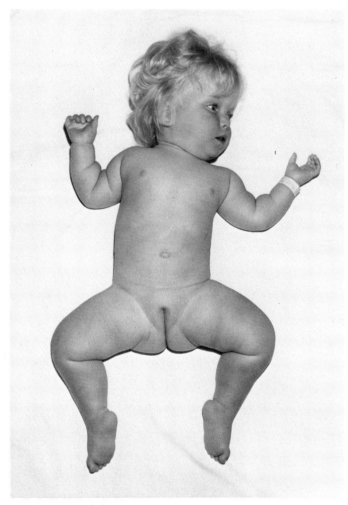

Fig. 7. Abduction-extension deformity of the hips. There is reflex innervation only from the sacral segments.

THE UNSTABLE HIP:
INFRA-ACETABULAR OSTEOTOMY

Earl Feiwell, M.D.

Femoral osteotomy is an integral part of the maintenance of hip reduction. The cause of paralytic hip dislocation is an imbalance of forces. A common result is bony deformity, first occurring in the femur and later in the acetabulum.

If congenital hip dysplasia is considered as a model because of its frequency and greater therapeutic experience, the problems become quite apparent. Here, the abductor muscle is normal physiologically, but functions poorly because of poor fulcrum or the lever arm (Fig. 1). The only way that normal hip development occurs is through a concentric reduction of the femoral head acetabular relationship. The normal muscle can then build strength and hold the reduction (Fig. 2). If a potentially normal muscle cannot create stability and normal development in the presence of dysplasia, how can we expect a transferred muscle with a much less potential strength and anatomic limitations to do a better job? Obviously, to obtain a stable hip concentric reduction must be obtained and forces directed to maintain this reduction.

Acetabular deformity occurs because of stress placed on improper areas of the acetabulum. Placement of pressure on the rim melts bone away. When the femur is in excessive

valgus and a strong abductor is lacking, the head remains on
the outer rim, leading to erosion (Fig. 3 & 4). The adducted
position of the femur in relation to the acetabulum can be
caused by any combination of valgus of the neck (Fig. 5a),
adducted position of the femur (Fig. 5b), or pelvic obliquity
(Fig. 5c). The nearer the angle between the neck of the
femur and the horizontal of the pelvis approaches 90 degrees,
the more unstable the hip will become.[4]

Excessive anteversion also acts to direct the head away
from the center of the triradiate cartilage (Fig. 6a).
External rotation of the limb has the same effect (Fig. 6b),
for as Menalaus points,[3] even after anteversion correction
has been performed, external rotation can occur with a lax
capsule leading to the same femoral head position in relationship to the acetabulum.

The femoral head can be centered and forces maintained
directed into the acetabulum, we can anticipate a good
reduction.[2] This occurs in the congenital hip with well-
balanced muscular forces about the hip and is anticipated in
the paralyzed child with appropriate transfers.

Abduction of the hip with mild internal rotation centers
the head in the acetabulum in a reducible hip. However, as
soon as the hips are brought back down to the weight bearing
position, weight is again placed on the outer rim of the
acetabulum.

The method of providing a persistent abduction position
of the femoral head and still allow weight bearing position
is by the varus osteotomy (Fig. 7). Our goal is 110 degrees,
but a 100 degrees to 120 degrees is satisfactory. Femoral
osteotomy at 110 degrees provides relative abduction and
forces that are sufficient to prevent recurrence of valgus,
particularly when the iliopsoas has been transferred to the

greater trochanter. This is reasonable in light of the previously mentioned study of Brookes and Wardle, which showed that the iliopsoas in its normal position tends to increase valgus whereas lateral forces on the greater trochanter tend to increase varus.[1] Also with the patient weight bearing on the superior portion of the femoral head, additional varus force is present. Osteotomies at 90 degrees or less can increase angulation tending towards danger of epiphyseal slip as well as fractures. Valgus of the neck much greater than 120 degrees does not accomplish an adequate abduction relationship and in addition may revert to a greater degree of valgus with growth.

TECHNIQUE

A preoperative x-ray of the hip is taken in the neutral position, that is with the knee slightly bent so that the patella is in the upright position. Maximum internal rotation is more accurate and relatively easy to perform. The external rotation position is extremely inaccurate, as it presents a definite increase in the valgus position thereby being exceedingly misleading to the surgeon in preoperative planning. A primary determination is made at the time of surgery when guide pins are in place.

A lateral incision is used to reach the proximal femur. A threaded Steinmann pin is inserted up the neck just short of the epiphysis then a second smooth Steinmann pin is inserted perpendicular to the lateral shaft of the femur below the site of the intended osteotomy (Fig. 8a). An x-ray is taken with the pin horizontal to the x-ray plate, thus two pins are used to determine the exact angle of valgus and the desired degree of correction. An estimate of the degree of anteversion can be made with the properly placed femoral

neck pin. We use a heavy threaded Steinmann pin in the
femoral neck because of the tendency of the pin to slip out
during manipulation at the time of osteotomy. A smooth, thin
pin readily frees itself and frequently falls out of the
soft porotic bone. If this happens once the osteotomy has
been made and the head-neck component becomes relatively
free, it is difficult to then accurately control the proximal
fragment.

A wedge of bone of the appropriate angle of correction
is removed if bilateral procedures are to be done. This
permits a closing wedge and more stable positioning (Fig.8b).
Early weight bearing can then be achieved with less fear of
an increasing varus deformity. Greater stability is achieved
if the lateral cortex and periosteum can be allowed to
remain relatively intact, the wedge is removed medially and
the lateral portion of the femoral cortex being snapped with
some bony integrity remaining.

A second type of osteotomy is also used (Fig. 8c).
Initially, this was done routinely in all our cases, but now
is used primarily in a unilateral procedure. The osteotomy
is performed by shifting the distal femur medially and
inserting the proximal fragment into the medullary canal of
the distal fragment (Fig. 8d). This procedure allows for
greater length of the femur achieving only about half the
loss of strength that a closing wedge osteotomy might cause.

Crossed Steinmann pins are placed across the osteotomy
site for fixation and the original pins are removed after
x-rays are taken (Fig. 8b & 8d). The crossed pins have been the
most satisfactory method in our hands. We have had difficulty
in using fixed angle pins for various reasons. Appropriate
sized nail plates are not readily available and then
difficulties encountered in placement of a nail plate of

correct length and width into the femoral neck without injuring the epiphysis is an additional problem. The crossed pin technique has been satisfactory. Compression plates have been useful only when rotational osteotomies have been performed and these have been sufficiently low on the shaft so that a proximal hold can be obtained with the plate. The plate and screw may lead to additional extensive future surgery for its removal.

Insertion of crossed Steinmann pins at the fracture site is at times difficult, and I can only say that the best way is whatever is most convenient. The pin should cross the cortex of one bone and the medial cortex of the second bone. At times this is accomplished by insertion through the greater trochanter and possibly may require passage of the pin through the skin rather than through the surgical incision itself. Passage of the pin through the distal fragment and then proximally may actually pass out of the femoral shaft and cross over medially and enter the femoral neck. In any case, the pin once inserted with even a moderately satisfactory hold should not be removed for perfect positioning since after one or two removals and reinsertions, satisfactory fixation becomes extremely diffi-cult. The pins are left long and cut off just below the skin for easier removal.

Sectioning of the iliopsoas tendon can be performed at the time of the osteotomy since it too is at the level of the lesser trochanter. An anterior iliopsoas transfer can be accomplished at the same time by extending the incision proximally a la Watson-Jones, freeing the iliopsoas tendon and iliacus from the proximal femur and passing it through a bony defect created between the sartorius and the rectus femoris and suturing it to the area of the greater trochanter.

Posterior transfers have been performed at the same time, but additional incisions have been necessary.

At the time of the osteotomy, a vertical lateral cortical cut is made prior to transecting the femur in order to allow proper identification of rotation. If some rotation correction is desired then this can be adequately measured by the change in position of the proximal cut to the distal cut. We primarily correct valgus and therefore when the pinning is carried out the two cuts are approximated.

The question of derotation for anteversion should be considered at this time. Menalaus,[3] in correcting for anteversion, repairs the anterior capsule because it was his feeling that if this was not done the laxity allowed a greater amount of external rotation since no internal rotation forces are present and the patient's femoral head position remained exactly as it was preoperatively even though bony correction of the anteversion had been performed. If it is felt that anteversion is a source of dislocation, correction can readily be made by a transverse cut, rotating the limb and then removing the varus wedge. Capsular reefing is probably indicated if significant rotation is carried out.

Postoperatively, the patients are placed in bilateral spica casts regardless of whether the procedure was unilateral or bilateral. I do not feel that a single spica cast is sufficient to maintain the reduction and it requires a higher hold on the chest. The so-called spica-and-a-half casts should not be used in these children as the exposed lower extremity is prone to fracture. The feet may be left free at the ankles. However, I prefer to utilize the plaster past the end of the toes in order to prevent any trauma to the exposed portions of the extremities. The plaster casts are very well padded, particularly around the sacral area.

We have attempted to make preoperative plaster casts in order to save surgical time. However, these frequently do not fit well following osteotomy. Bivalve casts were used for a period of time, but we had difficulties in attempting to replace the halves following removal. They also increase the tendency of patients to shift position in the cast causing heel ulcers.

At this time, the full plaster cast is applied and left in place. The sensitive areas still can be seen and checked, such as around the sacral area. Frequent turning, pronation and supination, and side to side are utilized to lessen localized areas of pressure on bony prominences.

The patient is started on upright weight bearing after three or four weeks depending on the apparent stability. The closing wedge osteotomy with good pin fixation can be started up relatively early, whereas the displacement osteotomy with questionable fixation would be watched much more closely and weight bearing delayed.

The effect of varus osteotomy was dramatically demonstrated in one patient who was seen in our clinic after surgical treatment in Texas. The patient had bilateral iliopsoas transplants in the posterior lateral method of Sharrard. One side was well reduced with the iliopsoas functioning and the opposite side did not appear to function and was subluxed. The side that was well reduced had had a spontaneous fracture of the intertrochanteric region prior to surgery, and had healed in a varus position of approximately 110 degrees. The opposite side had a natural valgus position. A varus osteotomy was performed. The iliopsoas transplant was freed and placed on greater tension on the femur. The muscle subsequently functioned and the hip has remained reduced.

This also points to the fact that any femoral osteotomy
that is carried out should be done before an iliopsoas
transplant or at the same time. If a varus osteotomy is
carried out after iliopsoas transplant has been performed, it
slackens the muscle by shortening the distance between the
greater trochanter and the origin within the ilium. The
tendon must be reimplanted under greater tension if the
osteotomy is performed. The only exception to this would be
if the patient had a fixed abduction contracture due to a
tight iliopsoas tendon and a varus osteotomy is performed to
bring the extremity into a more vertical position.

If an acetabular procedure is necessary as well as
femoral osteotomy and iliopsoas transplant, I prefer not to
do all the work at the same time, but will do the femoral
osteotomy and release the iliopsoas, possibly transfer it
proximally, tagging and lying free where it can be readily
found. Then I will wait two weeks and carry out the rest of
muscle transplant and acetabular procedure.

Femoral osteotomy to provide extension has a definite
place in our armamentarium.[3] Marked flexion contractures
tend to recur with soft tissue releases. Excessive capsular,
as well as muscle releases, may give limited flexion of the
hip. A wedge of bone taken just below the base of the neck
frequently including the lesser trochanter can give excellent
improvement of the patient's flexion contracture. Thirty
degrees of bone can be easily removed, at the same time
sectioning a tight iliopsoas tendon through the osteotomy
and releasing the sartorius through a small incision at the
anterior superior spine. With this method little capsular
scar tissue occurs and there is more permanent hip extension.
Preoperatively, the hip must be checked for a full range of
flexion for obviously if the hips can only come to 90 degrees

prior to surgery, the child will have less ability to sit
upright, postoperatively, since his hip flexion range has
been exchanged for extension. With 30 degrees of wedge of
bone removed and a section of the iliopsoas tendon freed and
· a tight sartorius released, 40 to 45 degrees of hip flexion
contracture can be readily corrected.

This procedure is carried out through a lateral incision.
The bone is exposed and a wedge removed with the apex forward
(Fig. 9). The wedge is closed and Steinmann pins are then
inserted through the lateral cortex into the femoral neck.
A directly transverse cut is made at the proximal portion
and the oblique wedge removed distally. The iliopsoas is
released at this time as the insertion is often attached to
the wedge. The varus wedge could also be performed at this
time if that were indicated. A tight sartorius should be
released through a small incision at the anterior superior
spine and a tight iliotibial band can be sectioned through
the lateral incision. Hips that are dislocated and have
significant flexion contractures may be treated in this
fashion so the patient can be ambulatory.

In summary, varus osteotomy is an effective method of
correcting the most significant femoral deformity and provide
satisfactory femoral acetabular relationships. The osteotomy
allows a similar relationship to that obtained by abducting
the femur to obtain a concentric relationship within the
acetabulum while maintaining the lower extremity in a vertical relationship to the body. A satisfactory femoral
acetabular relationship is necessary as a prerequisite to
any other muscle transplant about the hip. Extension
osteotomies of the femur are an effective adjunct in
relieving severe hip flexion contractures.

REFERENCES

1. Brookes, M. and Wardle, E.N.: Muscle action and the shape of the femur. *J. Bone Joint Surg., 44B*:398, 1962.

2. Harris, N.H., Lloyd-Roberts, G.C. and Gallien, R.: Acetabular development in congenital dislocation of the hip. *J. Bone Joint Surg., 57B*:46, 1975.

3. Menelaus, M.B.: Dislocation and deformity of the hip in children with spina bifida cystica. *J. Bone Joint Surg., 51B*:238, 1969.

4. Somerville, E.W.: Paralytic dislocation of the hip. *J. Bone Joint Surg., 41B*:279, 1959.

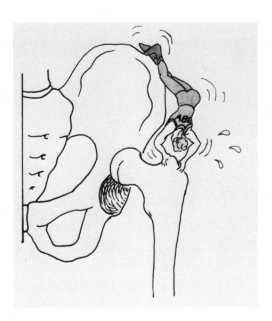

Fig. 1.

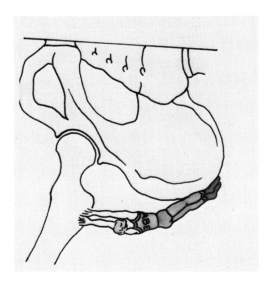

Fig. 2.

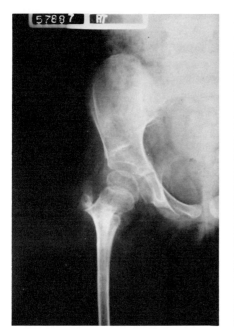

Fig. 3.   Femoral neck is in valgus
with imbalance of forces creating
subluxation. A shelf operation had
been performed above the
acetabulum.

Fig. 4.   Femoral head has slowly
eroded the edge of the acetabulum.
Arrow points to the original edge.

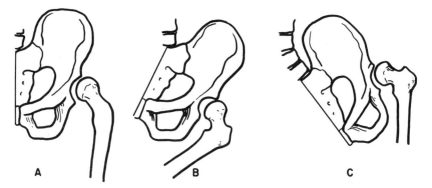

Fig. 5.   A. Relationship of femoral head to the acetabulum related to valgus
position of the femoral neck.
B. Femoral-acetabular relationship is the same if the femur is
adducted.
C. Femoral-acetabular relationship is the same if the pelvis is tilted.

550

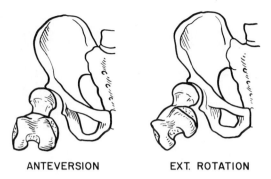

ANTEVERSION   **EXT. ROTATION**

Fig. 6. Femoral-acetabular relationship is the same
with increased anteversion or increased external
rotation.

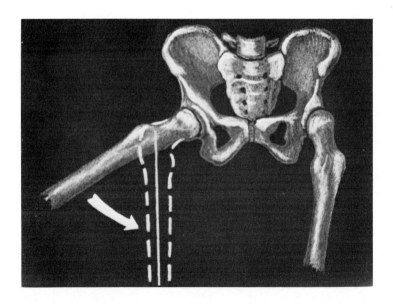

Fig. 7. Valgus neck with femur in weight-bearing position gives a poor
femoral-acetabular relationship. Abduction is necessary to center the femoral
head. Osteotomy (dotted lines) allows abduction position of the head and neck
but weight-bearing position of the femur.

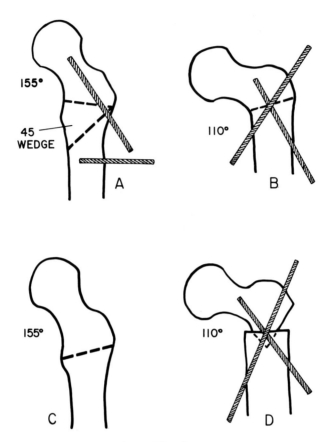

Fig. 8.

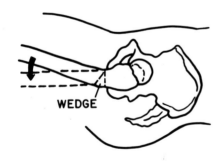 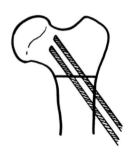

Fig. 9.

THE UNSTABLE HIP - SUPRA ACETABULAR
OSTEOTOMY

N. Carroll, M.D., BSc, F.R.C.S. (C)

Spina bifida children have many hip problems: muscle
weakness, muscle spasticity, muscle contracture, capsular
laxity, deficient acetabulum, saucer-shaped acetabulum, neck-
shaft malalignment and malrotation, and pelvic obliquity.

In neonates, our therapists exercise the hips to prevent
contractures. If an adduction contracture occurs, an
adductor tenotomy is performed. We avoid spica plasters,
similar to those used in congenital dislocation of the hip,
because flexion abduction and external rotation contractures
tend to develop. If an orthosis is required to keep the
neonate's hip in joint, it should be designed to maintain
abduction and internal rotation, so that the iliopsoas muscle
is not allowed to shorten. Aggressive hip surgery is usually
delayed until the child is about 18 months old, at which
time we have a good idea as to the child's potential. This
surgery is reserved for children whom we believe will be
household- or community-walkers.

Hip abductor-extensor paresis and beginning subluxation
can be managed by assuring adequate abduction and by an
iliopsoas tendon transfer. If the subluxation is more severe,
a capsulorrhaphy will be required. If the acetabulum is
saucer-shaped, the femoral head will be better contained if

the capsule is completely cleared from the lateral surface of
the ilium, and the cartilage model of the acetabulum levered
down over the head and held in position by a bone graft.

Spina bifida children present with three types of hip
dislocation. If the hip was dislocated *in-utero* (teratogenic
dislocation), it will be high and stiff - like that in an
arthrogrypotic child. The second type of dislocation
appears shortly after birth. If such a child presents at age
3-4 years, surgery may reveal that the acetabulum is small
and deficient; the only way of finding the true acetabulum is
to trace the ligamentum teres to its source. It is always
necessary to divide the transverse acetabular ligament.
Following adequate capsulorrhaphy, better stability can be
achieved by doing a Chiari osteotomy.[1] We rarely do an
innominate osteotomy[2] to stabilize the hip of a spina bifida
child because here we are dealing not with a mal-directed
acetabulum as seen in congenital dislocation, but with a
deficient acetabulum. If such an acetabulum is directed
anteriorly and laterally the femoral head will dislocate
posteriorly. We reserve the innominate osteotomy for treatment of congenital subluxation, congenital dislocation, and
Perthes Disease with subluxation; the prerequisites are head-
acetabular congruity, and a full range of motion.

In the third type of dislocation, the head was in joint
during the first or second year of life, but was gradually
dislocated due to adductor-flexor *vs.* abductor-extensor
imbalance. In this instance the acetabulum is saucer-shaped.
At the time of open reduction, capsulorrhaphy, and psoas
transfer, the cartilage model of the acetabulum is levered
down over the femoral head, and held by a bone graft to
assure better stability.

After surgery for these three types of hip dislocation, the hip is protected in a spica for 6 weeks.

REFERENCES

1. Chiari, K.: Ergebnisse mit der Beckenosteotomie als Pfannendach plastik. *Z. Orthop.*, *87*:14, 1955.
2. Salter, R.B.: An operative treatment for congenital dislocation and subluxation of the hip in the older child. IN Recent Advances in Orthopedics, A. G. Apley, (ed.), London, J. & A. Churchill Ltd., 1969, pp. 325.

FIXED PELVIC OBLIQUITY, TREATMENT BY
POSTERIOR ILIAC OSTEOTOMY

Richard E. Lindseth, M.D.

Pelvic obliquity frequently occurs in children born with myelomeningocele. Two primary reasons cause this high frequency: unequal muscle activity across the hip and pelvis, producing an adduction contracture of one hip and an abduction of the other, and uncompensated scoliosis due to bony deformity of the lumbosacral spine.

Uncompensated scoliosis due to fixed bony deformity of the lumbosacral spine is the most common cause of pelvic obliquity in the myelomeningocele clinic at Riley Children's Hospital. In a recent survey of one hundred patients over the age of ten years, 66 percent of these children had scoliosis. Of these children with scoliosis, 60 percent had uncompensated curves causing pelvic obliquity for an overall incidence of 40 percent.[2]

Pelvic obliquity also has a profound effect upon dislocation of the hip. Regardless of the level of paraplegia, 95 percent of the children over the age of ten with pelvic obliquity had dislocation or severe subluxation of the hip on the high side. The dislocation occurred in most of the children after the age of eight, at which time the pelvic obliquity was well established and the dislocation appeared to be caused by the pelvic obliquity rather than the pelvic obliquity caused by the hip dislocation. Pelvic obliquity

affected standing and sitting balance. Only fifteen out of
fifty children with this deformity were able to walk. When
sitting balance was lost as well, the children were forced to
use their hands to help sit, thereby decreasing their upper
extremity function. Ulceration beneath the prominent
ischium was also common. To the child already struggling to
remain functional, the presence of a progressive scoliosis,
pelvic obliquity, dislocation of the hip, lack of sitting
and standing balance, and ischial decubitus ulceration was
often overwhelming.

TREATMENT

The ideal treatment of pelvic obliquity is to prevent it
by correcting the muscle imbalance around the pelvis and
hips and by controlling the scoliosis by early detection,
aggressive brace treatment and surgical stabilization.
However, despite the above procedures, pelvic obliquity
continues to occur. In those cases where pelvic obliquity
could not be corrected by surgery on the spine or the hips,
a surgical procedure has been developed to produce a compensating deformity in the pelvis, much like the lumbar spine
often produces a compensatory curve in dorsal idiopathic
scoliosis. This compensatory deformity in the pelvis is
obtained by bilateral posterior iliac osteotomy with the
removal of a wedge from the low side of the pelvis and adding
it to the high side (Fig. 1). This procedure causes a
rotation of the sacrum within the pelvis without changing
the functional length of the iliac vessels or of the anterior
muscles crossing the hip joint (Fig. 2). Initial attempts
to perform the osteotomies anteriorly using the anterior,
approach to the ilium were unsuccessful, due to the inability
to achieve a satisfactory mobility of the pelvis.

Before this osteotomy is performed, it is important that
the spinal curvature has been fused to prevent further progression of the curve.   There also must be sufficient pelvis
remaining after any previous surgery for bone grafting or
muscle transfer such as an iliopsoas transfer through the
ilium.

PROCEDURE

It is necessary that satisfactory x-rays be obtained to
show the degree of correction desired, and that these x-rays
are present in the operating theater.   There may be confusion
at the time of surgery as to which side should be corrected,
and it is necessary to refer back to the x-rays to make sure
that the wedge is taken from the correct side.   The osteotomy
is performed similar to the procedures described by Lloyd-
Roberts[1] and O'Phelan[3] for extrophy of the bladder.

The child is prone during the procedure.   Bilateral
posterior incisions are performed, starting laterally at the
anterior-superior iliac spine, along the iliac crest to the
posterior-superior spine, then curving downward along each
side of the sacrum to the superior part of the sciatic notch.
In a child, the iliac apophysis is then split longitudinally.
The paraspinus muscle, the quadratus lumborum, and the iliac
muscle are taken with the inner half of the apophysis.   The
inner periosteum is divided laterally and it is stripped from
the medial table of the ilium.   The gluteal musculature is
taken with the outer half of the apophysis.   After the medial
origin of the gluteus maximus has been stripped from the
sacrum, the outer periosteum is divided longitudinally just
lateral to the sacroiliac joint and down to the sciatic
notch.   The periosteum is then stripped from the outer table

of the ilium, care being taken to avoid damage to the
superior and inferior gluteal artery and nerve. Soft tissues
are retracted down to the sciatic notch, both medially and
laterally, and an iliac osteotomy is performed using an
osteotome. The osteotomy is centered approximately one inch
lateral to the sacroiliac joint. Because of the oblique
direction of the sacroiliac joint, the osteotomy will just
miss the lateral margin of the sacrum at the inner table of
the pelvis. A bone spreader is then placed in the osteotomy
to insure that the osteotomy is complete. This osteotomy is
performed on both ilia. A wedge of bone is then removed from
the low or long side of the ilium (Fig. 1). This wedge is
usually one inch wide at the crest and zero to one-half inch
wide at the sciatic notch, but the size depends upon the
degree of correction desired, the size of the pelvis, and the
pre-operative x-rays. After the wedge of bone has been
removed, correction of the deformity is obtained by pulling
on the leg on the short side and pushing on the leg on the
long side (Fig. 2). This will usually close the osteotomy
where the wedge was removed, although there is often an
upper displacement of the ilium. If the osteotomy does not
close, insufficient bone has been removed from the sciatic
notch. A rongeur can be used to remove more bone until the
osteotomy closes. With the use of a spreader, the osteotomy
on the high side is opened sufficiently to receive the graft.
The graft is held in place by two Kirschner wires that are
drilled from the posterior ilium through the wedge into the
iliac table (Fig. 3). Occasionally it is easier to place the
pin in the opposite direction depending on the shape of the
ilium. We have not had difficulty with displacement of the
graft, although the pin placements occasionally take several
attempts. The closing wedge osteotomy can be held if

necessary by a non-absorbable suture through drill holes in the ilium. On the donor side, the projecting end of the ilium is removed to allow the iliac apophysis to be sutured together over it.

On the graft side, the iliac apophysis is closed in a "Z" fashion with the paraspinus muscles staying medially and the gluteal muscle joined laterally. After skin closure, the child is placed in a double long leg hip spica cast for eight weeks. This is usually sufficient time to allow healing of the pelvis. The Kirschner wires may be removed any time thereafter.

This procedure has been performed in nine children who have been followed for over one year since surgery. The mean degree of correction was 13 degrees with a maximum correction of 22 degrees. For the last five patients the correction has been better and has averaged 18 degrees. However, this indicates the importance of obtaining maximum correction of the scoliosis and stabilizing the spine early. Correction of the list was more successful with a mean correction of 70 percent and was completely corrected in five children. Consequently all the children had improvement in their sitting and standing balance. The hips have remained reduced in eight of nine children. There was no major complication from the surgery and the correction has remained up to six years, which is the longest follow-up.

CONCLUSION

A relatively simple and safe procedure has been developed for the correction of pelvic obliquity resulting from uncompensated scoliosis that cannot be corrected by standard procedures. Six year follow-up has shown that the correction is permanent without tendency for the obliquity to return.

REFERENCES

1. Lloyd-Roberts, C.G., Williams, D.I. and Braddock, G.T.F.:
    Pelvic osteotomy in the treatment of ectopia-vesicae.
    J. Bone Joint Surg., *41B*:751, 1959.

2. Mackel, J.L. and Lindseth, R.E.: Scoliosis in myelo-
    dysplasia. *J. Bone Joint Surg.*, *57A*:1031, 1975.

3. O'Phelan, E.H.: Iliac osteotomy in extrophy of the
    bladder. *J. Bone Joint Surg.*, *45A*:1409, 1963.

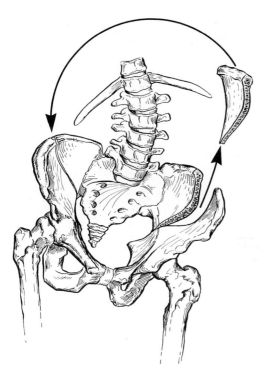

Fig. 1. The compensatory deformity in the pelvis is produced by removal of a wedge of bone from the posterior ilium on the low or long side and transferring it to a posterior iliac osteotomy on the high or short side. This causes a rotation of the pelvis around the sacrum so that the plane of the ischium and acetabulum is perpendicular to the long axis of the body and the head is centered over the pelvis.

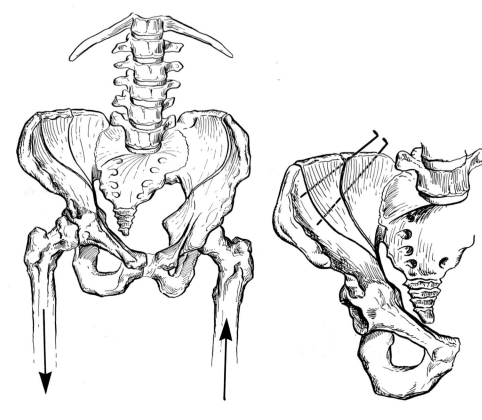

Fig. 2.   After the wedge of bone has been removed, the osteotomy is closed by pushing upward on the leg on this side. The osteotomy on the high side is opened to receive the graft by pulling on this leg and using a bone spreader.

Fig. 3.   The graft is held in place by one or two Kirschner wires which may be placed either from medial to lateral or lateral to medial, depending on which appears easier at the time of surgery.

PATHOPHYSIOLOGY OF SPINAL DEFORMITY
IN MYELOMENINGOCELE

Michael J. Rozen, M.D.

The increased longevity of the myelomeningocele patient
has exposed the complexity and magnitude of associated spinal
deformities. Initial orthopaedic care was aimed at the hips
and feet to increase ambulation, but as more of these
children survived infancy, progressive and frequently severe
spinal problems became the limiting factor. We have slowly
come to the realization that progression of spinal deformity
must be prevented in myelomeningocele as it is when associated with other diseases. The solution to this problem
has been more difficult with standard bracing and surgical
techniques not being effective. To understand the failure
of the standard modalities requires an understanding of the
pathophysiology of the spine in the myelomeningocele patient.

EMBRYOLOGY

The neural folds join to form the neural tube on or
before the nineteenth day of gestation. Tubalization begins
in the thoracic spine and proceeds both cephalad and caudad.
Around the neural tube align the segmentally formed mesodermal somites which during the fourth to the tenth embryonic
week go through a period of segmentation and reformation to
form the vertebral bodies.[6] The process involves the joining

of the caudal half of the superior somite with the cephalad
half of the lower somite to form the vertebral body. The
segmental artery thus comes to lie in the center of the
vertebral body. If the tubalization process is interrupted
and the neural folds remain separated, then the posterior
elements fail to fuse.[2]

CLASSIFICATION

    Raycroft and Curtis[9] divided spinal curvatures in myelo-
dysplasia into two large groups: congenital and developmental. The term "congenital" implied not only the absence
of posterior bony elements but also a primary structural
abnormality of the vertebral bodies. The deformity is
therefore similar to other forms of congenital scoliosis and
its prognosis can be anticipated. The vertebral body
abnormality can either be a failure of formation - either
complete (absent vertebrae) or partial (wedge shaped or hemi
vertebrae) or a failure of segmentation - either complete
(solid bony bar) or incomplete (a unilateral unsegmented bar).
Any combination can also occur (Fig. 1). The unilateral
unsegmented bar can be anticipated to progress and should be
fused early. The incidence of congenital scoliosis in
myelomeningoceles is 30% and almost 100% of these curves tend
to progress to a varying degree.

    Myelodysplastic children with spinal curvature who have
only dysgenesis of the posterior bony elements are termed
"developmental". These children characteristically have
straight spines at birth. Fifty percent of these children
with straight spines can be expected to develop curves. The
onset is usually before age five and seldom after age ten.[9]

    Hensinger and MacEwen[4] expanded this classification to
include lordosis and kyphosis. While no rigid classification

can be universally applied, it has been useful to follow
their schematic (Table 1.). However, it must be remembered
that combinations, for example, lordo scoliosis, are common.

DEVELOPMENTAL SCOLIOSIS

Developmental scoliosis must be viewed in relation to
the problems associated with myelodysplasia. Not only do
these children have varying levels of paraplegia, but also
hydrocephalus, muscle weakness and imbalance, soft tissue
contractures, and joint contractures or dislocations. Most
frequently, it begins in the lumbar spine and presents before
age five as a long "C" shaped paralytic type curve (Fig. 2).
It is most common in paralytic levels above L3-4 and
approaches 100% incidence in patients with thoracic levels.
Once progression has become established, it is usually rapid
and relentless. Mackel and Lindseth[8] found in 82 patients
with myelodysplasia that 66% had scoliosis. Of these
patients, 83% of the congenital curves and 36% of the developmental curves had progressed beyond 45 degrees by age ten.

The progression is accentuated not only by gravitational
forces but also by improper placement of support straps and
crutches for maintaining these children in the erect position.
This is especially true in developmental lordosis where
Kilfoyle[7] has shown that the child slopes forward with the
center of gravity passing anterior to the lumbar spine when
the child thrusts forward with the crutches out infront.
Biomechanical accentuation of the normal lumbar curve occurs
and result in a fixed hyperlordosis.

The occurrence of developmental scoliosis has been
related to pelvic obliquity. Raycroft and Curtis[9] found that
83% of their patients with developmental scoliosis had pelvic

obliquity and that 70% had a dislocated hip. The classic
pattern was for the curve to develop in the lumbar spine and
be convex to the low side of the pelvis with the hip on the
high side being dislocated (Fig. 3). They divided the
factors that lead to this pattern into suprapelvic, transpelvic, and infrapelvic groups (Table 2.). The suprapelvic
factors are imbalance of spinal muscles from asymmetrical
innervation, and soft tissue contractures from scarring
secondary to closure of the defect or repeated skin breakdown.

The psoas muscle is the prime transpelvic offender. It
is innervated by the Ll-2 nerve roots which are frequently
intact. When unilaterally unopposed, it will cause a hip
flexion-adduction deformity with subsequent pelvic obliquity.
In addition, it causes a forward tilt to the pelvis and
developmental lordosis with hip flexion contractures.

Infrapelvic factors are felt by Raycroft and Curtis[9] to
have the earliest influence on pelvic obliquity. A pattern
of adduction and internal rotation of one leg associated
with abduction and external rotation of the opposite leg
leads to a "windblown" posture and pelvic obliquity.
Sharrard[10] feels this is first seen in placeocephaly with
facial asymmetry (Figs. 4,5,6). The adduction results from
unopposed adductor muscles and the abduction from positioning
and muscle weakness. An unopposed iliopsoas greatly
increases the forces producing adduction internal rotation
deformity at the hip.

LORDOSIS

Lordosis, usually of the lumbar spine is the most
common developmental curve in myelodysplastic regardless of
whether or not associated with scoliosis (Fig. 7). It is
usually not present at birth and occurs secondary to fixed

distal contractures. Muscle imbalance of the hip flexors,
especially an unopposed iliopsoas produce a forward tilt of
the pelvis and an exaggeration of the normal lumbar lordosis
(Fig. 8). As mentioned earlier, a tripod stance with "swing
to" or "swing through" gait will accentuate the deformity.
Also, soft tissue scarring and fibrosis can produce a hyperlordosis. For an ill understood reason, there was a frequent
occurrence of a severe lordosis in patients with lumbar
peritoneal shunts. An increased incidence of lordosis in
patients with hydrocephalus has been noted and Sharrard[10]
feels the lordosis may be secondary to arachnoiditis. The
lordosis will progress and become severe unless the underlying factors are prevented or dealt with appropriately and
fixed contractures prevented.

KYPHOSIS

Banta and Hamada[1] found that 46 of their 457 myelomeningocele patients had kyphosis. They classified them into
flexible paralytic, congenital rigid lumbar, and kyphoscoliosis groups. The flexible paralytic kyphosis had gentle "C"
shaped curves which progressed an average of three degrees
per year. The congenital lumbar kyphosis progressed 8.3
degrees per year and the patients with kyphoscoliosis progressed 6.8 degrees per year.

CONGENITAL LUMBAR KYPHOSIS

An unique problem seen only in myelomeningocele is the
occurrence of congenital lumbar kyphosis (Fig. 9). It occurs
in the lumbar spine involving all vertebrae from the thoraco-
lumbar junction to the end of the sacrum. The apex of the
curve is at L2-3. The kyphosis is fixed and rigid and is
usually accompanied by complete paralysis below the level of

the lesion. The incidence varies between 12.5 and 27%.[5]
The etiology of this entity is not well understood. Barson[2]
feels that it is analogous to Arnold-Chiari malformation and
speculates the deformity is caused by retention or persistence of the primitive tailfold. Other explanations related
to differential rates of neural ectodermal vertebral mesoderm
have also been suggested.

Drennan[3,11] has noted the role of muscles in the
development of the kyphosis during intrauterine life. The
bony lesion is wider than in the usual myelomeningocele. The
lateral masses are more prominent and are pushed so far
lateral that their posterior surface faced forward. The
erector spinae and other posterior vertebral muscles are
carried laterally and become converted into flexors of the
trunk (Fig. 10). Once the deformity has occurred, it is
aggravated by the crura of the diaphragm and the hypertrophied psoas muscle. The vertebral bodies become wedge shaped
with contracture of the annulus fibrosis and the anterior
longitudinal ligament occurring (Fig. 11).

While the child is supine, frequent skin breakdown over
the apex with drainage and ulceration are common (Fig. 12).
When the child sits, he must use his hands for balance since
his trunk is well forward of his pelvis. The curve is
accentuated with gravity and progression even more likely.
A compensatory lordosis develops in the thoracic spine. The
rib cage encroaches further on the pelvic brim and the
thoracic cage is compromised as the abdominal contents are
forced against the diaphragm. At the present, no satisfactory method of treatment for this deformity exists. Bracing
has universally failed and should not be used. We have not
been happy with our results from resection of the kyphosis

and agree with Hensinger and MacEwen[4] that the best approach
may be anterior release with interbody fusion through a
combined thoraco abdominal retro peritoneal approach.

Developmental kyphosis is less of a problem and usually
is flexible. We have noted it more in sitters and have been
better able to control it with body jacket type bracing.

SUMMARY

In summary many patterns of spinal deformity can occur
in myelomeningoceles. Scoliotic curves can be described as
"congenital" or "developmental". Hyperlordosis frequently
occurs in these patients. Unique to the myelomeningocele
patient is the occurrence of congenital lumbar kyphosis.

As in spinal deformity associated with other disease
entities, the presence of a curve must be diagnosed early
and its progression prevented.

REFERENCES

1.   Banta, J.V. and Hamada, J.S.: Natural History of the
     Kyphotic Deformity in Myelomeningocele. Paper presented
     to Western Orthopaedic Association, 1975.

2.   Barson, A.J.: Spina bifida: The significance of the
     level and extent of the defect to the morphogenesis.
     Dev. Med. Child Neurol., *12*:129, 1970.

3.   Drennan, J.C.: The role of the muscles in the develop-
     ment of human lumbar spine. *Dev. Med. Child Neurol.*,
     Suppl. 22:33, 1970.

4.   Hensinger, R.H. and MacEwen, G.D.: Congenital anomalies
     of the spine. IN The Spine, Philadelphia, W.B. Saunders,
     1975, pp. 200.

5. Hoppenfeld, S.: Congenital kyphosis in myelomeningo-
    cele. *J. Bone Joint Surg., 49B*:276, 1967.

6. Kilfoyle, R.M.: Myelodysplasia. *Pediat. Clinic N. Am.,
    14*:419, 1967.

7. Kilfoyle, R.M., Foley, J.J. and Norton, P.L.: Spine
    and pelvic deformity in childhood and adolescent
    paraplegia. *J. Bone Joint Surg., 47A*:659, 1965.

8. Mackel, J.L. and Lindseth, R.E.: Scoliosis in myelo-
    dysplasia. *J. Bone Joint Surg., 57A*:1031, 1975.

9. Raycroft, J.F. and Curtis, B.H.: Spinal curvature in
    myelomeningocele: Natural history and etiology.
    IN American Academy of Orthopaedic Surgeons Symposium
    on Myelomeningocele, St. Louis, C.V. Mosby Co., 1972.

10. Sharrard, W.J.W.: Personal Communication, 1976.

11. Sharrard, W.J.W.: The kyphotic and lordotic spine in
    myelomeningocele. IN American Academy of Orthopaedic
    Surgeons Symposium on Myelomeningocele, St. Louis,
    C.V. Mosby Co., 1972.

TABLE 1.

Spinal Deformities of Myelodysplasia

   I. SCOLIOSIS

       A. Congenital Vertebral Anomalies

       B. Developmental

           1. Suprapelvic

           2. Intrapelvic

           3. Infrapelvic

  II. LORDOSIS

III. KYPHOSIS

       A. Congenital Lumbar

       B. Developmental

TABLE 2.

Pelvic Factors - Developmental Scoliosis

SUPRAPELVIC FACTORS

    Muscle Imbalance

    Asymmetrical Involvement

    Soft Tissue Contracture

TRANSPELVIC FACTORS

    Psoas Muscle - Hip Flexion Contracture

                Lordosis

INFRAPELVIC FACTORS

    Hip Abduction/Adduction

    "Wind-Blown"

        Dislocated Hip - High Side

        Exaggerated Spine Deformity

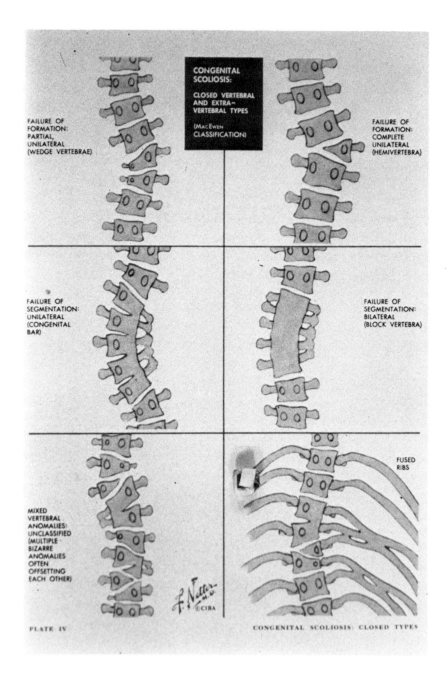

Fig. 1. Patterns of congenital scoliosis by Frank Netter, M.D.—Cibia Symposium—Scoliosis by Dr. Hugo Keim.

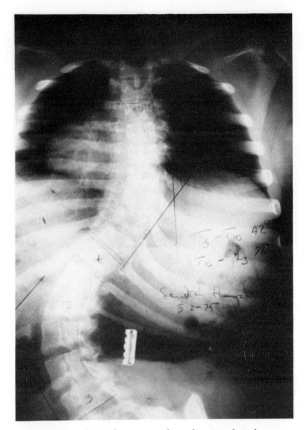

Fig. 2. Developmental scoliosis—lumbar curve—convex to the low side of the pelvis.

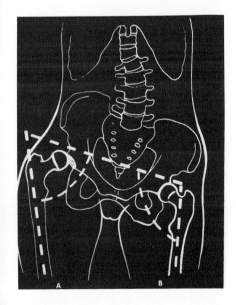

Fig. 3. Pelvic obliquity (from Tzimas, N.A.: Comprehensive care of the child with spina bifida manifesta, In Rehabilitation Monograph XXXI, New York Institute of Rehabilitation, N.Y.U. Medical Center, 1966).

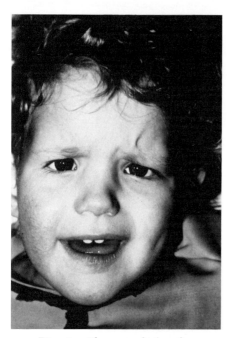

Fig. 4. Placeocephaly—from W.J.W. Sharrard.

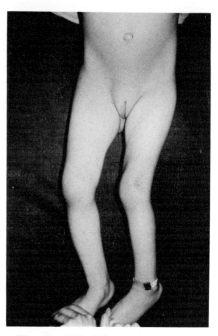

Fig. 5. Windblown deformity—from W.J.W. Sharrard.

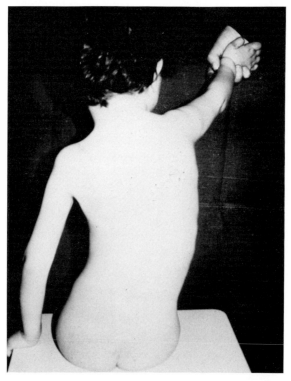

Fig. 6. Developmental scoliosis—from W.J.W. Sharrard.

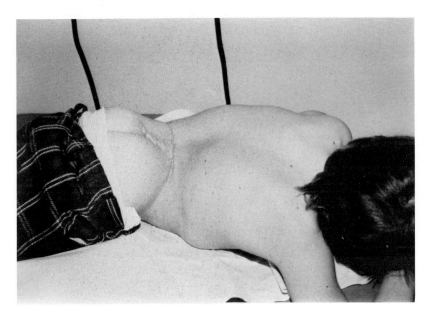

Fig. 7. Myelomeningocele patient with severe lumbar lordosis. Note associated pelvic tilt and pelvic obliquity.

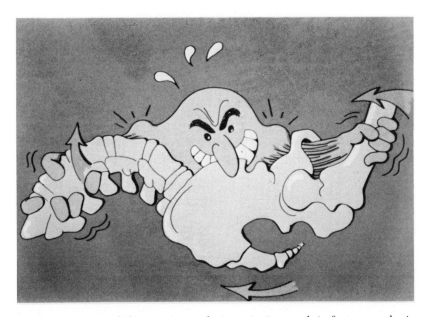

Fig. 8. Unopposed iliopsoas muscle is main intrapelvic factor producing lordosis and hip flexion contracture.

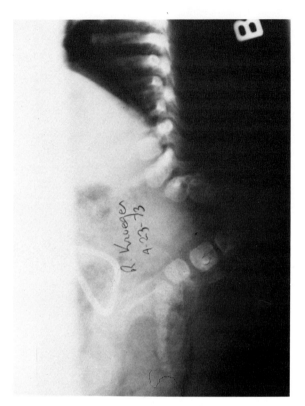

Fig. 9.   Congenital lumbar kyphosis.

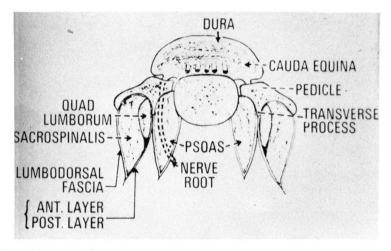

Fig. 10.   Diagram of transverse section of vertebrae and its muscles in kyphotic area. From Sharrard, W.J.W. and Drennan, J.C.: Osteotomy—Excision of the spine for lumbar kyphosis in older children with myelomeningocele. J. Bone and Joint Surg., 54B: 50, 1972.

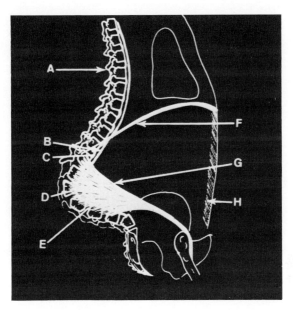

Fig. 11. Drawing illustrating the deforming forces
found in congenital lumbar kyphosis. A. Compensatory
dorsal lordosis. B. Contracted anterior longitudinal
ligament. C. Contracted annulus fibrosis. D. Wedge-
shaped vertebral bodies. E. Intervertebral discs
narrowed anteriorly with the nucleus pulposus shifted
posteriorly. F. Diaphragm attached to the apex of the
deformity. G. Psoas muscle is hypertrophied and
bowstrings across the curve. H. Anterior abdominal
musculature.[4]

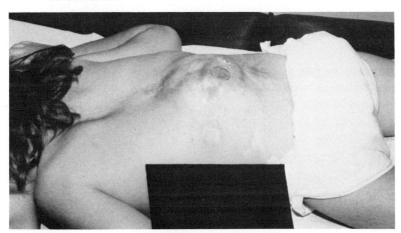

Fig. 12. Congenital lumbar kyphosis with ulceration, skin break-down, and
scarring.

579

SURGICAL TREATMENT OF SCOLIOSIS
IN MYELODYSPLASIA

John A. Odom, Jr., M.D. and
Courtney W. Brown, M.D.

INTRODUCTION

The number of children who survive with myelomeningocele
has risen markedly due to early closure of the dural sac and
improved urological care. Therefore, more patients with
spinal deformities are present for orthopaedic treatment than
in previous years. The majority of the spine deformities are
scoliosis but are frequently associated with kyphosis and
lordosis.

The myelodysplastic child with scoliosis is a far more
complex problem than the routine patient with idiopathic
scoliosis. The orthopaedic surgeon who operates on the
myelodysplastic patient must be competent in not only
approaching the spine posteriorly but also anteriorly.

The method of posterior instrumentation[4] was a significant help in attempting to obtain fusion in these patients,
but often failed due to lack of posterior elements. Anterior
approach to the spine with internal fixation[3] was a significant contribution to a variety of spinal deformities, but
particularly to the myelodysplastic spine with missing
posterior elements.

Several authors, Kilfoyle and Norton;[6] Sharrard;[8,9]
Brown, Bonnett and Perry;[2] Sriram, Bobechko and Hall;[10] Hull,

Moe and Winter[5] have written on this subject and contributed
significantly. However, Ashley, et. al.[1] and Lindberg,
Brown and Bonnett[7] were the first to emphasize anterior
fusion combined with posterior fusion.

MATERIAL

Twenty-six myelomeningocele patients with spinal
deformity underwent spinal fusion from 1971-1975. Twenty-
one were treated at Denver Children's Hospital and five at
other hospitals. The follow-up ranges from one to five years.
The level of neurological deficits ranged from T-8 to L-3.
All patients had multiple lower extremity deformities severe
enough for treatment.

Twelve patients had scoliosis with moderate associated.
lordosis or kyphosis. Nine patients had pure kyphosis of
the lumbar or thoracolumbar spine with no associated
scoliosis. Four patients had kyphosis as the primary
deformity with only moderate scoliosis. One patient had a
severe lumbar lordosis with no other associated deformity.

SURGICAL APPROACH

A variety of different approaches was carried out in the
beginning of this series. The complications and problems
that occurred are discussed. Halo-femoral traction is
reserved only for the severest of curves.

Generally curves are over 50 degrees and are progressive
before bracing is abandoned for surgical intervention. It is
preferred that the patient be over ten years of age before
surgery. However, the patient may be operated much earlier
if the curve progresses too rapidly (Fig. 1A, 1B, 1C).

Our present approach is:

1) Admit the patient two days prior to surgery for
completion of a thorough work-up.

2) An anterior fusion with Dwyer instrumentation for
lordosis and scoliosis is carried out (Fig. 1B), or an
anterior rib strutt graft is performed for kyphosis and
scoliosis. Vertebral body resection may or may not be
carried out.

3) The use of pre-operative and post-operative I.V.
Keflin for 36 hours is routine.

4) A pulmonary internist helps manage the patient postoperatively for three or four days.

5) A posterior fusion with Harrington instrumentation
is done two or three weeks after anterior fusion (Fig. 1C).

6) The patient is mobilized in plastic body jacket
(Fig. 2A, 2B, 2C) seven to ten days following posterior
fusion. Long leg braces can be attached to the body jacket
for ambulation.

7) The body jacket is discontinued six to twelve months
following posterior fusion.

COMPLICATIONS

INFECTION

Four of the 26 patients (15.3%) developed post-operative
wound infections. All of the infections were superficial and
all were in patients with kyphosis as the primary deformity.

PRESSURE SORES

Six of the patients (23%) developed some type of
pressure sores during their post-operative immobilization.
All of these patients with pressure sores had post-operative
plaster immobilization.

FRACTURES

Six patients (23%) sustained fractures of their lower

extremities soon after removal of the casts for immobilization of their spines. All patients who had spine fusions
followed by casts that included the lower extremities, had
one to four fractures following removal of plaster.

One patient sustained a fracture at her distal femur
through a pin tract where she had had halo-femoral traction.
There were no fractures in the patients who had an anterior
and posterior approach and were mobilized early in the upright position with a body cast or a plastic body jacket.

PSEUDOARTHROSIS

Seven patients (26.9%) of this series developed pseudoarthrosis. Each of these patients had only a posterior
approach. Every patient (13%) who had both anterior and
posterior approaches went on to solid union.

PROGRESSION OF CURVES AFTER ANTERIOR FUSION ALONE

Three patients initially had Dwyer instrumentation with
spinal fusion with no posterior approach. Each of these
patients had primarily a thoraco-lumbar curve with a minimal
thoracic curve above. After the original surgery to correct
the thoracolumbar curve, the thoracic curve was much improved
also. However, in one case the upper curve progressed enough
that it had to be fused posteriorly at a later date. Both
of the other patients had progression of their upper thoracic
curves but have not yet been operated.

DEATH

One of the patients died seven days post-operatively due
to respiratory complications following a Dwyer instrumentation. He had a left thoracic curve of 148 degrees and a
right lumbar curve of 144 degrees and was 44 years old.
Needless to say, it is better to surgically treat all of
these   curves   while   they   are   not   so   severe

and before they get out of their teenage years.

DISCUSSION

In this small series of myelodysplastic patients with
spinal deformities, pseudoarthrosis occurred when the patient
had only a posterior fusion. This occurred in spite of the
fact that the patients were well immobilized in plaster postoperatively for nine months.

Three patients had Dwyer instrumentation alone and went
on to solid union. However, anterior fusion alone, in the
author's hands, has gone on to pseudoarthrosis in other
incidences. One cannot achieve immobilization as rigidly
with Dwyer instrumentation as one can with Harrington rods.

An inherent defect in Dwyer instrumentation is not being
able to fuse comfortably from neutral vertebra above to
neutral vertebra below. The anterior fusion is almost
invariably too short. If the patient does not have an
extended posterior fusion secondarily, the curve will progress above and below the anterior fusion in many cases.

One of the primary problems in any paralytic scoliosis,
particularly myelodysplasia, is pelvic obliquity. All
patients in this series with scoliosis had pelvic obliquity.
With Dwyer instrumentation the pelvic obliquity is not
completely corrected. When Harrington instrumentation, using
a sacral-alar hook, is carried out as a second stage after
Dwyer instrumentation, the pelvis is leveled or more nearly
leveled. If one leaves pelvic obliquity with a solid fusion
of the spine to the sacrum, the incidence of pressure sores
on the lower ischium may increase.

For all the above reasons, it appears logical that an
anterior fusion followed two to three weeks later by a
posterior fusion is the treatment of choice for myelomeningo-

cele scoliosis.   Using this method the surgeon can 1) more
nearly guarantee solid fusion, 2) minimize the chances of
curve progression, 3) level the pelvis better, and 4)
mobilize the patient earlier.

SUMMARY

Twenty-six myelomeningocele patients with spinal
deformity are discussed.   Twelve had scoliosis, nine had
pure kyphosis, four had kyphosis as the primary deformity
with only moderate scoliosis and one had severe lumbar
lordosis.

The high incidence of complications including infection,
pressure sores, fractures of the lower extremities following
cast removal, pseudoarthrosis, progression of the curve, and
death are discussed.

The recommended method of treatment is anterior fusion
followed two to three weeks later by posterior fusion.   Seven
to ten days later the patient is mobilized in a plastic
removal body jacket.

REFERENCES

1. Ashley, R.K., Larsen, L., James, P. and Gilbert, R.:
    Combined Surgical Approach to Spinal Deformity.
    Delivered at the Ninth Annual Meeting of Scoliosis
    Research Society, San Francisco, 1974.

2. Brown, J.C., Bonnett, C., Perry, J.:   The Surgical Treat-
    ment of Spinal Deformity in the Juvenile and Adolescent
    Myelodysplastic Patient.   Delivered at the Sixth Annual
    Meeting of Scoliosis Research Society, Hartford, 1971.

3. Dwyer, A.F., Newton, N.C. and Sherwood, A.A.: An anterior approach to scoliosis. *Clinical Orthopaedics and Related Research, 62*:192, 1969.

4. Harrington, P.R.: Treatment of scoliosis. *J. Bone Joint Surg., 44A*:591, 1962.

5. Hull, W., Moe, J. and Winter, R.: The Surgical Treatment of Spinal Deformities in Myelomeningocele. Delivered at the Ninth Annual Meeting of Scoliosis Research Society, San Francisco, 1974.

6. Kilfoyle, R.M., Foley, J.J. and Norton, P.L.: Spine and pelvic deformity in childhood and adolescent paraplegia. *J. Bone Joint Surg., 47A*:659, 1965.

7. Lindberg, C., Brown, J.C. and Bonnett, C.: The Surgical Management of Spinal Deformities in Myelodysplasia. Delivered at the Tenth Annual Meeting of the Scoliosis Research Society, Louisville, 1975.

8. Sharrard, W.J.W.: Spinal osteotomy for congenital kyphosis in meningomyelocele. *J. Bone Joint Surg., 50B*:466, 1968.

9. Sharrard, W.J.W. and Drennan, J.C.: Osteotomy-excision of the spine for lumbar kyphosis in older children with myelomeningocele. *J. Bone Joint Surg., 54B*:50, 1972.

10. Sriram, K., Bobechko, W.P. and Hall, J.E.: Surgical management of spinal deformities in spina bifida. *J. Bone Joint Surg., 54B*:666, 1972.

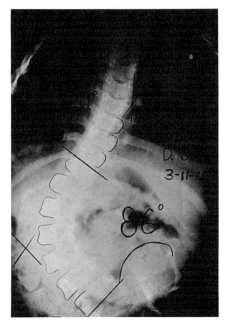

A

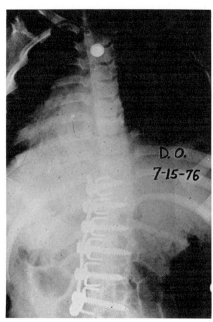

B

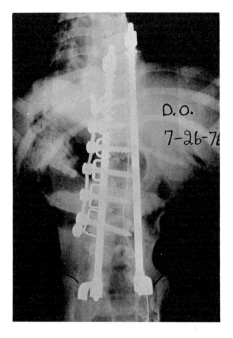

C

Fig. 1. A. X-rays showing five year old T-10 myelodysplastic with progressive scoliosis not responding to bracing. B. Immediate post-operative Dwyer instrumentation. C. After posterior Harrington instrumentation to the sacrum.

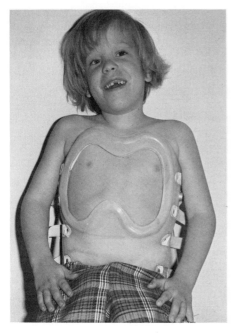

A

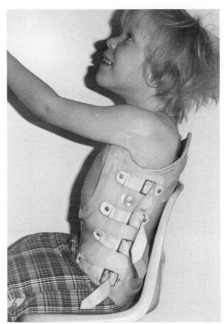

B

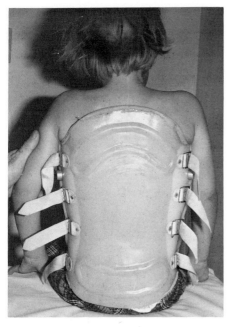

C

Fig. 2. A polypropylene removal jacket for holding patient post-operative. A. Front view. B. Side view. C. Rear view. This brace can be attached to long leg braces.

LORDOSIS AND LORDO-SCOLIOSIS
IN MYELOMENINGOCELE

W.J.W. Sharrard, M.D., F.R.C.S.

Scoliosis associated with abnormal vertebral formation
such as hemivertebrae or unsegmented bars is recognisable
from infancy and is a recognised cause of progressive
scoliotic deformity in a proportion of children in the
course of growth. Where the vertebral bodies are normal and
the defect is confined to absence of spinous processes and
laminae, no specific spinal deformity may be present during
the first five years or more of life. After this time, it
may be apparent that lumbar or thoraco-lumbar scoliosis
(Fig. 1) is developing especially in a child who has fairly
severe lower limb paralysis and spends a lot of his or her
time sitting (Fig. 2). From the age of nine onwards, lordotic
or lordo-scoliotic deformity is liable to increase extremely
rapidly so that a curve (Fig. 3) which, up to that time, has
not measured more than 30 or 40 degrees may increase by more
than 100 percent in the course of a year.[1,4]

ETIOLOGY

Absence of posterior skeletal elements appear to be the
important factor in the development of this deformity, which
results from growth of the vertebral bodies combined with
absence of growth of the posterior bony elements and extensive
scarring at the site of the primary closure of the myelo-

591

meningocele lesion. That this is not the only factor is
suggested by the fact that children suffering from congenital
or acquired hydrocephalus without myelomeningocele may
develop progressive lordosis after the tenth year of life.[5]
Some of these patients have been treated by shunts inserted
between the spinal theca and the peritoneum during the first
two years of life and it was thought possible that the
laminectomy required to perform this procedure had been the
irritating factor responsible for the later development of
deformity. However, some cases have been seen in which
lordosis has developed in congenital hydrocephalus treated by
ventriculo-atrial or ventriculo-peritoneal shunt in the
presence of a completely intact vertebral column. There may,
therefore, be some association between the presence of hydrocephalus and the liability to develop lordosis in myelomeningocele patients as well.

The part played by muscle imbalance or perverted muscle
action is difficult to analyse. Paralysis extending up to
the eighth thoracic neural level and associated with severe
weakness or complete paralysis of lumbar and abdominal
muscles is likely to produce a collapsing type of spinal
deformity similar to that found in poliomyelitis. Unbalanced
activity of trunk muscles, particularly in association with
hemimyelocele, together with abnormal vertebral body formation makes the possibility of increasing lordo-scoliosis
even greater. Once deformity has increased to more than 50
to 60 degrees, gravity aggravates the progression of the
deformity.

Deformity at the hip influences the posture of the
pelvis and lumbar spine. Flexion deformity of one or both
hips aggravates a tendency to lordosis and adduction or
abduction deformity aggravates pelvic obliquity and a

liability to scoliosis. Hip deformity alone in the absence
of primary factors in the spine does not initiate fixed
lordosis or lordo-scoliosis nor does pelvic obliquity from
the hip causes alone produce a scoliosis but the combination
may act to aggravate any lordo-scoliosis that is already
developing. In this respect, the activity of the iliopsoas
may be a factor in the production of both hip and spine
deformity.

THE EFFECTS OF PROGRESSIVE LORDOSIS AND LORDO-SCOLIOSIS

The most important effect of progressive lordosis and
lordo-scoliosis is deterioration in trunk stability and
balance. The child finds it increasingly difficult to sit
without toppling over and has to put his hands on either side
to maintain himself upright. Increasing obliquity of the
pelvis results in more and more pressure being put on one
buttock and ischial tuberosity so that, eventually, a serious
ulceration (Fig. 4) over the ischial tuberosity may develop
and become very intractable. The ribs on the concave side
of the deformity pass downwards into the pelvis on the inner
side of the iliac crest and the abdominal contents become
compressed. Cardiac, respiratory and intra-abdominal function
may be affected and the ureters may become kinked and compressed. Occasionally pain is a presenting symptom. When
deformity becomes severe, it becomes ugly and even grotesque
and adolescent children who are already conscious of handicap
and deformity in the limbs become even more conscious of a
deformity that they did not previously have. Whether standing
or sitting, the vertical height of the child is significantly
diminished.

Treatment by Milwaukee Brace has a very limited place
in the management of lordo-scoliosis in spina bifida even

with the greatest care in design and application, pressure
sores over the sacral and ischial regions are almost impossible to prevent and traction on the neck is likely to
disturb shunts for hydrocephalus. Plaster or polythene
jackets are also difficult to use and also tend to cause
pressure over the outer side of the hip and in the axilla.
Lordosis, in particular, is almost impossible to control by
any type of jacket.

The only satisfactory method of treatment is operative.
Correction and fusion of lordotic spinal deformities by the
posterior route in patients with myelomeningocele is difficult, hazardous and often ineffective.[4] The posterior
approach is hampered by scarring and contracture, by the
presence of the spinal membranes and neural structures beneath the skin, by the depth of the spine, and by difficulty
of access because of the proximity of the rib cage to the
iliac crest. Correction of the deformity by stretching the
posterior structures is limited by the shortness of dural and
nervous structures and, in a child who has some lower limb
innervation, increased paralysis may result. Maintenance of
correction by Harrington rods is limited by the feasibility
of skin closure over the rods and, even if the skin can be
closed, secondary ulceration may occur weeks or months after
operation. The absence of posterior skeletal elements gives
an inadequate bone surface for fusion and bone grafts must
be placed laterally between the transverse processes which
are themselves poorly developed.

In view of these daunting factors, the posterior
approach has been abandoned. An anterior approach[2,3] to the
lordotic lumbar and lower thoracic spine gives excellent
access to the affected vertebral bodies. Removal of the
wedge-shaped intervertebral discs and the adjoining portion

of the vertebral bodies at multiple levels allows a good
correction to be made of a severe deformity and avoids
tension on nervous structures. The problem of fixation of
the corrected deformity has been resolved by the introduction
of Dwyer staple and cable apparatus.

Before operation, assessments need to be made of the
state of control of hydrocephalus and the function of any
ventricular shunt, renal function by electrolyte estimation
and intravenous pyelography, and of respiratory function by
spirometry and blood-gas analysis. Any fixed hip deformity,
particularly hip flexion deformity, needs to be corrected by
soft tissue release or osteotomy or attempts to correct
spinal deformity by traction will fail.

A considerable amount of correction of spine deformity
can be obtained by a period of one month of traction (Fig.5).
Our preference has been for the use of simple Crutchfield
tongs applied to the skull and by pins inserted through the
lower ends of the femora or upper ends of tibia. The patient
can be nursed on a Stryker frame with regular turning and
the average weight applied is 9 to 10 kg to the head and an
equal total weight to the lower limbs. Correction of pelvic
obliquity can be encouraged by the application of unequal
weights to the two limbs. Alternative methods such as halo-
pelvic traction have been tried but have not been found to
be very satisfactory in patients with hydrocephalus and
severe lower limb paralysis. The traction apparatus is
released two days before operation.

A possible complication after spinal operations in
children with hydrocephalus is the development of a blocked
shunt or an aggravation of hydrocephalus. For this reason,
it is always advisable to perform a cranial burr hole as a
precaution against the need for ventricular aspiration during

or after operation. There has been some indication that the
need for a long period in the horizontal position may pre-
dispose to shunt blockage. The cranial burr hole usually
made in the parietal region can be done at the time when the
skull traction is applied or immediately preceding the spinal
operation. Any deterioration in neurological function in the
lower limbs during the period of traction would suggest the
need for cessation of further attempts to correct deformity
by this means though, in our experience, this has never
occurred.

OPERATIVE TECHNIQUE[1,2,3]

The patient is anaesthetised using intubation and intravenous infusion is commenced early, it being of the greatest
importance to ensure adequate blood replacement which may be
considerable. The patient is placed with the convex side of
the curve upwards, lying almost directly on the side and the
operating table is broken over the region of the curve so
as to open up the side of the abdomen to be operated upon
(Fig. 6). The rib chosen for entry to the chest is related
to the intended upper limit of spine fusion, the aim being to
expose at least one vertebra above the first vertebra to be
included in the fusion. Distally, the spine should be
exposed if possible to a level one vertebra below the lower
vertebra to be included. For fusion commencing proximally
at the tenth, eleventh or twelfth thoracic vertebra, the rib
to be removed should be the eighth, ninth or tenth rib
respectively. If the spine needs to be exposed more proximally than this, a second rib can be removed more proximally
and, if the occasion requires it, the posterior ends of
intervening ribs can be divided together with their intercostal vessels and nerves to allow a flap of chest wall to be

mobilised forwards. In this way it is possible to extend the
proximal level as far as the fifth or sixth thoracic vertebra
but this has rarely been needed.

The rib is removed up to the costal cartilage anteriorly
and posteriorly as close as possible to the costo-transverse
joint. The chest is entered through the rib bed. The skin
incision is continued obliquely across the upper abdomen
towards the mid-line distal to the umbilicus. The abdominal
muscles are divided obliquely and the spine exposed extra-
peritoneally, the kidney, suprarenal glands and ureter being
mobilised medially. The peritoneum is separated from the
under surface of the diaphragm so that the diaphragm can be
divided about 1 inch from its periphery and the abdominal and
thoracic exposures combined. The lumbar spine can be exposed
distally to the level of the fourth or, with division of
ilio-lumbar vessels to the fifth lumbar vertebral body. When
there has been a previous operation for urinary diversion,
distal exposure may be difficult because of extensive adhesions containing the ureter but, with care, the whole
conduit can be mobilised to allow distal exposure of the
lumbar vertebrae. The aorta and inferior venacava do not
give any difficulty since they are displaced to the concave
side of the scoliotic spine.

The vertebrae are exposed subperiosteally, the lumbar or
intercostal vessels being divided and cauterised or ligated
as they cross the middle of the vertebral bodies. It is
important that the vertebral bodies should be exposed laterally to the level of the intervertebral foramina but with care
to avoid dissection in the region of the foramen which tends
to precipitate bleeding. The intervertebral discs and a thin
portion of the adjoining surfaces of the vertebral body are
removed as a wedge with the aim of correcting lordosis and

scoliosis. The removal of bone towards the posterior part of
the vertebral body is best achieved by a lateral-cutting burr.
Each vertebral body should be demonstrably mobile at the end
of this phase of the operation and, if necessary, transverse
processes or rib heads may need to be removed to achieve
this degree of mobility.

Final correction and fixation is achieved by the application of Dwyer staples and cable. Staples of correct width
are applied to each vertebral body and held in place by a
large coarse-thread screw passed across the vertebral body
obliquely so that the tip of the screw penetrates the opposite
posterior or postero-lateral cortex of the vertebral body,
preferably entering the pedicle on the opposite side. Firm
fixation of the staple and screw is vital and if a vertebral
body proves to be too fragile to obtain a secure hold, that
vertebral body can be by-passed.

Fixation of adjoining screws and staples by a wire cable
under tension is done progressively and carefully. Correction is aided by reversing the break in the operating table
to bring the ribs on the convex side towards the iliac crest
and by pressure by assistants on the spine laterally whilst
the vertebrae are being held together. At the completion of
fixation, the curvature should be substantially if not
completely corrected in both planes (Fig. 7).

The abdomen is closed, the diaphragm sutured and the
chest closed with two drains connected to underwater seals.
Blood loss should be anticipated to be between 50 percent
and 200 percent of the blood volume and a watch needs to be
kept for signs of hypocalcaemia by estimates of blood
potassium, plasma oxygen and plasma carbon dioxide during
operation as necessary. The patient is nursed in an intensive
care unit for two or three days, the thoracic drain tubes

being removed after 48 hours. After this, normal nursing
on a Stryker frame continues until fusion is sound at three
months. When walking or sitting is resumed, a temporary
light plastic jacket may be needed for a few weeks.

RESULTS

In our own series, there have been no neurological
consequences of the operation and any muscle activity in the
lower limbs that was present before operation has been
retained. Recovery immediately after operation has been
remarkable with the absence of shock or prolonged debility.
There have been no deaths at the time of operation. In two
patients out of thirty operated upon, acute hydrocephalus
has developed due to a blocked shunt more than two weeks
after operation. In one instance, replacement of a shunt
was uneventful. In another, acute cardiac arrest occurred,
which was fatal.

Fusion of the vertebral bodies has proved to be reliable
and has only failed on two occasions, one at the proximal end
and the other at the distal end of the curve but this has not
affected the overall result. The degree of correction
obtained has ranged between 25 and 60 degrees. It has not
always been appropriate to aim to correct the curve completely
because the presence of a second curve proximal to the
corrected curve precludes any attempt to correct the thoraco-
lumbar curve completely - the spine should come unbalanced
in the opposite direction. If the curve is initially 60
degrees or less, correction to less than 20 degrees can be
anticipated. Curves as great as 130 degrees before operation
can be corrected to 70 degrees with considerable improvement
in the clincial state. A striking feature of the results
is the greatly improved stability and balance and a

noticeably improved appearance and increase in height.

Provided that the spine fusion has extended to one vertebra beyond the end of the curve proximally and distally, no relapse has occurred, but where it has not proved possible to extend the fusion proximally to a sufficient level, further progress of the deformity is liable to develop and to require a second fusion either intra-thoracically or posteriorly if posterior elements are present. It is not possible to extend the fusion beyond the level of the fifth lumbar vertebra distally and even this proves to be difficult in many patients so that the lowest level that can be fused is between the third and fourth lumbar vertebra. It has been suggested that, if there is significant pelvic obliquity, fusion should continue to the sacrum and that this part of the spine should be fused separately through a postero-lateral approach. Our experience has been that, if the main curve is corrected sufficiently, the pelvic obliquity will be corrected with it (Fig. 8) and it is then useful to retain a degree of mobility in the lumbosacral spine. If correction of the lumbar curve has not been as good as had been hoped, progressive recurrence of pelvic obliquity may then be an indication for a second limited fusion in the lumbosacral spine. The best timing for operative correction and fusion must be an individual matter for each patient. The vertebrae must be of sufficient size and strength to accommodate the Dwyer apparatus and this usually implies that it cannot be performed below the age of eight years. On the other hand, the smaller the curve at the time of correction, the more satisfactory will be the result.

REFERENCES

1. Baker, R.H. and Sharrard, W.J.W.: Correction of lordo-scoliosis in spina bifida by multiple spinal osteotomy and fusion with Dwyer fixation: A preliminary report. *Dev. Med. Child Neurol., Suppl. 29, 15*:12, 1973.

2. Dwyer A.F., Newton, N.C. and Sherwood, A.A.: An anterior approach to scoliosis. A preliminary report. *Clin. Orthop. & Related Research, 62*:192, 1969.

3. Dwyer, A.F. and Schafer, M.F.: Anterior approach to scoliosis. *J. Bone Joint Surg., 56B*:218, 1974.

4. Sriram, K., Bobechko, W. and Hall, J.E.: Surgical management of spinal deformities in spina bifida. *J. Bone Joint Surg., 54B*:666, 1972.

5. Steel, H.H. and Adams, D.J.: Hyperlordosis caused by the lumboperitoneal shunt procedure for hydrocephalus. *J. Bone Joint Surg., 54A*:1537, 1972.

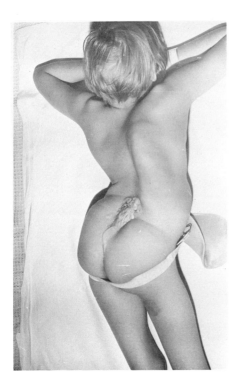

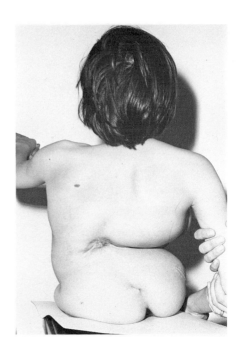

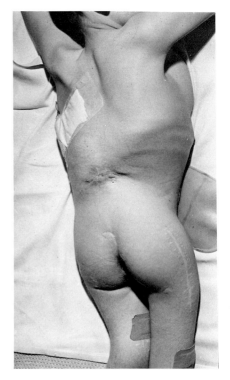

Fig. 1.   Lordoscoliosis in
myelomeningocele.

Fig. 2.   Severe lordoscoliosis in
myelomeningocele. A (*top right*).
Before correction. The chest wall on
the right is approximate to the pelvis
and pelvic obliquity is marked. B
(*bottom right*). After correction.
Trunk balance has been restored and
appearance much improved.

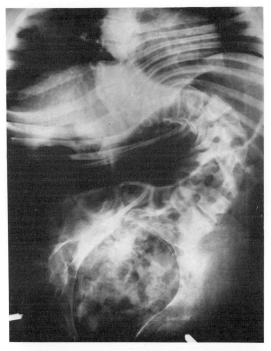

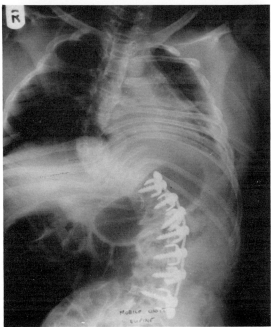

Fig. 3. Radiograph of lordoscoliosis of patient in Fig. 2.
A (*top*). Before correction. B (*bottom*). After multiple
vertebral osteotomy and Dwyer cable and stapling.

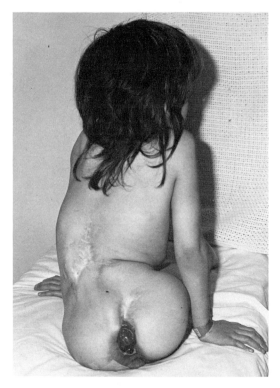

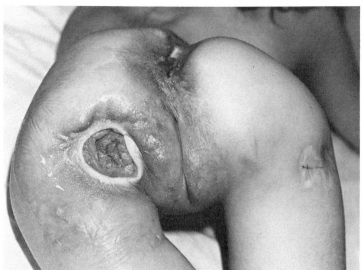

Fig. 4. Effects of lordoscoliosis in myelomeningocele. The patient was paraplegic with complete bladder and bowel incontinence. A (*top*). Sitting posture. B (*bottom*). Ischial pressure sore.

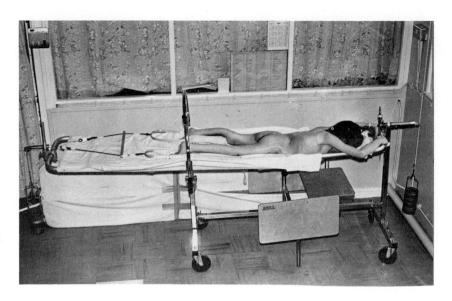

Fig. 5.   Skull-femoral traction on a Stryker frame.

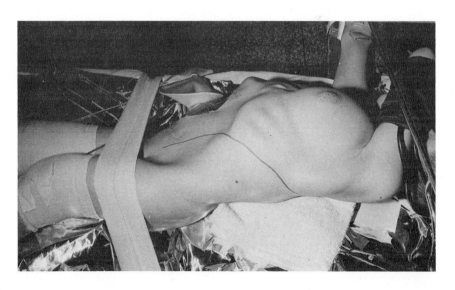

Fig. 6.   Multiple vertebral osteotomy. Operative position and line of skin incision.

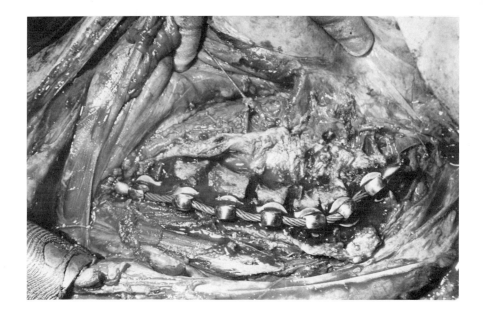

Fig. 7. Multiple vertebral osteotomy. Dwyer cable and staples at the end of operative correction.

Fig. 8. Radiographs of lordoscoliosis.

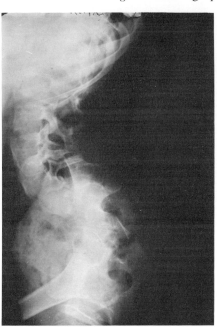
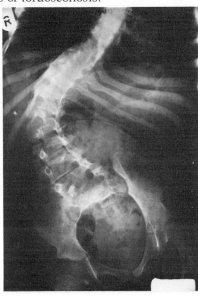

A. Before correction. Note Pelvic obliquity and severe lordotic deformity.

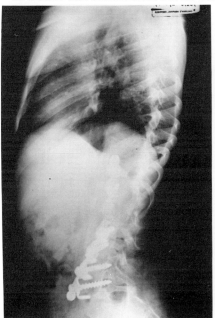
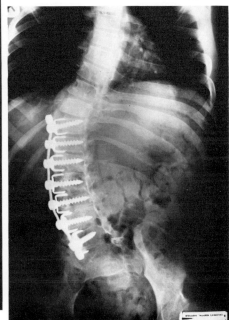

B. After correction. Pelvic obliquity has been substantially corrected and lordosis restored to normal.

607

THE KYPHOTIC SPINE IN
MYELOMENINGOCELE

Robert A. Dickson, Ch.M., F.R.C.S.
and Kenton D. Leatherman, M.D.

INTRODUCTION

Congenital lumbar kyphosis is the least common spinal deformity encountered in patients with myelomeningocele. It differs from the usual paralytic curvature by being rigid, structural from the outset, and present at birth. This latter characteristic makes closure of the overlying sac extremely difficult. Notoriously resistant to any form of conservative therapy all congenital kyphoses are the subject of surgical intervention. It is tempting to approach these posterior deformities from the back, and indeed, the early results from doing so may appear rewarding. Unfortunately, there is an innate tendency for these lumbar kyphoses to progress despite posterior surgery. This is because the basic pathology exists anteriorly and unless the operative procedure is performed with this in mind, results are likely to continue to be disappointing.

PATHOLOGY

The excellent work of Hoppenfield,[2] although frequently referred to, is often overlooked. In a meticulous study involving clinical and radiographic investigations correlated with cadaver dissections he clearly demonstrated the true

deforming forces. Figures 1 and 2 show these anterior basic
mechanisms. The apical vertebral body is wedged anteriorly
and often appears 'rounded off'. The vertebrae above and
below share in this structural bony deformity but to a lesser
extent. Frequently, as in a high level neurological lesion,
there is extensive loss of the posterior elements which
complements the anterior changes. Soft tissues are an
integral part of the anterior deforming forces, in particular
tight annuli fibrosi and a contracted anterior longitudinal
ligament. Indeed when Hoppenfield divided these in cadaver
specimens he could obtain a good correction. To these must
be added three sets of muscles which are also offenders. Due
to posterior bony element rotation the paraspinal muscles
convex to exert a flexor effect on the already deformed
spine. The crura of the diaphragm and the psoas musculature
are the others responsible. It is hardly surprising, therefore, that surgical intervention from the back is attended
by poor results when the problems exist in front.

CLINICAL FEATURES

Myelomeningocele with kyphosis is always associated with
severe lower limb paralysis and in Sharrard's experience the
commonest situation is paralysis of all muscles below the
third lumbar neural segment. Many, however, have neurological
levels of thoracic twelve or above with associated hydrocephalus and, therefore, have no walking potential.

The clinical appearance of the characteristic deformity
is shown in Figure 3. The typical short-segment kyphosis
confined to the lumbar spine can be clearly seen in this
five year old, Figure 3-A. The overlying skin is always
scarred and of poor quality, Figure 3-B. In this instance
the integument is intact but frequently skin breakdown with

super-added infection lead to ulceration which may resist
conservative treatment. Infection may then spread to the
cerebro-spinal fluid and threaten the neurological level or
even life itself.

While the most severe deformities are accompanied by a
compensatory thoracic lordosis, the most usual situation is
that the entire spine above angulates further forward as the
kyphosis progresses until chest and thighs meet which may be
the only factor preventing the child from toppling over.

MANAGEMENT

There is no place for bracing alone in the management
of these individuals whose deformities are rigid and progressive. Surgery is the only solution to this problem. It
would seem logical to correct the spinal lesion at the same
time as the defect is closed on the first day of life and,
indeed, Sharrard[5] has developed a technique of neonatal
osteotomy-resection for this purpose. This may be helpful
by enabling good skin cover to be achieved from the outset
and would lessen the tendency to recurrent breakdown and
ulceration which would otherwise occur in the poor quality
skin stretched by the kyphotic deformity. All too frequently,
however, the child reaches the spinal center long after this
latter situation has developed. The surgeon is then driven
into operative treatment for two reasons - 1) to prevent or
definitively treat the overlying skin problem, and 2) to
prevent or correct the underlying deformity and so enable
the child to be an independent sitter.

The surgical approaches to these two problems are
totally different and it is extremely important that this
point be appreciated. While we pay particular attention to
skin asepsis in spinal surgery this may be extremely

difficult or even impossible to achieve. Indeed the excision
of an overlying septic skin ulcer may be the only route of
approach to the underlying deformity. For this reason the
amount of exposure and quantity of implant materials inserted
must be kept to a minimum. Figure 4 illustrates such a case.
A 140 degree lumbar kyphosis was associated with overlying
skin ulceration resistant to non-operative local treatment.
The spine was approached posteriorly by excising the
ulcerated skin and the redundant spinal cord ligated and
excised. A wedge excision of the apical vertebral body was
then performed and compression hooks were used for fixation
(Fig. 4-B). A good correction was obtained and the overlying
wound healed uneventfully in an area of now good quality skin.
When the child attempted to sit, the spine above collapsed
forward, the compression hooks tented the skin and had to be
removed. The deformity is recurring, (Fig. 4-C), and the
child is still unable to sit. This must be the expectation
when only a local fusion is performed after wedge excision
with limited fixation from the back when the deforming forces
exist in front.

When the deformity is not associated with an overlying
skin problem then definitive corrective surgery can be
performed, bearing in mind the pathological anatomy in these
spines. Figure 5 illustrates this point. This child with a
100 degree lumbar kyphosis was unable to sit without an
anterior support to prevent his toppling over (Fig. 5-A). A
two stage surgical procedure was performed. In the first
stage the kyphosis was approached anteriorly, the tight
anterior longitudinal ligament and annuli fibrosi divided,
the deformed vertebra removed, and an anterior rib strut
graft inserted. At a second operation two weeks later the
spine was approached posteriorly, the wedge excision closed

with a compression system, and an extensive posterior fusion
was performed with Harrington distraction rods extending from
the middle of the thoracic spine to the sacrum. The lateral
radiograph (Fig. 5-B) shows the position of the anterior
strut graft and a good correction of the deformity achieved.
At follow-up four years later (Fig. 5-C) the correction has
been maintained, the anterior graft has been incorporated,
there is a solid posterior fusion with hooks and rods holding,
and the patient can sit upright independently with a straight
spine.

DISCUSSION

Congenital lumbar kyphosis in myelomeningocele is
characterized by its severity, rigidity, and progression.
Superimposed on the structural vertebral changes are strong
anterior soft-tissue deforming forces. The sitting potential
of the child, already a non-walker, is in serious jeopardy
as his center of gravity is drawn further anteriorly.
Furthermore, problems concerning the quality of the skin
overlying the deformity are an ever-present threat to life,
there being a high incidence of cerebro-spinal infection in
these individuals. Neonatal osteotomy-resection of the
deformed vertebra may solve the immediate problem of providing a good quality to the overlying integument and this must
be the initial treatment of choice. Recurrence of deformity
and non-union are known complications, however, but this
procedure affords the only means of preventing skin sepsis.
With healthy skin cover the child can then await the definite
corrective surgery he will require when more mature to
prevent recurrence of deformity which is a sine qua non of
gravity's further adverse influence on the anterior deformity
forces.

Unfortunately, many of these children do not have the opportunity for this type of surgery at birth and present much later to a spinal center with established skin ulceration. Local posterior wedge excision of the apex of the deformity should be performed in order to allow satisfactory skin healing.[6] Such a procedure cannot be expected to prevent progression of deformity and it would, therefore, appear more prudent not to further endanger the situation by introducing a foreign body (wire, screw, staple) which in any event will produce no beneficial effect. The introduction of an implant should await the definite corrective two stage procedure which can be performed when the skin is healthy and the spine more mature. A two stage anterior and posterior approach has already proved itself effective in the treatment of other severe, rigid, spinal deformities[1,3,4] and is the only method of dealing with the anterior deforming forces. Both anterior and posterior fusions are essential in producing stability in paralytic spinal disorders and in order to prevent the spine from collapsing above and below the corrected kyphosis, a solid posterior fusion is necessary extending well above the deformed area down to the sacrum.

The suggested management of kyphosis in myelomeningocele is summarized in Table 1.

REFERENCES

1. Dickson, R.A. and Leatherman, K.D.: Spinal deformity in adults - changing concepts. *J. Bone Joint Surg.*, *58A* In press, 1976.

2. Hoppenfield, S.: Congenital kyphosis in myelomeningocele *J. Bone Joint Surg.*, *49B*:276, 1967.

3. Leatherman, K.D.: Resection of vertebral bodies.
    J. Bone Joint Surg., *51A*:206, 1969.
4. Leatherman, K.D.: The management of rigid spinal curves.
    Clin. Orthop, 93:215, 1973.
5. Sharrard, W.J.W.: Spinal osteotomy for congenital
    kyphosis in myelomeningocele. *J. Bone Joint Surg.*,
    50B:466, 1968.
7. Sharrard, W.J.W. and Drennan, J.C.: Osteotomy-excision
    of the spine for lumbar kyphosis in older children with
    myelomeningocele. *J. Bone Joint Surg.*, *54B*:50, 1972.

TABLE 1.

Congenital Kyphosis in Myelomeningocele

Management		
Neonatal Osteotomy-Excision	–	On the first day of life to aid sac closure and provide adequate skin cover
Posterior Wedge Excision	–	To provide healthy skin cover when ulceration of the integument overlies the kyphosis
The Two Stage Procedure	–	Necessary in all cases to provide definitive correction of the deformity

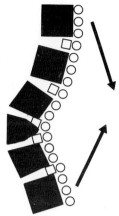

■   VERTEBRAL BODY

□   ANNULUS FIBROSUS

○   ANTERIOR LONGITUDINAL
         LIGAMENT

Fig. 1.   The anterior deforming forces.

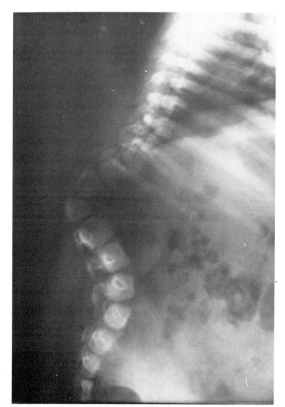

Fig. 2.   Lateral radiograph of a congenital lumbar
kyphosis.

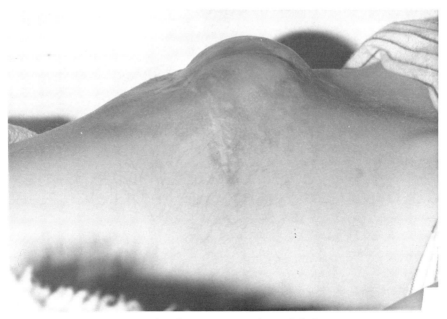

Fig. 3A. The characteristic clinical deformity.

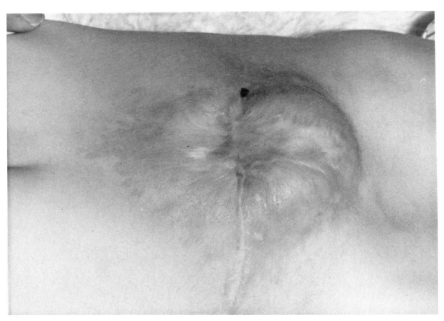

Fig. 3B. The overlying skin is scarred and of poor quality.

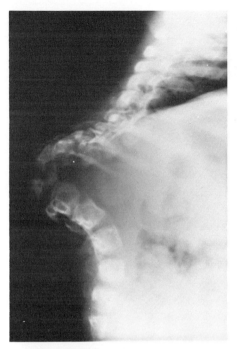

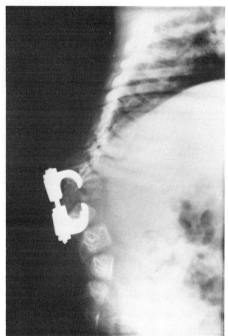

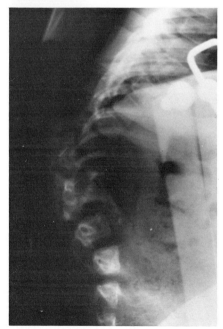

Fig. 4A (top left). Pre-operative lateral radiograph of a severe 140 degree congenital lumbar kyphosis.

Fig. 4B (top right). Lateral radiograph after posterior wedge excision and internal fixation with compression hooks. A good correction has been achieved.

Fig. 4C (bottom left). When the spine collapsed forward above the kyphosis, the hooks had to be removed to prevent skin breakdown. The deformity is recurring and the child cannot sit.

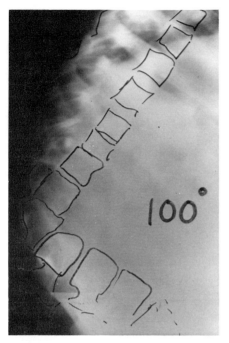

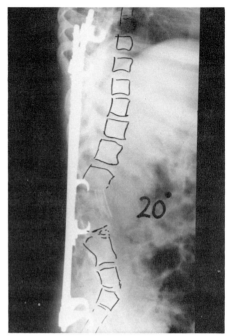

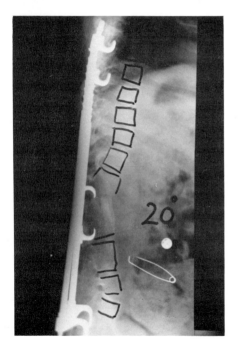

Fig. 5A (top left). Pre-operative lateral radiograph of a severe 100 degree congenital lumbar kyphosis.

Fig. 5B (top right). Lateral radiograph showing the excellent correction achieved by a two-stage procedure—anterior soft tissue release, vertebral body resection, and posterior fusion·with rods.

Fig. 5C (bottom left). Lateral radiograph four years later. Hooks and rods are holding and there has been no loss of correction.

VERTEBRAL BODY RESECTION FOR SPINAL DEFORMITY IN MYELOMENINGOCELE

Robert A. Dickson, Ch.M., F.R.C.S.
and Kenton D. Leatherman, M.D.

INTRODUCTION

The management of scoliosis, kyphosis, and lordosis in relation to myelomeningocele has already been well described in previous chapters. However, the axial skeleton in spina bifida may not just be the site of a progressive collapsing type of deformity. It is in the spine of the myelodysplastic that some of the most severe problems exist which are among the most challenging in the entire field of spinal surgery and which warrant the most exacting operative intervention. The two-stage vertebral body resection and posterior fusion with Harrington instrumentation[3,4] is the only satisfactory method of dealing with the most complex situations.

THE CONCEPT OF VERTEBRAL BODY RESECTION

The removal of a vertebral body is not a new operation. It was pioneered many years ago in Hong Kong by Professor Hodgson for tuberculous spinal disease,[2] and in Louisville for the management of rigid spinal deformities.[3,4] Its importance in the management of severe deformities in spina bifida is only now being appreciated in other centres. Fig. 1 shows the frequency of the various different operative procedures used to deal with myelomeningocele spines in our

centre. It can be seen that almost two-thirds of the
procedures performed involved excision of a vertebral body.
Posterior fusion with rods, by far the most popular operation
for idiopathic scoliosis, was used in less than one-third of
our patients. But why the apparent concentration on vertebral body resection, a procedure for rigid deformities, when
the basic lesion is supposed to be a paralytic collapsing
type of curve? In our experience of over 50 cases of spinal
deformity in myelomeningocele 47 percent had associated
congenital abnormalities, the most common being a unilateral
unsegmented bar. A rigid spinal curvature, therefore,
frequently complicates the issue, and requires a more
aggressive approach than if the deformity was merely
paralytic in origin.

PATIENTS

Eleven patients underwent vertebral body resection for
deformities excluding congenital lumbar kyphosis. The mean
age of these individuals at operation was 13.4 years and the
mean follow-up period of 3.5 years. Fig. 2 shows the various
deformity types. Six patients had scoliosis as the sole
deformity, three had an associated lordosis, and two an
associated kyphosis.

MANAGEMENT

Table 1 shows the various operative procedures of which
vertebral body resection was an integral part. Vertebral
body resection alone was only performed in two cases. Seven
patients underwent a second-stage posterior fusion with rods
(usually with posterior osteotomy), and one required Dwyer
instrumentation in addition. In one individual with a double
structural curvature two vertebral body resections were

performed, and the posterior fusion with rods was the finale
of a three-stage adventure. The two-stage vertebral body
resection followed by posterior fusion with Harrington
instrumentation was, therefore, the most usual performed.
The value of this procedure developed in Louisville is
illustrated by Fig. 3. This five year old has a typical
pre-operative radiographic appearance, Fig. 3-A. This is a
supine film of a child unable to sit. A lower left thoracic
unilateral unsegmented bar has given rise to this severe
132 degree deformity. The left costal margin is tucked under
the left iliac wing which has migrated superiorly due to the
marked degree of pelvic tilt. At the first stage the apical
vertebral body is approached through the bed of the rib above
the apex on the convex side, in this instance the right
eighth rib. This vertebral body is then removed, Fig. 3-B.
At the second stage, usually performed two weeks later, the
posterior bony elements, if present, corresponding to the
level of the body excised, are then removed and this area is
closed with a compression system. An extensive posterior
fusion is then performed from the middle of the thoracic
spine right down to the sacrum, Fig. 3-C. The deformity, now
corrected to 87 degrees is maintained by means of a distraction rod which must extend well above the congenital component of the deformity and right down to the sacrum to get
below the paralytic component. The special sacral alar hook
is ideal for this purpose and obviates the need for the
troublesome sacral bar. The pelvic tilt has been markedly
reduced. At follow-up eighteen months later this child,
with no leg function, is an independent sitter.

Sometimes it is necessary to be even more aggresive,
particularly when two severe rigid curvatures exist in the
same spine. Fig. 4 illustrates such a case. This three

year old girl has an upper left thoracic unilateral unsegmented bar giving rise to a severe 110 degree deformity, Fig. 4-A. Below this there is a 112 degree thoraco-lumbar curve which radiographically defies precise classification but whose absence of movement on lateral bending confirms its rigid character. A severe pelvic tilt is again present in this non-sitter. At the first stage, Fig. 4-B, the upper apical vertebral body was removed through the bed of the right fifth rib. Two weeks later at the second stage, Fig. 4-C, the lower apical body was excised subpleurally and retroperitoneally via the eleventh left rib. At the third stage two further weeks later, Fig. 4-D, an extensive posterior spinal fusion with Harrington instrumentation was performed. The site of the upper body resection was closed with a compression system on the convex side. Two distraction rods were used to jack up the concavity of the lower curve, it being technically extremely difficult to fit a compression system into non-existent posterior elements. At follow-up one year later, Fig. 4-E, hooks and rods are holding, there has been no loss of correction, and the child can sit with a clinically straight spine.

It is tempting when excision of a vertebral body has given rise to a good correction to omit the second stage. This temptation must be resisted. Fig. 5 serves as the necessary warning. A severe 100 degree curvature, Fig. 5-A, could only be corrected to 60 degrees by halo-femoral traction, Fig. 5-B. The third lumbar vertebral body was then removed and the patient retained in traction. The deformity was, thereby, further corrected to 37 degrees, Fig. 5-C, and a spontaneous interbody fusion occurred. No second stage was performed but two years later the curvature has increased to 60 degrees, Fig. 5-D.

Another   operation   was   clearly   indicated.

<u>RESULTS</u>

Table 2 summarizes the results of vertebral body
resection for spinal deformity in myelodysplasia in our
centre. The mean pre-operative curvature of these patients
was 97 degrees and operative treatment corrected this to 55
degrees (a 43 percent correction). In one individual the
wound took four weeks to heal, and one case progressed again
after surgery. There were no infections, no cases of
increased neurological loss and no deaths in this series.
The absence of infection we believe to be due to our policy
of prophylactic antibiotics, urinary sterilization, and
meticulous pre- and per-operative skin care.

Although operative technique is particularly important
in spinal surgery, the operation itself is only a part of
the overall management of these children. The resection of a
vertebral body may appear to be a formidable procedure but,
performed properly, it is not attended by a high complication
rate. We have looked very carefully at the post-operative
course of patients undergoing spinal surgery for deformities
associated with myelodysplasia and have painstakingly
documented the important variables. It can be seen from
Table 3 that with regard to our two-stage procedure the first
stage (vertebral body resection) was associated with a blood
loss of 600 cc's, less than half of that associated with
posterior fusion with rods. This we believe to be due to
removing the vertebral body slice by slice with a chisel and
then immediately covering the raw surface with bone wax.
By this means bleeding is kept to a minimum from this
extremely vascular cancellous bone. Furthermore, if blood
loss is replaced as it occurs we have never found it

necessary to infuse additional blood in the post-operative
period following vertebral body resection. In contradistinction even when blood loss is replaced during posterior
fusion with rods we have found it necessary in one-third of
all cases to give an additional unit on the third post-
operative day. This is based arbitrarily on not allowing
the haemoglobin to fall below 10 G. in the post-operative
phase.

It is important to realize that in these children with
abnormalities of function involving many systems, post-
operative problems are more likely to arise than if the
child was otherwise normal. It is the early complications,
if not promptly treated, that are life-threatening. Table 4
is taken from our study of all spinal surgery performed on
children with spina bifida,[1] not just the ones who have
undergone body resection. With the exception of the one case
of prolonged cerebro-spinal fluid leak in an individual who
underwent excision of a diastematomyelia in addition to
spinal stabilization, all these early complications are
those associated with surgery in general, not just spinal
surgery. Our surgical forefathers have warned us that any
of these may be associated with a rise in temperature in the
post-operative phase. However, all patients undergoing
spinal surgery for myelodysplasia have a post-operative
pyrexia with a mean maximum temperature of 101.7 degrees
Fahrenheit and mean duration until this falls to normal of
eight days. The mean maximum temperature of those who
developed early post-operative complications did not differ
significantly from those who had uneventful post-operative
courses, nor was there any significant trend for the
temperature to be elevated above the mean. The time taken
for the temperature to revert to normal was not dissimilar

in the two groups. Repeated careful clinical examinations
of all post-operative patients are, therefore, mandatory as
inspection of the temperature chart is unreliable.

CONCLUSIONS

These are some of the most aggressive forms of surgical
intervention that can be performed on the spine. We believe
that there is a world of difference between being condemned
to a supine life and being an independent wheel-chair
operating sitter. The pleasure of retained eyesight is one
of the few remaining functions in these individuals but a
twenty-four hour a day inspection of the ceiling of their
room can hardly be described as visual satisfaction. An
axial skeleton which points upwards on sitting allows the
quality of life to assume a new dimension in these most
unfortunate children.

REFERENCES

1. Dickson, R.A. and Leatherman, K.D.: Spinal Deformity in
    Myelomeningocele - Surgical Treatment. In press, 1976.

2. Hodgson, A.R.: Correction of fixed spinal curves.
    J. Bone Joint Surg., *47A*:1221, 1965.

3. Leatherman, K.D.: Resection of vertebral bodies.
    J. Bone Joint Surg., *51A*:206, 1969.

4. Leatherman, K.D.: The management of rigid spinal curves.
    Clin. Orthop., *93*:215, 1973.

TABLE 1.

Type of Procedure

Body Resection and Posterior Fusion with Rods	7
Body Resection Only	2
Two Body Resections and Posterior Fusion with Rods	1
Body Resection, Dwyer, and Posterior Fusion with Rods	1

TABLE 2.

Vertebral Body Resection

Mean Preop. Curve	97
Mean Postop. Curve	55
Early Complications - Delayed Wound Healing	1
Late Complications - Pseudarthrosis/Marked Loss of Correction	1
Infections	0
Increased Neurological Loss	0
Deaths	0

TABLE 3.

Blood Loss

Body Resection	Posterior Fusion With Rods
600 cc's	1340 cc's
No Additional Blood Required	Additional Blood Frequently Required on Third Day

TABLE 4.

Early Complications

Delayed Wound Healing	3
Haematoma	1
Vaginal Discharge	1
Urinary Infection	1
Atelectasis	1
Pneumothorax	1
C S F Leak	1

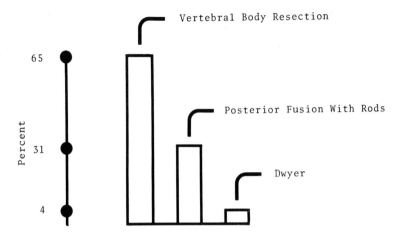

Fig. 1. The frequency of the various operative procedures.

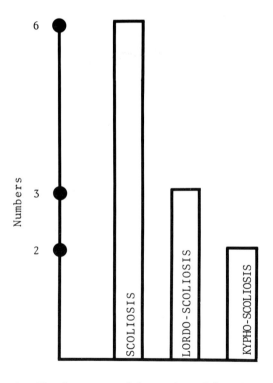

Fig. 2. The frequency of the various deformity types.

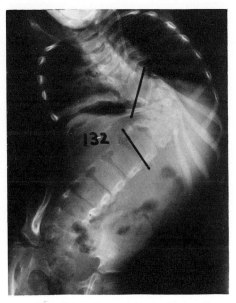

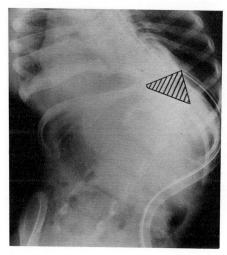

Fig. 3B. Antero-posterior radiograph after removal of the apical vertebral body.

Fig. 3A. Antero-posterior radiograph of a 132 degree deformity associated with a unilateral bar.

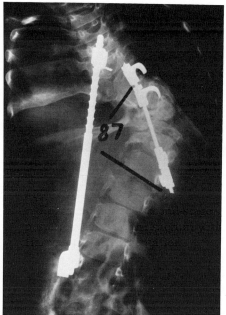

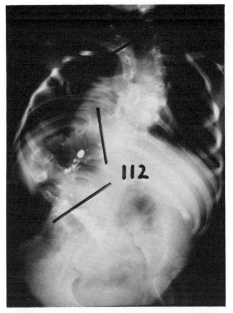

Fig. 3C. Antero-posterior radiograph after the second-stage posterior fusion to the sacrum with Harrington instrumentation.

Fig. 4A. Antero-posterior radiograph showing severe double structural curves with a unilateral bar and marked pelvic tilt.

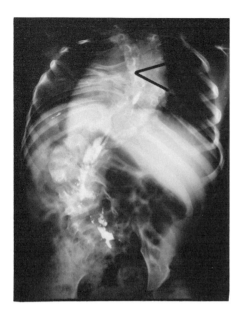

Fig. 4B. Antero-posterior radiograph after excision of the lower apical vertebral body.

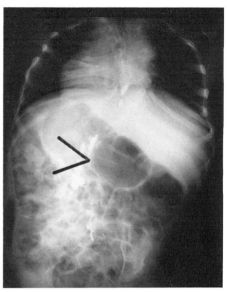

Fig. 4C. Antero-posterior radiograph after excisis of the lower apical vertebral body.

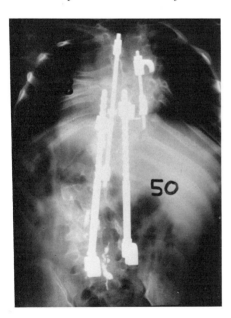

Fig. 4D. Antero-posterior radiograph after the third-stage posterior fusion with rods. The curves are markedly reduced, the chest is much more symmetrical, and the pelvic tilt is almost completely corrected.

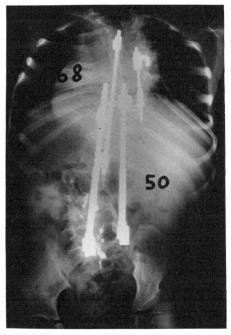

Fig. 4E. Antero-posterior radiograph at follow-up, one year later. Hooks and rods are holding and there has been no loss of correction.

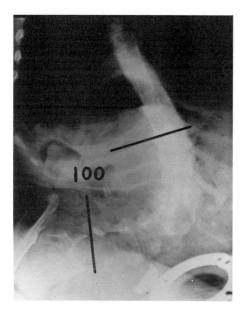

Fig. 5A. Antero-posterior
radiograph showing a severe 100
degree paralytic curvature with
marked pelvic tilt.

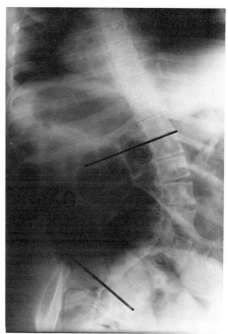

Fig. 5B. Antero-posterior
radiograph after halo-femoral
traction. The curvature has been
reduced to 60 degrees.

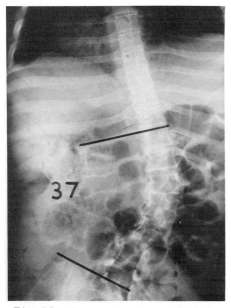

Fig. 5C. Antero-posterior
radiograph after excision of the third
lumbar vertebral body. The
curvature has been reduced further
to 37 degrees and a spontaneous
interbody fusion has occurred.

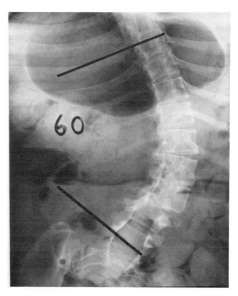

Fig. 5D. Antero-posterior
radiograph two years later. The
deformity has regressed to 60
degrees.

Part IV
UROLOGY

Participants

William E. Bradley, M.D.
Baylor University Medical Center, Houston, Texas
A. Estin Comarr, M.D.
University Medical Center, Loma Linda, California
Joseph A. Cox, M.D.
University of Cincinnati, Cincinnati, Ohio
Ananias C. Diokno, M.D.
University of Michigan Medical Center, Ann Arbor, Michigan
Arthur T. Evans, M.D.
University of Cincinnati Medical Center, Cincinnati, Ohio
Casimir F. Firlit, M.D., Ph.D.
Children's Memorial Hospital, Chicago, Illinois
Robert D. Jeffs, M.D.
Johns Hopkins Hospital, Baltimore, Maryland
George T. Klauber, M.D.
University of Connecticut, Newington, Connecticut
Daniel C. Merrill, M.D.
University of California at Davis, Martinez, California
Lester Persky, M.D.
Case-Western Reserve School of Medicine, Cleveland, Ohio
Pramod R. Rege, M.D.
University of Cincinnati Medical Center, Cincinnati, Ohio
F. Brantley Scott, M.D.
Baylor University Medical Center, Houston, Texas
David B. Shurtleff, M.D.
University of Washington School of Medicine, Seattle, Washington
Emil A. Tanagho, M.D.
University of California, San Francisco, California

NEUROLOGY OF MICTURITION

William E. Bradley

INTRODUCTION

The physiology of the urinary bladder has undergone
considerable change in understanding during the past decade
as the result of the efforts of anatomists, physiologists,
pharmacologists and clinical investigators. The breadth and
scope of this understanding has been derived from comparative
and human studies into urothelium, connective tissue,
vascular supply and neural pathways of the detrusor muscle
and urethra.

The two functions of the urinary bladder are those of
1) storage and 2) expulsion of urine. All elements colla-
borate to attain this end with the impermeability of the
urothelium assuring the efficiency of the underlying contrac-
tile mechansim.

Urine storage capability is assured by the distensibility
of the transitional epithelium and the impermeability of the
epithelium assuring no intrinsic change in osmolality of the
stored urine. The accommodation of intramural structures
is a function of the elastic properties of smooth muscle,
collagen, elastic fibers and mucopolysaccharides and is
non-neural in origin. However, recent experiments in the
laboratory animal utilizing electrical stimulation of the
sympathetic innervation have suggested these nerves play a

role in change in accommodation. Accommodation may be
measured by plotting the slope of the tonus limb of the
cystometrogram. This slope may be increased by detrusor
fibrosis secondary to recurrent infection and depressed by
rupture of the tissue elements secondary to overdistention.
So the storage phase is largely a passive event during which
there is an increasing generation of sensory impulses in
tension endings localized principally in the collagen layers
surrounding the smooth muscle fasicles and in small part to
stimulation of volume receptors in the individual smooth
muscle fasicles. The buildup in sensory impulses which
travel in the spinal cord to the brain stem are proportional
to the intravesical volume. These sensory impulses are
necessary to induce a reflex contraction of the detrusor
muscle as was shown a long time ago when section of the
sacral, dorsal or sensory roots permanently abolished the
detrusor reflex. With gradually increasing sensory impulses
there is greater excitation at many levels of the nervous
system to produce the second and possibly more complicated
function of the urinary bladder, the expulsion of intravesical content.

The portions of the central nervous system responding
to the intravesical sensory impulses generated by filling
include 1) The cerebral cortex, 2) thalamus, 3) basal
ganglia, 4) limbic system, 5) hypothalamus, 6) brain stem
reticular formation, 7) cerebellum and 8) spinal cord.
Within these areas there is separation of the neuron pools
concerned with innervation of the detrusor muscle and the
periurethral striated muscle.

As the detrusor muscle and urethra are midline axial
structures there is bilateral representation at many levels
as well as crossing of fibers. This crossing occurs at the

level of the brain stem and in the lumbar portion of the spinal cord and in the peripheral innervation. Hence, unilateral interruption of cortical, brain stem or spinal innervation produces no discernable alteration in detrusor or urethral function.

CEREBRAL CORTEX AND INNERVATION OF THE DETRUSOR MUSCLE AND URETHRA

The cerebral cortex is divided arbitrarily into four lobes: frontal, parietal, occipital and temporal. Years of clinical observation and laboratory research have established that certain specific sensory and motor functions are localized within each of these lobes. Frequently, these functions such as vision or hearing are localized to gyri within the lobes which are demarcated from other gyri by involution or fissures called sulci.

The detrusor motor and sensory areas in the cerebral cortex are separate and distinct from those concerned with the periurethral striated muscle. These have been localized to superiomedial portion of the frontal lobe, the anterior portion of the cingulate gyrus and the genu of the corpus callosium in both man[1] and the experimental animal (Fig. 1). In man this localization has been determined by examination of patients with extensive lesions affecting these areas. In the experimental animal this has been decided by studying the effect of stimulation upon the detrusor reflex[6] and by stimulation of the pelvic and pudendal nerves and recording the evoked responses in these areas.[5]

The cerebral cortical representation of the periurethral striated muscle has been localized to the supero-medial portion of the sensori-motor area caudal to the Rolandic fissure.

The layers of the cerebral cortex have a horizontal and a vertical organization. The horizontal organization is manifested as layers of lamina, 6 in number. The most important cell of these layers is located in lamina V and is a pyramidal shaped cell giving rise to an efferent projection fiber (Fig. 2). Pyramidal shaped cells in the detrusor motor cortex are the origin of projection fibers traveling to the detrusor motor center in the brain stem. Similar projection fibers from the pudendal portion of the sensori-motor cortex pass via the corticospinal tract and travel in the spinal cord to synapse on the anterior horn cells in the pudendal nucleus. The pyramidal cell derives its name from the shape of the cell body consisting of cell body, dendrites, and axon.

There is also a vertical organization of the cells of the cerebral cortex. A cylinder or column of neurons is activated by one and only one specific sensory stimulus. Distension of the detrusor muscle or contraction of the detrusor muscle or contraction of the muscle fibers generates sensory impulses which ascend in the spinal cord and brain stem to terminate on the dendrites of the pyramidal cells in the detrusor portion of the cerebral cortex. Similarly a cylinder or column of neurons in the pudendal area of the sensori-motor cortex is activated by impulses generated in sensory endings in the periurethral striated muscle and anal sphincter. The single long apical dendrite of the pyramidal cell ascends vertically through the cortical mantle to terminate in the most superficial layer. Through its length synaptic contacts are made by sensory endings.

The efferent or projection fiber from the pyramidal cell projects into the white matter of the cerebrum and ends in a 1) association, 2) commissural, or 3) projection fiber.

Association fibers are those axons of the pyramidal cells connecting the detrusor motor portion of the cerebral cortex to the pudendal portion of the sensori-motor cortex. Reciprocal axonal pathways are also present.

The commissural or interhemispheric fibers are the axons of pyramidal cells that interconnect the detrusor motor center in the frontal cortex of one hemisphere to the detrusor motor center in the contralateral hemisphere by commissural projection fibers in the corpus callosium. Similar commissural fibers interconnect the pudendal area of the sensori-motor cortex of one hemisphere to the corresponding area in the contralateral hemisphere. In patients in whom section of the corpus callosium have been made for control of a convulsive disorder there have been no reports of bladder dysfunction. Therefore, these commissural pathways are not of crucial significance in control of bladder function.

Finally, the projection fibers to and from the detrusor and sphincter areas in the cerebral cortex include:

1. Cortico-reticular fibers arising from pyramidal cells in the detrusor motor portion of the frontal cortex. These fibers pass through the internal capsule and synapse in the non-specific thalamic nuclei and basal ganglia and ultimately end by synaptic termination on neurons of the pontine-mesencephalic reticular formation. From this nucleus arises the axons of the reticulo spinal tract which travel in the lateral columns of the spinal cord to end by synapses on the interneurons of the detrusor nucleus in the lumbar and sacral spinal cord.

2. The descending pathway from the pudendal portion of the sensori-motor cortex, the cortical spinal tracts, passes in the internal capsule and the brain stem and as the

cortico-spinal tract in the lateral columns of the spinal
cord to terminate on the anterior horn cells in the pudendal
nucleus of the sacral gray matter. The corticospinal tracts
extensively decussate and cross to the contralateral side in
the caudal end of the medulla.

3. Ascending fibers from sensory endings in the detrusor muscle ascend in the spinothalamic tracts and posterior
columns to synapse on neurons in the ventral and basal aspect
of the thalamus and ultimately terminate on dendritic pews
in the detrusor portion of the cerebral cortex.

4. Ascending impulses from sensory endings in the
periurethral striated muscle which travel in the posterior
columns to the cerebellum. After synapses there they travel
rostrally and after synapsing in the thalamus terminate in
the pudendal portion of the sensori-motor cortex.

Both ascending and descending tracts from the cerebral
cortex condense in the internal capsule. This anatomical
site is a frequent area of arterial occlusion in cerebro-
vascular disease.

THALAMUS

The thalamus is the principal relay center for projection fibers to and from the cerebral cortex. Each thalamic
nucleus projects to an area of the cerebral cortex and in
turn receives projection fibers from it. The thalamic
nuclei, therefore, are integral parts of corticothalamic
systems as well as of ascending sensory systems. Each
sensory pathway terminates in a specific thalamic nucleus.
For the periurethral striated muscle the sensory pathways
synapse in ventralis posteromedialis. The synaptic termination of the proprioceptive endings in the detrusor muscle
are unknown but most probably end in nucleus dorsalis

medialis. The thalamus is a processing station for inputs
from widely differing areas within the brain. Other thalamic
nuclei receive inputs from the reticular formation and
project widely to the cerebral cortex. These are referred
to as nonspecific thalamic nuclei.

The thalamic nuclei receive both afferent input from
sensory fibers and from the cerebral cortex through projection fibers. The output from these thalamic relay nuclei
passes in the white matter to terminate in specific areas of
the cerebral cortex. Detrusor sensory pathways relay from
the thalamus and thence to the prefrontal region of the
frontal lobes and from periurethral striated muscle thalamic
relay nucleus to the pudendal portion of the periurethral
striated muscle. Lesions in these nuclei result in the same
reflex disturbance as cortical lesions.

THE BASAL GANGLIA

The basal ganglia consist of the caudate nucleus, red
nucleus substantia nigra, putamen and globus pallidus (Fig.3).
The evidence that these nuclei control voiding is overwhelming and include clinical reports of urinary incontinence in
Parkinson disease[6] as well as evidence from the experimental
animal. The Parkinson patients have been examined cystometrically and have demonstrated detrusor hyperreflexia or
uninhibited bladder contractions.

The input to the basal ganglia is derived from the
frontal lobe. The output is directed to the brain stem
reticular formation including the detrusor motor nucleus.
Stimulation of the globus pallidus and substantia nigra in
the experimental animal have shown detrusor reflex suppres-
sion whereas ablation resulted in detrusor hyperreflexia.[5]

THE LIMBIC SYSTEM (Fig. 4)

The limbic system has input from all sensory pathways and influences the autonomic nervous system by its effect on the hypothalamus and brain stem. The nuclei comprising the limbic system include the amygdala, the hypocampal formation and the cingulate gyrus. The hypocampal formation projects fibers to the anterior thalamus and hypothalamus. Stimulation of the limbic system in the experimental animal has been shown to affect the detrusor reflex. In patients with limbic system seizures, urinary incontinence and detrusor contraction have been reported as pre-ictal events.

THE HYPOTHALAMUS

The hypothalamus is located at the base of the thalamus and functions in two broad areas: 1) The maintenance of a relatively constant interval body environment, 2) Behavior patterns including micturition.

The hypothalamus derives its principal input from the brain stem reticular formation and can be regarded as a rostral extension of that area. The hypothalamus is an intermediate zone between the brain stem and cerebral cortex. The hypothalamus may be anatomically divided into four areas: 1) Pre-optic and 2) Supra-optic areas, 3) Tuberal area and 4) Mamillary area. In the anterior hypothalamic nuclei the parasympathetic excitatory role has been localized including micturition. Neurons in the posterior hypothalamus have been identified in the experimental animal as responding to bladder distention.

THE CEREBELLUM (Fig. 5)

The cerebellum acts to modulate motor activity initiated in other parts of the central nervous system.[2] The cerebellum

receives sensory impulses from both the detrusor muscle and
periurethral striated muscle in the experimental animal.
Stimulation of the anterior vermis in the experimental animal
has been shown to depress detrusor reflex contractions.
Ablation of the anterior vermis results in detrusor hyperreflexia. In patients the data on bladder contractions
following cerebellar lesions is conflicting since cerebellar
lesions are frequently associated with brain stem compression
or invasion of brain stem structures.

THE RETICULAR FORMATION (Fig. 6)

The reticular formation is the intricate neural network
of cells which forms most of the brain stem tegmentum. The
reticular activating system is the functional system
utilizing the reticular formation as its neural substrate.
The reticular formation is organized into reticular nuclei
and into 1) diffuse ascending reticular pathways and 2) descending reticular pathways. The ascending reticular pathways
pass to the thalamus and cortex and are involved with the
state of alertness of the individual and activation of the
cortical areas concerned with detrusor contraction. The
descending reticular pathways pass in the reticulo spinal
tracts in the spinal cord to innervate the detrusor motor
areas in the lumbar and sacral spinal cord. The reticulo
spinal tracts also connect to the gamma efferent system
innervating muscle spindles in the periurethral striated
muscle and anal sphincter.

The reticular formation is organized into a lateral and
a medial portion. The descending spinal portion has its
neurons in the medial areas and the ascending portion in the
lateral areas. The lateral area is essentially a sensory
zone receiving input from higher centers and from the spinal

cord.   This sensory region projects its output to the medial
brain stem reticular formation where the detrusor motor
center is located.

The input to the brain stem reticular formation is
derived from the spinal cord, from the cerebral cortex and
from the cerebellum.   The input from the spinal cord includes
the spino reticular tracts and the spino-thalamic tracts.
Descending input from the cerebral cortex includes the
cortico-bulbar and cortico-reticular tracts.   There is also
input from the basal ganglia, limbic system and hypothalamus.

The output of the reticular formation is directed to the
thalamic nuclei and the hypothalamus to the cerebral cortex
and basal ganglia.   The descending spinal pathway connects
to the detrusor nuclei in the lumbar and sacral spinal cord
and to gamma and alpha motor neurons in the pudendal nucleus.[3]

SPINAL CORD[7] (Fig. 7)

The spinal pathways concerned with the detrusor and
urethra include sensory pathways from detrusor muscle and
from the periurethral striated muscle.   The descending motor
pathways include the reticulo spinal tracts to innervate the
detrusor nuclei in the lumbar and sacral spinal cord and the
cortico spinal tract to innervate the pudendal nucleus.
Ascending sensory impulses proprioceptive in nature ascend
in the posterior columns from free unspecialized endings in
the detrusor muscle and from muscle spindles in the periurethral striated muscle and anal sphincter.

The descending pathways include the reticulo spinal
tracts and the cortico spinal tracts.   The medial pontine
reticulospinal tract originates in the medial pontine
tegmentum and descends as an uncrossed reticulo-spinal tract
to end on detrusor motor neurons in the intermedio-lateral

cell column of the lumbar and sacral gray matter. The
lateral medullary reticulo spinal tract descends largely as
an uncrossed tract and ends in a manner similar to the above.

The detrusor motor neurons in the spinal cord concerned
with innervation of the smooth muscle cells of the detrusor
are located in the intermedio-lateral cell column of the
lumbar and sacral spinal cord. The motor neurons concerned
with innervation of the periurethral striated muscle and anal
sphincter are located in the anterior horn cells of the
sacral gray matter.

The longitudinal distribution of detrusor motor neurons
has been plotted by electrophysiological and morphological
techniques in the experimental animal and man. The longitudinal distribution of the lumbar input is from the tenth
thoracic to the first lumbar segment. The longitudinal
distributional of the sacral input is from the second to the
fourth sacral areas.

There is no sensory input to these neurons at a segmental level. Rather the sensory impulses from the bladder are
"long routed" to the detrusor motor center in the brain stem.
These travel to and from the brain stem in the reticulo-
spinal tracts. There are in addition peripheral sensory
afferents in the sacral nerves that evoke a response in the
lumbar motor neurons.

There is rostral displacement of the pudendal spinal
nucelus from autonomic motor neurons by at least one spinal
segment. Sensory input to the pudendal nucleus is from
spindle endings in the periurethral striated muscle and anal
sphincter. Counts of these endings have shown them to be
sparse in the periurethral muscle and frequent in the anal
sphincter. There is extensive crossing of spinal innervation
at the L1 level leading in some patients to an asymmetric

functional input. There is also extensive input to the
pudendal nucleus from afferent sensory endings in the detrusor muscle.

One of the most important elements in spinal organization of innervation of the detrusor muscle and periurethral
striated muscle is the presence of recurrent inhibition.
This recurrent inhibition provides for termination of the
detrusor reflex as well as localization of detrusor motor
function in the detrusor motor nucleus.

The central innervation of the bladder and urethra can
for purposes of clinical application be simplified into
closed neural circuits or loops.[4]

Loop I (Fig. 8) consists of to and fro pathways from
the frontal lobes to the detrusor motor nucleus in the
pontine-mesencephalic reticular formation. This pathway
relays to the nuclei of the basal ganglia and the thalamus.
The cerebro-cortical area constituting the rostral end
station of this loop has been already defined and includes
the supero-medial portion of the mid-portion of the frontal
lobe, the anterior portion of the cingulate gyrus and the
genu of the corpus calloseum. The limbic system and the
hypothalamus influence the output of this loop by its effect
upon the detrusor motor center in the brain stem.

Loop II consists of neural pathways from sensory endings
in the detrusor muscle terminating on the detrusor motor
nucleus with pathways to the detrusor nucleus in the sacral
gray matter (Fig. 9). This loop is the prerequisite for the
development of a coordinated detrusor reflex of sufficient
temporal duration to produce total evacuation of intravesical
content.

The third loop (Fig. 10) is that composed of afferent

sensory fibers from the detrusor muscle which impinge synaptically on pudendal motor neurons. The effect of impulse
generation in this loop is to produce exclusive depression of
pudendal nerve activity with resultant relaxation of the
periurethral striated muscle.

The fourth loop consists of supraspinal and segmental
components of the innervation of the periurethral striated
muscle (Fig. 11). Since the periurethral striated muscle
in the male is heavy and in the female is a rudimentary
structure this loop is of more significance in male continence than female. The supraspinal components of this loop
are the sensory pathways in the posterior columns and the
motor tracts arising in the sensori-motor cortex and traveling to the pudendal nucleus in the cortico spinal tracts.
The segmental arc consists of muscle spindles or stretch
receptors in the sphincter whose input ends synaptically on
the pudendal motor neurons. From there alpha motor fibers
arise to innervate the muscle.

PERIPHERAL INNERVATION OF THE DETRUSOR MUSCLE AND URETHRA

Spinal Innervation of the Detrusor Muscle, Urethral
Smooth Muscle, Periurethral Striated Muscle and Uroepithelium.
INNERVATION OF THE GANGLIA (Fig. 12)

There are lumbar and sacral contributions to the pre-
ganglionic input to the pelvic ganglia. In man the lumbar
input is from T-10-L1 and the sacral S3 and S4. There is no
clear demarcation between sympathetic and parasympathetic
innervation as cholinergic and adrenergic fibers have been
identified in lumbar pathways and adrenergic as well as
cholinergic in sacral pathways. Afferents affecting lumbar
output are in sacral pathways but no influence through spinal
tracts has been demonstrated by lumbar stimulation.

The pre-ganglionic input terminates principally on the dendrites of ganglionic neurons. Here excitation occurs by release of acetylcholine. By utilizing electrical stimulation in the experimental animal an inhibitory inter-neuron has been demonstrated.

The ganglia have been indicated to be either exclusively innervated by lumbar, sacral or combined input. They are principally located in the interstices of the detrusor muscle.

Post ganglionic motor neurons innervate the detrusor muscle by stimulation of either alpha or beta adrenergic receptors or cholinergic receptors. These receptors are selectively distributed through the detrusor muscle and urethra. The receptors are located in the muscle and sub-mucosa. There is extensive cross over of the peripheral motor fibers.

The alpha receptors are excited by norepinephrine release from axonal varicosities. These varicosities consist of thinning of the Schwann layer with appearance of vesicles in the axonal swelling. The vesicles are of three different size groupings and different morphological appearance. With appearance of the post ganglionic action potential a process called exocytosis occurs in the varicosity. This consists of mobilization of transmitter and release into a cleft where it passes to depolarize a cell or pacemaker cell. With depo-larization of the pacemaker cell there is stimulation of surrounding cells by passage of current through low resistance intrasynaptic pathways called tight junctions. Stimulation of a receptor produces depolarization and contraction. Stimulation of B receptors produces hyperpolarization and relaxation.

Stimulation of cholinergic receptors produces uniform

depolarization and contractions. There are equally
contradictory communications as to whether the transmitter
released by sacral nerve stimulation is acetylcholine or not.
There is atropine resistance to blockade of neuromuscular
transmission in the bladder. One investigator has attributed
this to the intimate adherence of the neuromuscular junction.

The neuromuscular bundle consists of 12-15 muscle fibers
enclosed in a collagen capsule. This is the equivalent of
the signal skeletal muscle fiber. With induction of contraction there is swelling of the collagen capsule and induction
of tension. This tension development is coordinated to
produce evacuation of intravesical content into the proximal
urethra.

The motor innervation of the periurethral striated
muscle consists of a neuromuscular junction in a manner
similar to that in skeletal muscle (Fig. 13). The mean time
of contraction of the periurethral striated muscle are those
of slow twitch muscle. However, in contrast neuromuscular
transmission in periurethral striated muscle is resistant to
blockade by tubocurarine.

SENSORY INNERVATION OF THE DETRUSOR MUSCLE, UROTHELIUM AND URETHRA

Free and unspecialized sensory nerve endings are present
within the detrusor muscle and submucosa. There is extensive
cross over of these sensory nerve endings in a manner similar
to post-ganglionic motor nerve endings. This cross over is
up to 40% in amount.

Sensory innervation of the periurethral striated muscle
is by way of spindles. Spindle counts in the periurethral
striated muscle are scanty but abundant in the anal sphincter
These in turn are innervated by gamma motor fibers

accounting for tension and bias of the spindle, i.e.,
sensitivity to stretch.

URETHRAL FUNCTION

Opening of the proximal urethra normally occluded by the
inherent tonicity of collagen and elastic fibers occurs by
widening and shortening during detrusor reflex owing to the
mode of insertion of the detrusor muscle fibers. Two loops
formed of smooth muscle fibers compose the bladder neck.
These are (1) the trigonal loop and (2) the detrusor loop
(Fig. 14). The detrusor muscle fasicles are arranged in
groups with insertion into these loops.

The smooth muscle of the urethra is distributed in two
layers: (1) an inner longitudinal layer, continuous with the
detrusor muscle, and (2) an outer circular layer. The latter
circular muscle is responsible for urethral sphincter action
of the smooth muscle and for regulating urethral resistance.
No sphincteric action has been attributed to the inner layer.

The striated muscle portion of the urethra contributes
significantly to urethral resistance. This resistance is
applied to the mid-urethral segment. The striated muscle
component of the urethra has dynamic characteristics which
permit rapid adaptation for changes in urethral resistance.
A few seconds before voiding and preceding detrusor contraction, there is a drop in urethral resistance and it becomes
equivalent to intravesical pressure. This has been attributed to pelvic-floor relaxation. With contraction of the
fasicles, the loops pull apart, permitting expulsion of the
urine into the proximal urethra.

IN SUMMARY

Central and peripheral neural elements contribute to the

regulation of storage and evacuation phases of micturition. There are many gaps in our knowledge of this process in man.

REFERENCES

1. Andrew, J. and Nathan, P.: The cerebral control of micturition. *Proc. Roy. Soc. Med., 58*:553, 1965.

2. Bradley, W.E. and Teague, C.T.: Cerebellar regulation of the micturition reflex. *J. Urol., 101*:396, 1969.

3. Bradley, W.E. and Teague, C.T.: Spinal cord organization of micturition reflex afferents. *Exp. Neurol., 22*:504, 1968.

4. Bradley, W.E., Timm, G.W. and Scott, F.B.: Innervation of the Detrusor Muscle and Urethra. IN Urologic Clinics of North America, Vol. 1, J. Lapides (ed.), Philadelphia, W.B. Saunders Co., 1974.

5. Lewin, R.J., Dillard, G.V. and Porter, R.W.: Extra-pyramidal inhibition of the urinary bladder. *Brain Research, 4*:301, 1967.

6. Murgnahan, G.F.: Neurogenic disorders of the urinary bladder in Parkinsonism. *Brit. J. Urology, 33*:403, 1961.

7. Oliver, J.E., Bradley, W.E. and Fletcher, T.F.: Spinal cord representation of the micturition reflex. *J. Comp. Neurol., 137*:329, 1969.

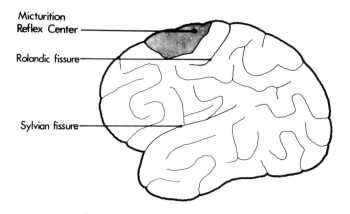

Fig. 1. Detrusor motor center in frontal lobe.

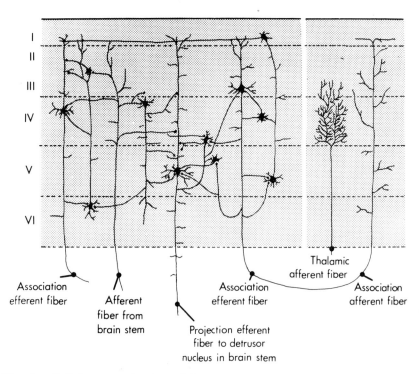

Fig. 2. Cellular organization of detrusor motor center in the frontal cortex.

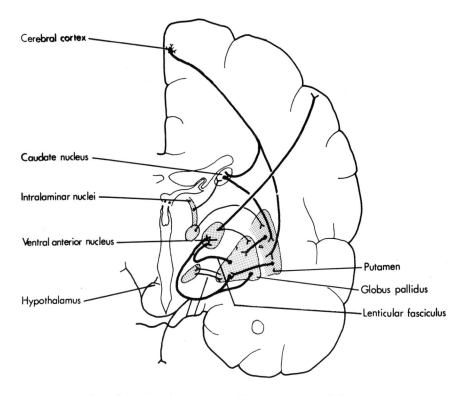

Fig. 3. Nuclei of the basal ganglia and organization of the detrusor motor center.

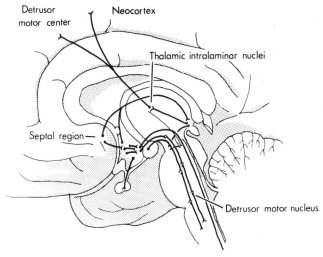

Fig. 4. The connections of the limbic system to the detrusor motor centers in the cerebral cortex and brain stem.

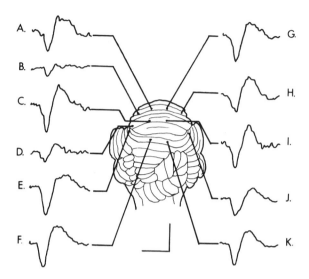

Fig. 5. Responses (A–K) evoked in the anterior vermis of the cerebellum by stimulation of the pelvic detrusor nerves in the experimental animal.

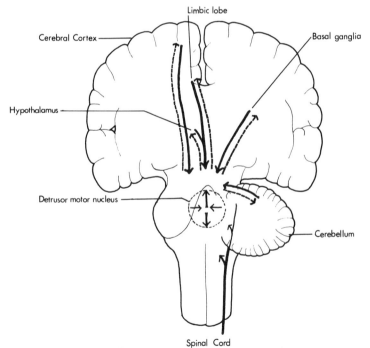

Fig. 6. Connections of cerebral cortex, basal ganglia, limbic system, and cerebellum to the detrusor motor nucleus in the brain stem.

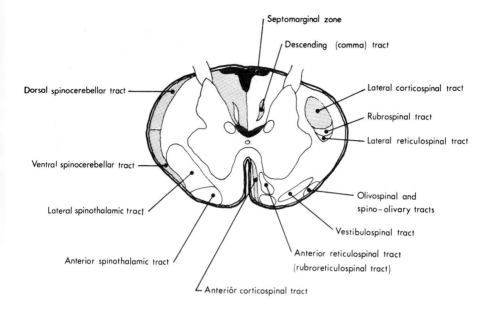

Fig. 7. Ascending and descending tracts in the spinal cord. The reticulospinal tracts are those connecting the detrusor motor center in the brain stem to the detrusor motor nuclei in the intermedio-lateral cell column of the sacral gray matter.

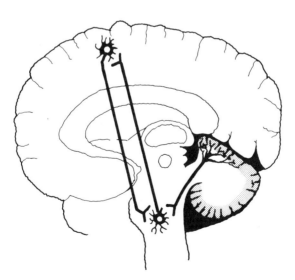

Fig. 8. Loop I. See text for description.

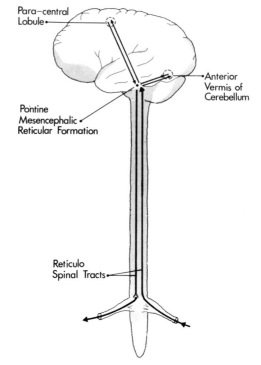

Fig. 9.   Loops I and II.

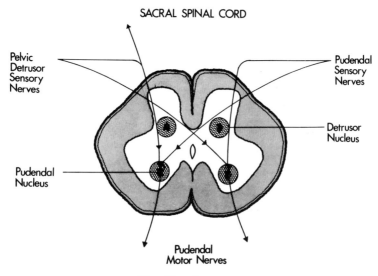

Fig. 10.   Loop III.

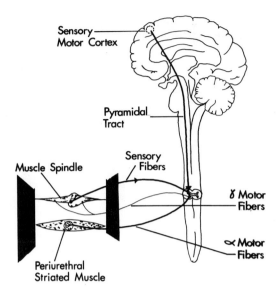

Fig. 11.   Loop IV.

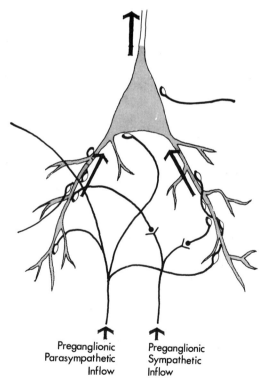

Fig. 12.   Motor innervation of a pelvic ganglion.

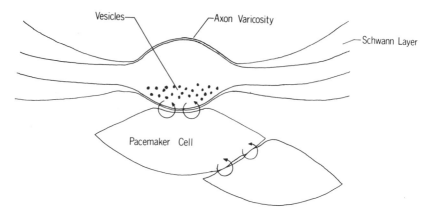

Fig. 13. Post-ganglionic motor innervation of detrusor smooth muscle.

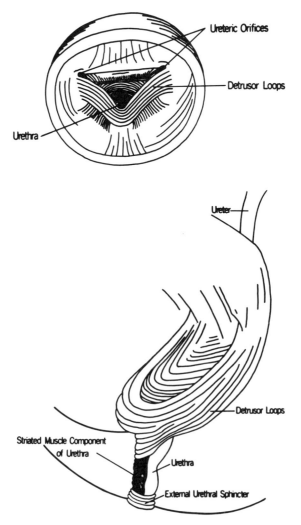

Fig. 14. Organization of detrusor muscle bundles.

PATHOPHYSIOLOGY OF INCONTINENCE:
ANATOMICAL AND FUNCTIONAL
CONSIDERATIONS

Emil A. Tanagho, M.D.

Embryologically, the bladder and urethra make up one
continuous tubular structure surrounded by a uniform mass of
mesenchyme. Later, this mesenchymal mass will assume a
different shape -- its top part becomes formed into a detrusor or a bladder by expansion and sacculation, its lower
segment, remaining tubular, becomes the sphincter. There is,
however, no actual differentiation between what is the
bladder and what is the urethra, except probably some constriction where the 2 units meet.

Male and female develop in the same manner, the only
difference being that, in the male, the prostatic gland buds
out from urogenital sinus around the mullerian tubercle,
incorporating within itself most of the sphincteric muscle
fibers.

From this embryologic basis the entire urethral structure can be defined as a muscular tube merely continuing
with the bladder wall above. The latter acts as a reservoir
and the former as its sphincteric mechanism. The muscles
are directly continuous, with the same origin and the same
nerve supply.

Anatomically, the urethral sphincteric segment is
composed of 2 layers -- an inner longitudinal coat of smooth

muscle fibers which are in direct continuation with the inner
longitudinal coat of the bladder, and an outer semicircular
coat directly continuing with the detrusor outer longitudinal
coat.   These fine delicate urethral muscle fibers are embed-
ded in dense collagen tissue preventing their separation or
attenuation under distension and stretch.

To this smooth sphincteric muscular unit a voluntary
component of striated muscles is added -- wrapped around the
middle third of the female urethra and the membranous segment
of the male urethra.   These skeletal muscle fibers are part
of the genitourinary diaphragm and receive their innervation
from the sacral plexus via the pudendal nerve.

Like most other investigators we studied the female
sphincteric mechanism, since it is much simpler to understand
and evaluate than its male counterpart.   Our discussion will
be limited to this female sphincter.

FUNCTIONAL CONSIDERATIONS

What does the anatomical arrangement of the urethral
sphincter signify from the functional viewpoint?   The
activity of its muscular components can be easily measured
and recorded.   In our laboratory, we use a 4-channel catheter
to record intravesical pressure and 2 urethral pressures,
the 4th channel being used for bladder filling.   We also
simultaneously record intra-abdominal pressure, anal sphincteric pressure, as well as urine flow rate and total volumes
voided.   When pressure is recorded above the entire length
of the sphincteric segment it is termed urethral pressure
profile.   On observing pressure profiles we see that maximum
closure pressure is not found at the level of the internal
meatus but further down, at about the middle third of the
(female) urethra.

We have done detailed studies on the activity of the 2
muscular components of the sphincteric mechanism: We can
stimulate the pelvic parasympathetic nerve fibers and excite
active contraction from the smooth muscular component of the
urethra; we can also stimulate the pudendal nerve and excite
active contraction from the skeletal component. These
studies can be done in the static state or in the active
state, when the urethra is open and urine flow is in progress.

In addition, it is also possible to eliminate muscular
activity of the urethral sphincter by pharmacological
blockade of each component. Skeletal muscle activity is
easily inhibited by administration of curare and any response
to pudendal nerve stimulation is thus abolished. Smooth
muscle activity is almost totally abolished by administration
of atropine, with the consequence that response to pelvic
nerve stimulation is minimal if at all present.

We are able to measure total bladder outlet resistance,
gradually eliminate the contribution of each muscular component, then measure what activity remains: In such a manner
we can quantitate the contribution of the voluntary component
and that of the involuntary component; what is left behind
is the effect of the physical properties of the urethral
tube with its collagenous and elastic elements. Roughly 50
percent of the activity of the sphincteric mechanism is due
to the tonus of the skeletal component, while the other 50
percent is primarily a function of the smooth involuntary
component. The collagenous elastic element produces a
minimal resistance under normal conditions.

Continence. The combined activity of the 2 muscular
components of the urethra constitutes the basic mechanism for
continence. It provides constant closure pressure -- which
is the difference between total pressure within the urethra

and intravesical pressure. Normally, this closure pressure
is positive, thus maintaining the urine within the bladder
cavity. For voiding to take place bladder pressure has to
exceed this urethral pressure. It would be unphysiological
for the bladder to have to contract excessively in order to
overcome this relatively high urethral resistance. Thus, in
the normal voiding act, there is synchronism between the
activity of the detrusor and that of the sphincter: A few
seconds before the onset of detrusor contraction, a progressive, precipitous drop in urethral resistance takes place,
which is usually followed by detrusor contraction sufficient
to permit voiding with the least amount of work on the part
of the bladder.

If the mechanism of urethral pressure drop is at fault,
the bladder must generate a very high pressure to force the
urethra open. Once it is open, a slightly lower pressure
has to be sustained to permit continuous voiding.

As we mentioned, the 2 sphincteric elements of the urethra normally provide constant adequate closure pressure to
maintain continence. However, this closure pressure varies
according to circumstances: 1. It is augmented by
progressive bladder filling; 2. It is higher when the upright position is assumed; 3. It is maintained or augmented
also whenever the bladder is subjected to stress in the form
of increased intra-abdominal pressure, which is always
reflected as increase in intravesical pressure. This
increase in intra-abdominal pressure might be sharp, as with
coughing or sneezing; or it can be slow and sustained, as
with beardown effort and Valsalva's maneuver. Closure
pressure augmentation partly reflects activity and partly
direct transmission of intra-abdominal pressure. All these
changes can be detected and quantitated; any weakness of any

of the sphincteric elements can be detected by detailed urodynamic studies.

Urinary stress incontinence. The basic normal features of the sphincteric activity can be altered in a variety of diseases. Most commonly encountered are the changes associated with stress incontinence, which we feel is attributable to weakness of the pelvic floor support of the bladder -- since, once the bladder is properly supported and restored to its normal position, function is completely recovered. Also, in conditions of iatrogenic damage to the delicate urethral musculature, whether by resection and instrumentation, or from surgical dissection or mobilization from the outside, intrinsic weakness of the sphincteric musculature of variable degree is unavoidable. Finally -- and this condition is that which most concerns us here -- there is the neuropathic muscular involvement interfering, not only with the sphincter's synchronous activity, but also with its tonus and responsiveness to the needs and demands to which it is subjected. This last possibility can be a major factor in loss of the normal responses and mechanisms of continence.

PRACTICAL UROLOGICAL EVALUATION OF
THE NEUROGENIC BLADDER IN
MYELOMENINGOCELE

Robert D. Jeffs, M.D.

Deterioration of renal structure and function is the
hallmark of the paraplegic whether due to congenital or
acquired causes. At birth, the child with meningomyelocele
usually has no serious defect in renal function or drainage.
However, urological evaluation should establish a baseline
of structure and function in the neonatal period and should
establish a plan of action to protect the kidneys of that
child.

NEONATAL INVESTIGATION

Prenatal bladder function or dysfunction usually has not
produced serious hydronephrosis, reflux or trabeculation at
the time of birth. However, when the meningocele and cord
structures are exposed to the air and following closure of
the meningocele by surgery, changes in bladder and sphincter
innervation may occur which lead to disordered urodynamics
and consequent deterioration. Our evaluation of the neonatal
child with meningomyelocele by pyelogram and retrograde
cystogram in a consecutive series of 50 newborns revealed
normal renal function and drainage on intravenous pyelogram
in 93%. There was also absence of reflux in 91% indicating
that prenatal neurogenic dysfunction has little effect on

drainage or vesicoureteral reflux prior to birth.

NEUROLOGICAL EVALUATION PERTAINING TO BLADDER FUNCTION

In the newborn with meningomyelocele, the level of the
lesion, the degree of paralysis and the sensory level, give
a rough indication of what type of bladder to expect.
However, the incompleteness and the patchy nature of the
spinal lesion make it necessary to examine in detail the
innervation of the bladder and its sphincters in order to
establish proper management. Full urodynamic investigation
may not be possible in the neonatal period, however, serial
observation of the child during the first 6 weeks of age will
establish, by observation alone: 1) the presence or absence
of detrusor contraction, 2) the ability to manually express
through the bladder outlet and sphincter, 3) the presence
or absence of perineal sensation, and 4) the activity in the
anal sphincter.

Even without detailed urodynamic evaluation, this will
allow the clinician to roughly categorize the bladder defect
and group the patients according to their expected problems
and degree of risk.

CLASSIFICATION OF PATIENTS WITH NEUROGENIC BLADDER
DYSFUNCTION

The largest group of patients with neurogenic bladders
in the meningomyelocele patients have absent detrusor
contraction and flaccid insensitive external sphincters.
These bladders are easily expressed and develop little
trabeculation and tend to have less problem with residual
infection and reflux. The immediate surgical closure of the
meningocele in the first few hours of life has lead to
sparing of some bladder and sphincter nerves, so that fewer

children have this complete lower motor neuron lesion typical
of this group. The second group predictably will develop
trouble with retention and infection. In clinical evaluation,
there is no evidence of detrusor contraction and yet one can
detect active tone and contraction in the anal sphincter,
either under reflex or voluntary control. These bladders
tend to be distended and they are difficult to express. The
third grouping include those with function which is near-
normal and those who have complete interruption of the long
spinal tracts, sparing the spinal reflexes below, which allow
more or less automatic detrusor and sphincter function. The
degree of coordination between the bladder contraction and
the sphincter function will determine whether these patients
empty well and have little risks or are functionally
obstructed with consequent damage of residual infection and
hydronephrosis.

INITIAL INVESTIGATION

Intravenous pyelogram should be performed within the
first 2 weeks of age. Careful and repeated neurological
examination, clinical assessment of ability to void and to
empty the bladder and regular urinalyses and cultures should
indicate which patients are at risk, which have satisfactory
bladder emptying and therefore will be stable as far as
infection and obstruction are concerned. Voiding cysto-
urethrogram is not ordered routinely in the newborn period
to reduce the risk of lower tract contamination. Voiding
cystourethrograms should be ordered, however, to further
explain unusual bladder configuration, ureteral dilatation
and to detect reflux following the onset of urinary tract
infection.

URINARY ANTISEPTICS AND ANTIMICROBIALS IN EARLY MANAGEMENT

The bladder of the newborn meningomyelocele child
frequently will empty only with increased abdominal pressure
or expression. The neurosurgical treatment of the back
lesion often dictates a prone position, making expression
difficult and at the same time restricting the normal
muscular activity of the child. During this initial period,
the antimicrobial therapy may be useful to prevent complicating urinary tract infection. When the back has healed and
initial urological investigation is completed, the need for
antimicrobial treatment to cover the imperfections of
bladder emptying can be assessed. The aim of investigation
and early management should be to establish the routine of
care which, with or without, suppressive medication will
maintain sterile urine in the ureters and kidneys on a
continuing basis.

BLADDER EVACUATION

At the time of discharge from the hospital, the infant
should be emptying the bladder. This may be by normal
detrusor or reflex detrusor activity or by increased
abdominal pressure consequent on crying and other activities.
The frequent finding of a distended bladder which empties
sluggishly or incompletely, indicates the need for additional
measures to promote bladder evacuation. In some, manual
expression may be effective if infection or reflux are not
present. Some bladders can be stimulated reflexly by
abdominal or perineal touch or pressures. Intermittent
catheterization may have to be instituted in early infancy
when it is apparent that none of the above methods of bladder
evacuation are effective. Occasionally, when intermittent
catheterization is not practical or effective, early urinary

diversion by vesicostomy may be required.

BLADDER MODIFICATION

Those patients who are unable to empty the bladder and require intermittent catheterization or those who show trabeculation and early ureteral dilatation should be studied in detail urodynamically. The possibility of simplifying the routine of care or of preventing deterioration through bladder modification should be assessed. Urethral dilatation, urethrotomy, bladder or sphincter denervation or implantation of artificial detrusor stimulator are some of the means by which detrusor activity can be modified. Detailed knowledge of anatomical and neurological status of the bladder is required so that individualized treatment can be prescribed. Sexual function in later life must also be kept in mind so that all useful sensation and function is preserved.

VESICOURETERAL REFLUX

In the neurogenic bladder, vesicoureteral reflux is seldom present at birth, but it may develop in response to bladder infection or in response to high intravesical pressure and trabeculation. With control of infection and improved bladder emptying, reflux may disappear. Persistent reflux, particularly when in association with infection which is difficult to clear or is recurrent, may have deleterious effects on the upper tract. Reimplantation of the ureter to correct reflux can be successfully carried out in the neurogenic bladder if cases are properly selected, prepared and well followed after surgery. Antireflux surgery should be avoided in the hyperactive bladder showing many uninhibited contractions and progressive trabeculation. In those patients not responding to conservative measures to provide

good bladder drainage to clear infection or to correct
reflux, must be considered for urinary diversion. The
manner in which diversion is carried out will be selected
according to the needs of the individual case. Direct
ureteral drainage, vesicostomy or small or large bowel
interposition will be selected appropriate to the problem at
hand.

MANAGEMENT OF INCONTINENCE

     The outlet resistance in many meningomyelocele children
improves as they get older and particularly in the teenage
period. The child who is apparently completely incontinent
without significant dry interval in the preschool period may
develop useful resistance in teenage years. The development
of useful control depends on many factors, including bladder
innervation, sphincter innervation, effective bladder
capacity and hormonal changes occurring in the urethra and
prostate at puberty. A child who has a measurable dry
interval after evacuation of the bladder in the preschool
years can expect an increase in the length of the dry interval as he gets older which may bring satisfactory continence.
The addition of Probanthine and Imipramine can help to
increase bladder capacity and the administration of Ephedrine
may help to increase bladder neck resistance. Patients who
can be expected to manage their incontinence without surgery
or without the application of internal or external devices,
need repeated study to document the improvement that is
occurring and also need repeated encouragement to adhere to
their routine of care. Control that is useful, but not
perfect, may be supplemented by disposable pads, incontinence
clamps and the male incontinence device in selected patients.

The child with relatively high resistance and consequent
high residual may wet in an overflow manner. The institution
of intermittent catheterization in such a patient may make
him completely dry and afford a means of long term management.
The completely incontinent child and those who can empty
themselves well or can be made to empty completely and yet
have no useful dry interval, can be considered for implantable incontinence devices of the mechanical or hydraulic
variety. Urinary diversion is not now considered a first
line approach to the management of the incontinent neurogenic
bladder, but rather is reserved for the management of
incontinence associated with obstruction and infection or for
those who fail to respond to the other measures mentioned
above.

BOWEL MANAGEMENT

This subject will be considered elsewhere, but it is
mentioned to emphasize that effective and regular bowel
evacuation is essential to provide good bladder evacuation
and satisfactory bladder filling and capacity.

ROUTINE OF FOLLOWUP

The urinary tract of the meningomyelocele child as
indicated should be fully assessed during the neonatal
period. Thereafter urinalysis and urine culture should be
carried out at least every three months to insure the success
of the program which has been laid out. A repeat intravenous pyelogram six months later will confirm the success
of the program and thereafter, yearly pyelograms should be
sufficient for long term followup. When the urine becomes
infected or if hydroureter or other pyelographic abnormality
is noted on the intravenous pyelogram, a cystogram should be

performed looking for reflux, diverticuli and the condition
of the bladder outlet.

Events special to the lives of these children may change
the character of urinary drainage and thus increase the need
for special surveillance of the urine and the pattern of
urine emptying. These events include changing neurological
involvement, episodes of acute hydrocephalus, intermittent
infections and infectious diseases, operations with hospitalization and special brace and cast immobilization.
Changes with growth, the onset of kyphoscoliosis and the
pubescent changes may alter outlet resistance of the bladder.
The routine of care may also be upset by changing supervision,
changes in school and school grades and during holidays at
camp. Many of these problems can be anticipated and measures
undertaken to prevent ill-effects on the bladder and bowel
evacuation.

SEXUALITY

It is difficult to predict the presence or absence of
reflex or psychogenic erection from neurological examination
in the young child. The fact that many of these paralyzed
individuals make satisfactory sexual adjustments in adulthood indicates a need for preservation of all possible nerve
supply. In considering bladder modification through
denervation procedures and in considering urinary diversion,
subsequent sexual function should be kept in mind.

URINARY DIVERSION

The ileal conduit has been the standard for urinary
diversion in patients with neurogenic incontinence and/or
associated progressive renal damage for the past 20 years.
Imperfections of this method of diversion in late followup

have become apparent and are sufficiently alarming to caution against the wholesale use of the ileal conduit as a panacea for neurogenic dysfunctions in every child with meningomyelocele. Individual consideration of each patient weighing alternatives available will select those patients who have, or may develop useful continence or who may be considered for incontinence devices. It is obvious that urinary diversion will still be required when conservative treatment fails and when incontinence is unmanageable. The method of diversion selected, ideally, should have a non-refluxing stoma and an antireflux feature between ureter and the bowel conduit. The colon conduit with antirefluxing ureteral intestinal anastomoses would appear to fill the need, but long term results with regard to safety, and renal preservation must be accumulated and compared with the ileal conduit. The stoma at the site of diversion deserves meticulous care and must be fitted with a non-porous ring and bag. The supervision by an experienced ostomy therapist is invaluable in teaching the application of the bag, the care of the equipment and in supervising long term followup. The diverted urinary tract requires the same long term supervision as the undiverted neurogenic bladder. These patients must be followed regularly to detect changes in stomal size and caliber, changes in residual urine and bacterial flora. Intravenous pyelogram must be obtained at least yearly and changes in function and drainage should be investigated thoroughly to correct deficiencies in loop drainage before serious renal damage has occurred.

SUMMARY

The problems faced by the child with meningomyelocele are varied and complex. The child and his parents must seek

advice from many disciplines and opinions expressed are
usually best coordinated by regular visits to a multidisci-
plined clinic where medical, psychosocial and educational
needs can be assessed in the light of changing growth,
development and medical findings.

Constant encouragement and regular reevaluation are
needed to provide successful, physical and emotional
rehabilitation.

MYELOMENINGOCELE
TREATMENT MODALITIES IN PERSPECTIVE

Pramod R. Rege, M.D.

The majority of children with myelomeningocele who die succumb to renal failure after the first year of life.[10] The main aim of treatment in this condition is obviously to preserve renal function. Urinary infection and incontinence comprise the two main problems.

Ideally one would wish a continent child:

a. capable of periodically emptying the bladder completely.

b. to maintain low bladder pressure, especially during voiding.

c. to have a smooth walled bladder with normal capacity.

d. to have a bladder free from infection.

These ideals may not be attainable in the majority of these children. One must thus aim at rehabilitating the bladder as far as possible, using measures requiring minimal mechanical manipulation and yet permitting the bladder to function as a reservoir emptying intermittently.

In the affected children bowel function too is impaired by the neurologic deficit.[84] Constipation is common and hard feces may displace the bladder neck forward preventing complete emptying. The proximity of the constipated colon to genitourinary structures may allow bacteria to enter the excretory tract.[59] For this reason bowel care is of prime

importance. Stools should be kept in semisolid state and
periodic evacuation assured.

Kirkland, Eckstein, Lister found it impossible to corre-
late bladder function with the degree of neurologic or lower
limb competence.[12,34,43] The difficulty stems partly from the
complexity of the cord lesion[73] and in part is a reflection of
such secondary factors as overdistension of bladder which
may modify function even before birth. Damage to the nerve
or the cord itself during birth or operative intervention may
influence the overall neurologic status at birth. During
first few weeks of neonatal life, the neurologic deficits due
to concussion or contusion of the nerve or the cord will
recover. On the other hand late maturation of sensory nerve
tracts may permit perception of bladder fullness in late
childhood.[2] In the male however, the development of the
prostate at puberty, may permit the spontaneous achievement
of urinary continence. In the female an increased resistance
to outflow may result from hormonal influences. In view of
these possibilities, treatment should be conservative during
childhood.[86] Aggressive measures may be necessary to preserve
renal function by controlling urinary tract infection,
avoiding bladder and ureteric distension and reducing intravesical pressure.[28] In the course of caring for these patients
periodic assessment of bladder and the upper urinary tract
function is essential in planning and updating the treatment
choice of treatment depends upon:

a. the functional status of the urinary tract.

b. the patient's intellect and the coping capacity of
the family.

c. the extent of physical handicap.

d. evidence of motivation in both child and parents.

e. the socioeconomic background of the patient.

f. the facilities available.

Available therapeutic modalities are here described.

TO ASSURE URINARY TRACT DRAINAGE
CREDE' MANEUVER (Suprapubic Pressure)

"Crede'" has been considered a standard method to assist bladder evacuation in these children.[18] It is a reasonable approach if it's aim is achieved allowing the bladder to empty completely intermittently without generating high intravesical pressure. Patients amenable exhibit no vesico-urethral reflux and have minimal outflow resistance presumably because of a flaccid urethral sphincter.[60] The procedure should be carried out frequently depending upon the patient's age and susceptibility to infection.

If crede' maneuver is performed in children with competent or rigid pelvic floor, high intravesical pressure will be generated resulting in trabeculation, diverticulum formation and vesicouretheral reflux. As is well known urinary infection and elevated calyceal pressure will destroy renal parenchyma.

Pelvic floor flaccidity at birth is often a result of nerve contusion. After several weeks a deeply set anus (natal cleft) may reflect excessive activity of the pelvic floor. A careful evaluation is required to assess changing neurologic patterns during the initial post-natal period.[74] Crede' maneuver should not be employed in children with hyperactive pelvic floor.

Electromyography of the anal sphincter is helpful in detecting which patients have pelvic floor activity. Documentation of the electrical activity in striate muscle surrounding the urethra is more precise.[5,6] If combined with uroflowmetry dyssynergistic activity of striate muscle may be

detected.   Obviously the crede' maneuver is contraindicated
in this situation.

DILATATION OF URETHRA

Johnston has suggested dilatation of urethra as a means
of reducing outflow resistance in the infant with an exces-
ive activity in the pelvic floor and high intravesical
pressure.[29] In male children this can be accomplished through
perineal urethrostomy.[29]   This may be repeated after interval
of some weeks. Johnston has reported that this permits adequate bladder emptying and reduction in intravesical
pressures. If vesicoureteral reflux is minimal it may disappear spontaneously after urethral dilatation.[29]

INTERMITTENT CATHETERIZATION

Sterile intermittent catheterization was used by Guttman
in individuals with paraplegia with satisfactory results.[24]
Lapides has popularized clean technique in this country. It
may be used in children with myelomeningocele if incontinence
or inadequate bladder emptying exists. Infection may be
avoided since complete intermittent emptying of the bladder
by the catheter prevents overdistension and maintains adequate blood supply to the vesical urothelium.[38,39]

Catheterization may also be utilized as a method of
avoiding the threat of vesicoureteral reflux. The imminence
of such reflux can be gauged roughly by noting bladder
capacity at the point vesicoureteral reflux occurs in the
course of cinecystography. In cases in which the reflux
exists, control of infection and intermittent catheterization
may cause the vesicoureteral reflux to disappear 25-40% of
cases.[44]

In children with persistent and marked reflux, despite
a bladder with adequate capacity and smooth wall, the ureter
may be reimplanted. Reimplantation has been advocated as a

means of converting upper tract bacteruria to the one which
predominantly affects the lower urinary tract.[44]   Jeffs has
reported unsatisfactory results with ureteral reimplantation
in hyperactive neurogenic bladder. He advocated the procedure only in presence of atonic large capacity bladder. High
intravesical pressure may be the basis for the poor results
experienced in hyperactive or spastic bladders. The use of
anticholinergic drugs or alpha adrenergic blocking agents
may reduce intravesical pressures satisfactorily. Other
procedures such as "Y-V plasty" or external sphincterotomy
may be useful in certain cases and deserve consideration.

Intermittent catheterization may be carried out through
a perineal urethrostomy in a young male child thus avoiding
urethral trauma and the possibility of stricture formation.[29,35]

In order to increase bladder capacity permitting an
adequate volume of urine to accumulate between catheteriza-
tions various modalities may be used e.g. anticholinergic
medication, neurosurgical procedures (anterior rhizotomy of
the dominant sacral root) or other surgical measures (ileo-
cystoplasty, colocystoplasty, etc.).

INDWELLING FOLEY CATHETER

This is not a very satisfactory approach since bacterial
infection readily establishes itself in the bladder. In the
male the additional hazard of urethral trauma exists.[13] The
hyperactive bladder, moreover, remains incontinent despite
the indwelling catheter.

MEDICATIONS

Cholinergic and beta-adrenergic neuroreceptors pre-
dominate in the body of the bladder; here alpha receptors are
absent appearing only in the bladder base, the outlet, and
the urethra. Beta receptors also exist at the outlet and in
the urethra as do cholinergic receptors. The bladder base

has a rich supply of cholinergic and alpha-adrenergic
neuroreceptors.[31]

    In cases with uninhibited bladder contractions or in
those with hyperactive bladders, anticholinergic medication
may be useful, e.g. probanthine, tincture of belladona,
ditropan.[7] This serves to provide improved bladder reservoir function. Intermittent catheterization may also aid in
emptying the bladder and avoiding overdistension. In cases
in which intermittent catheterization fails to control incontinence an alpha-adrenergic stimulator, e.g. ephidrene
sulfate, or imipramine, may be of value.[8,31,32,45] Dibenze-
lene (alpha-adrenergic blocker) may be useful in cases with
high intravesical pressure secondary to outflow resistance
at the bladder neck or nearby urethra.[33,37,75,76] Cholinergic
drugs (urecholine) have been recommended when a significant
residual remains after the crede' maneuver.[18]

NEUROSURGICAL PROCEDURES

    Anterior rhizotomy of the dominant sacral root has been
utilized to relieve the hyperactive bladder syndrome. A
preliminary temporary nerve block should be performed to
evaluate the efficacy of this approach.[77] The procedure
should be undertaken only when a conservative medical regimen
has failed.

    Pudendal block and pudendal neurectomy may reduce out-
flow resistance in children with urethral sphincter spasm,
but results have not been too satisfactory.[15,77] External
sphincterotomy in boys may achieve the same goal and has
proven to be more reliable.[41,46,57,65,86]

URINARY DIVERSION

    Diversion if performed should be carried out proximal to
the incompetent segment of urinary tract. Unfortunately,
the results of ileoconduit diversion have been far from

satisfactory in the children.[66],[71] Stomal problems are common:
concretions, prolapse may develop. Stomal stenosis has been
reported in as many as 45 of patients.[19] Enlargement by
growth of the proximal blind pouch creates difficulty due to
reabsorption of electrolytes, and may require surgical
correction. Renal calculi usually of infection have occurred
as complications and have been difficult to treat.[62] An
incidence of 30% has been encountered.[9],[47] For these
reasons long term (15 years) results of ileoconduit diversion
have been poor.[49],[66] Another factor may be the high
pressures generated in the conduit which are transmitted to
the renal pelvis by ileo-ureteral reflux.[52]

The techniques employed to minimize the failure rate aim
to prevent reflux and avoid increased intra-loop pressure.
These have included "plug excision" and myotomy (Cleveland
Clinic).

Matheson has devised a method of fashioning an ileal flap
to avoid reflux at the point of uretero-ileal anastomosis;[48]
this requires continuing evaluation in the experimental animal.
In time the ileal flap used to construct a nipple may undergo
fibrotic stenosis or by some other mechanism allow recurrence
of reflux with the passage of time.[63],[72]

Utilizing the sigmoid colon instead of an ileoconduit is
a feasible procedure and may more likely avoid damage to the
upper urinary tract so often observed with long functioning
ileoconduits. The large stoma of the sigmoid conduit reduces
the incidence of stenosis. In the case of the decompensated
upper urinary tract rehabilitation of the bladder may not be
feasible; in such instances sigmoid conduit may be preferable.[11],[30],[53],[54],[55]

Terminal ureterostomy may facilitate the drainage of
the upper urinary tract in children with dilated ureters in

which peristalsis is present.[85] Construction of a skin flap
may avoid the problem of stomal stenosis.[78]

Cutaneous vesicostomy has not proved to be a satisfactory method except in the hands of its innovators.[40]

CONTINENCE

In so far as is possible the child should be permitted
to attend regular school sessions. Most Cincinnati schools,
unfortunately, are not equipped to serve handicapped children.
Urinary incontinence comprises a large percentage of students
unacceptable to other than special schools. I have a strong
conviction that major surgical procedures should not be
performed merely because of social pressure. Until age 5
years is attained diapers available are adequate to avoid
unpleasant ammoniacal odors. Among older children, however,
conservative measures will usually suffice if special diapers
are available for school attendance in this age category.
So-called marsupial pants (Kanga pants) are constructed with
an adequate pouch containing disposable absorbent pad (e.g.
cellulose to absorb and stabilize the urine). Such manufacturers as Proctor & Gamble or Johnson & Johnson may utilize
their special talent to develop aids of this nature.

Periodic bladder emptying by the crede' maneuver or by
intermittent catheterization may allow child to be continent,
when necessary drugs which modify the autonomic function of
the bladder may be helpful.

Continent vesicostomy has certain merits and intermittent catheterization may be carried out via the vesicostomy.
Such an approach, though promising, requires further
evaluation in the neurogenic bladder.[67]

In female children external devices prove to be unsatisfactory. In boys devices of this nature may serve a useful

purpose; the size of the phallus is a determining factor.
Boys with prominent fatty pubic region or with small external
genitalia may require delay in usage until puberty or later.

Pubic pressure urinal works best for younger children,
since the bag lies high enough to be worn under short
trousers. Tight groin straps may, however, cut into the
skin. In older children and adults, a condom type of sheath
is often preferable.

Ideally the foreskin should be retained to protect the
glans and the external urethral meatus. If too redundant,
partial circumcision may avoid ulceration.

SURGICAL PROCEDURES

Increasing urethral resistance: operative procedures
using urethral suspension, urethral compression or urethral
reconstruction are inadvisable in children with neurogenic
bladder.[1,17,42] Interest in their usage has been rekindled
recently as adjunct to intermittent catheterization.[79]

Prosthesis for incontinence: Scott has advocated a
modified Y-V plasty in girls to assure total incontinence
prior to inserting an artificial sphincter. Implantation of
a hydraulic device to achieve continence has appeal. A
silastic prosthesis developed by Scott et al, has been in use
for several years and results are said to be encouraging.[69,70]
Mechanical problems do arise and as with other prostheses
infection poses a significant threat. Prior to implanting
this device, one should be certain that the bladder empties
completely, functions well as a reservoir and is not susceptible to uninhibited contractions.

An inflatable silicone prosthesis devised by Rosen
contains a three contact area urethral occluder which avoids
full pressure occlusion of the urethra.[64] The design incorporates a single push pump and release mechanism, controlled

by a diaphragm valve. The prosthesis is implanted in the
perineum and is presently undergoing evaluation in the
United States.

Timm and Bradley are seeking a mechanism more akin to
normal reflex action by stimulating the detrusor to empty;
the sensory side of the reflex arc is replaced by a volume
sensor on the bladder wall; the urethra is occluded with an
inflatable plastic cuff powered by metal bellows.[83]

ELECTRONIC METHODS

Electrical stimulation of pelvic floor muscle may
reinforce reflex muscle response in patients with minimal
function in this area. Stimulation may be achieved by anal,
vaginal or implanted electrodes. Glenn and Caldwell have
claimed satisfactory results although Merrill has not had
this experience.[4,20,21,50]

Pelvic floor electric stimulation may induce inhibition
of contractility, thus permitting reduction of vesical
hyperactivity and causing the bladder to improve its reservoir function.[22]

Katona and Eckstein have evolved a unique concept of
creating new micturation reflexes by transmitting electrical
pulses into the bladder via a urethral catheter electrode.
Stimuli were applied several hours each day with clinical
success in initiating normal emptying. A controlled trial,
however, yielded disappointing results.[3]

There has now accumulated considerable experience with
electronic stimulators, especially with the "Mentor" apparatus.
This comprises specially designed electrodes, wound into a
double helix and buried bilaterally; they deliver biphasic
impulses to the detrusor muscle. Transmission of the
impulses to neighboring skeletal muscles causes stimulation
of the pelvic floor. The child may then void despite high

intravesical pressures and a contracted urethral sphincter.
If sensory capacity is preserved, the child may complain of
suprapubic pain. Unfortunately these stimulators do not wear
well and Caldwell, Sussett, Bradley and other have found
them to be unsatisfactory.[3,51]

More promising in cases with upper motor neuron lesions
is direct stimulation of the sacral cord, a procedure which
could produce a coordinated reflex bladder emptying. Though
Nashold et al and Grimes et al have infused enthusiasm for
this approach, experimental work performed by Tanagho et al
does not support this optimism.[23,58,80,81]

Edward and Malvern summed up the present situation by
concluding that cases benefited by electrical devices are
those most likely to achieve continence by other means.[14]

UNDIVERSION

Long term results of ileoconduit are poor. Because of
this, Dr. Hendren advocates reestablishing integrity of the
urinary tract in those with ileoconduit diversion. He
implants distal end of the ileoconduit into the bladder using
antirefluxing technique.[25,26] Though initially he did not
advocate this procedure for children with neurogenic bladder,
this approach has merits especially if it is combined with
intermittent catheterization.[36]

INFECTION CONTROL

Most patients in whom bacteruria is encountered in what
appears to be an otherwise normal upper urinary tract, the
organism stems from the bladder.[61] Frailey technique or
immunofluorescent staining against IgG coating of bacteria
may help to diagnose upper urinary tract bacteruria.[16,82]
Utilizing oral antibiotic agents prophylactically tends to
cause superinfection which may in turn require the

administration of other potentially dangerous antibiotic
drugs. With urinary tract drainage assured, single installation of antibiotic solution e.g. (0.2% Neomycin Solution)
for 45 minutes may suffice in controlling vesical bacteria.
If necessary this can be repeated at intervals.

Bacteruria which is symptomatic or else from upper
urinary tract, may be treated with a short course of an
appropriate antibacterial substance. Should renal deterioration become apparent to intravenous pyelography, long term
prophylactic therapy may be justified using nitrofurantoin;
sulfisoxazole or in the older child a combination of sulfi-
methoxazole and trimethoprim.

In individuals with ileoconduit urinary diversion it is
important that bacteria which alkalinize the urine (proteus
mirabilis; pseudomonas pyocyneus, etc.) be controlled.
Infection with these organisms may quickly initiate calculus
formation in alkaline urine.[9,62] Brief course of appropriate
antibiotic agents and proper monitoring of urine cultures
obtained from the conduit will contribute to achieving this
aim. If necessary Neomycin can be installed in the ileoconduit for 45 minutes for the topical effect. Absorption
of Neomycin from the ileoconduit is minimal.

SUMMARY

Urinary infection and incontinence are the main problems
in children with myelomeningocele. Under such circumstances
one's major purpose is to preserve renal function. Aggressive
treatment is administered to control bacteruria and high
intravesical pressure. Since neurourologic phenomena may
alter with growth, surgical measures should be utilized with
restraint. Should supravesical urinary diversion be required,
the construction of a sigmoid conduit is recommended.

Facilitatory electrical stimulation of the pelvic floor needs further evaluation. Prosthesis for incontinence may be utilized in selected older children.

REFERENCES

1. Bates, C.P., Loose, H. and Stanton, S.L.R.: The objective study of incontinence after repair operations. *Surg. Gynecol. Obstet., 136*:17, 1973.

2. Bradley, W.E., Timm, G.W. and Scott, F.B.: Innervation of the detrusor muscle and urethra. IN The Urologic Clinics of North America, Symposium on Neurogenic Bladder, Vol. 1, J. Lapides (ed.), 1974.

3. Bradley, W.E., Timm, G.W. and Chou, S.N.: Decade of experience with electronic stimulation of micturition reflex. *Urol. Intern., 26*:283, 1971.

4. Caldwell, K.P.S.: The treatment of incontinence by electronic implants. *Ann. Roy. Coll. Surg., 41*:447, 1967.

5. Cook, W.A., Firlit, C., Stephens, F.D. and King, L.R.: Urodynamic evaluation of children. Read at the meeting of the American Academy of Pediatrics, Urological Section, Chicago, 1976, pp. 21.

6. Diokno, A.C., Koff, S.A. and Bender, L.F.: Periurethral striated muscle activity in neurogenic bladder dysfunction. *J. Urol., 112*:743, 1974.

7. Diokno, A.C.: Intermittent Catheterization. Proceedings meeting on total care of M.M. child, Cincinnati, 1976.

8. Diokno, A.C. and Taub, M.: Ephedrine in the treatment of urinary incontinence. *Urology, 5*:624, 1975.

9. Dretler, S.P.: The pathogenesis of urinary tract calculi occurring after ileal conduit diversion. I. Clinical

study. II. Conduit study. III. Prevention. *J. Urol.*, *109*:204, 1973.

10. Duckett, J.W. and Raezer, D.M.: Neuromuscular dysfunction of the lower urinary tract. IN Clinical Pediatric Urology, P.P. Kelalis and L.R. King (eds.), Philadelphia, W.B. Saunders Co., 1967, pp. 401.

11. Dybner, R., Jeter, K. and Lattimer, J.K.: Comparison of intraluminal pressures in ileal and colonic conduits in children. *J. Urol.*, *108*:477, 1972.

12. Eckstein, H.B.: The neurogenic bladder and urinary diversion. IN Paediatric Urology, D.I. Williams (ed.), London, Butterworths, 1968.

13. Eckstein, H.B.: Urology in childhood. IN Encyclopedia of Urology, Vol. XV, D.I. Williams (ed.), Berlin, Springer, 1974.

14. Edwards, L. and Malvern, J.: Electronic control of incontinence: A critical review of the present situation. *Brit. J. Urol.*, *44*:467, 1972.

15. Engel, R.M.E. and Schirmer, H.K.A.: Pudendal neurectomy in neurogenic bladder. *J. Urol.*, *112*:57, 1974.

16. Fairley, K.G.: The routine determination of the site of infection in the investigation of patients with urinary tract infection. IN Renal Infection and Renal Scarring, P. Kincaid-Smith and K.F. Fairley (eds.), Australia, Mercedes Publishing Services, 1970, pp. 165.

17. Flocks, R.H. and Boldus, R.: The surgical treatment and prevention of urinary incontinence associated with disturbance of the internal urethral sphincteric mechanism. *J. Urol.*, *109*:279, 1973.

18. Forrest, D.: Management of bladder and bowel in spina bifida. IN Spina Bifida for Clinician, G. Brocklehurst (ed.), Philadelphia, J.B. Lippincott Co., 1976, pp. 122.

19. Glenn, J.F., Small, M.P. and Boyarsky, S.: Complications of ileal segment urinary diversion in children. *Urol. Int., 23*:97, 1968.

20. Glen, E.S.: Effective and safe control of incontinence by the intra-anal plug electrode. *Brit. J. Surg., 58*: 249, 1971.

21. Godec, C., Cass, A.S. and Ayala, G.F.: Electrical stimulation for incontinence - technique, selection and results. *Urology, 7*:388, 1976.

22. Godec, C., Cass, A.S. and Ayala, G.F.: Bladder inhibition with functional electrical stimulation. *Urology, 6*:663, 1975.

23. Grimes, J.H., Anderson, E.E. and Currie, D.P.: Surgical management of the neurogenic bladder. *Urology, 2*:500, 1973.

24. Guttman, L. and Frankel, H.: *Paraplegia, 4*:63, 1966.

25. Hendren, W.: Reconstruction of previously diverted urinary tracts in children. *J. Pediatric Surg., 8*:135, 1973.

26. Hendren, W.: Urinary tract refunctionalization after prior diversion in children. *Ann. Surg., 180*:494, 1974.

27. Hodgkinson, C.P.: Stress urinary incontinence - 1970. *Amer. J. Obstet. Gynecol., 108*:1141, 1970.

28. Johnston, J.H. and Farkas, A.:. Congenital neuropathic bladder. *Urology, 6*:719, 1975.

29. Johnston, J.H. and Kathel, B.L.: The obstructed neurogenic bladder in the newborn. *Brit. J. Urol., 43*:206, 1971.

30. Kelalis, P.P.: Urinary diversion in children by the sigmoid conduit: Its advantages and limitations. *J. Urol., 112*:666, 1974.

31. Khanna, O.P.: Disorders of micturition:

Neuropharmacologic basis and results of drug therapy.
Urology, 8:316, 1976.

32. Khanna, O.P., Elkouss, G.C., Heber, D.L. and Gonick, P.:
    Imipramine hydrochloride: Pharmacodynamic effects on
    lower urinary tract of female dogs. *Urology, 6*:48, 1975.

33. Khanna, O.P. and Gonick, P.: Effects of phenoxybenza-
    mine hydrochloride on canine lower urinary tract:
    Clinical implications. *Urology, 6*:323, 1975.

34. Kirkland, I.: Urinary tract problems in spina bifida.
    Dev. Med. Child Neurol., 4:314, 1962.

35. Klauber, G.T., Jefferies, J.D. and Ridlon, H.C. et al:
    Intermittent catheterization by parent and child in the
    management of neurogenic bladder. Read at the meeting
    of the American Academy of Pediatrics, Urological
    Section, San Francisco, 1974, pp. 7.

36. Klauber, G.: Personal communication.

37. Krane, R.J. and Olsson, C.A.: Phenoxybenzamine in
    neurogenic bladder dysfunction. II. Clinical considera-
    tions. *J. Urol., 110*:653, 1973.

38. Lapides, J., Diokno, A.C., Silber, S.J. and Lowe, B.S.:
    Clean intermittent self-catheterization in the treatment
    of urinary tract disease. *J. Urol., 107*:458, 1972.

39. Lapides, J., Diokno, A.C., Lowe, B.S., et al: Followup
    on unsterile intermittent self-catheterization. *J.
    Urol., 111*:184, 1974.

40. Lapides, J., Koyanagi, T. and Diokno, A.: Cutaneous
    vesicostomy: 10-year survey. *J. Urol., 105*:76, 1971.

41. Lendon, R.G. and Zachary, R.B.: A histological study of
    the external sphincter in the male infant. *Dev. Med.
    Child Neurol., 16*:32, 1974.

42. Leadbetter, G.W. and Fraley, E.E.: Surgical
    correction for total urinary incontinence:

5 years after. *J. Urol.,* 97:867, 1967.

43. Lister, J.: The urinary tract in myelomeningocele.
IN Recent Advances in Paediatric Surgery, 2nd ed., A.W.
Wilkinson (ed.), London, Churchill, 1969.

44. Lyon, R.P., Scott, M.P. and Marshall, S.: Internal
catheterization rather than urinary diversion in
children with meningomyelocele. *J. Urol.,* 113:409, 1975.

45. Mahony, D.T., Laferte, R.O. and Mahoney, J.E.: VI.
Observations on sphincter-augmenting effect of imipramine in children with urinary incontinence. *Urology,*
1:317, 1973.

46. Malament, M.: External sphincterotomy in neurogenic
bladder dysfunction. *J. Urol.,* 108:554, 1972.

47. Malek, R.S., Burke, E.C. and DeWeerd, J.H.: Ileal
conduit urinary diversion in children. *J. Urol.,* 105:
892, 1971.

48. Mathisen, W.: New method for uretero-intestinal anastomosis. *Surg. Gynecol. Obstet.,* 96:255, 1953.

49. Mebust, W.K., Foret, J.D. and Valk, W.L.: Fifteen years
of experience with urinary diversion in myelomeningocele
patients. *J. Urol.,* 101:177, 1969.

50. Merrill, D.C.: The treatment of urinary incontinence by
pelvic floor stimulation. IN Myelomeningocele-Proceedings
of a Multidisciplinary Symposium, Cincinnati, 1976.

51. Merrill, D.C.: Clinical experience with Mentor bladder
stimulator. II. Meningomyelocele patients. *J. Urol.,*
112:823, 1974.

52. Minton, J.P., Kiser, W.S. and Ketchman, A.S.: A study
of the functional dynamics of ileal conduit urinary
diversion with relationship to urinary infection. *Surg.
Gynecol. Obstet.,* 119:541, 1964.

53. Mogg, R.A.: Urinary diversion using the

colonic conduit. *Brit. J. Urol.*, *39*:687, 1967.

54. Mogg, R.A. and Syme, R.R.A.: The results of urinary diversion using the colonic conduit. *Brit. J. Urol.*, *41*:434, 1969.

55. Spence, B., Esho, J. and Cass, A.: Comparison of ileac and colonic conduit urinary diversions in dogs. *J. Urol.*, *108*:712, 1972.

56. Mulholland, S.G., Yalla, S.V. and Raezer, D.M. et al: Primary external urethral sphincter hyperkinesia in a boy. *Urology*, *4*:577, 1974.

57. Nanninga, J.B., Rosen, J. and O'Connor, V.J.: Experience with transurethral external sphincterotomy in patients with spinal cord injury. *J. Urol.*, *112*:72, 1974.

58. Nashold, B.S., Friedman, H. and Boyarsky, S.: Electrical activation of micturition by spinal cord stimulation. *J. Surg. Research*, *11*:144, 1971.

59. Neumann, P.Z., deDomenico, I.J. and Nogrady, M.B.: Constipation and urinary tract infection. *Pediatrics*, *52*:241, 1973.

60. Pekarovic, E., Zachary, R.B. and Lister, J.: Indications for manual expression of the neurogenic bladder. *Brit. J. Urol.*, *42*:191, 1970.

61. Rabinovitch, H.H.: Bladder evacuation in child with myelomeningocele. *Urology*, *3*:425, 1974.

62. Rege, P.R., Levine, M.S., Oppenheimer, S. and Evans, A.T.: Renal calculi and bio-chemical abnormalities in children with myelomeningocele and ileo-conduit diversion. *Urology*, *5*:12, 1975.

63. Rege, P.R., Malik, I.K., Wendel, R.G. and Evans, A.T.: Muscular nipple uretero-ileal anastomosis to prevent reflux. *Urology*, *4*:402, 1974.

64. Rosen, M.: A simple artificial implantable sphincter.

Read at the meeting of American Urologic Association, Las Vegas, 1976.

65. Scott, F.B.: The management of neurogenic bladder in patients with myelomeningocele: Sphincterotomy, bladder flap, urethroplasty, and the artificial sphincter. IN Myelomeningocele - Proceedings of a Multidisciplinary Symposium, Cincinnati, 1976.

66. Schwarz, G.R. and Jeffs, R.D.: Ileal conduit urinary diversion in children: Computer analysis of followup from 2 to 16 years. *J. Urol.*, *55*:285, 1975.

67. Schneider, K.M., Reid, R.E., Fruchtman, B. and Levitt, S.B.: Continent vesicostomy: Surgical technique. *Urology, 6*:741, 1975.

68. Scott, F.B.: Treatment of urinary incontinence by implantable prosthetic sphincter. *Urology, 1*:252, 1973.

69. Scott, F.B., Bradley, W.E. and Timm, G.W.: Treatment of urinary incontinence by implantable prosthetic sphincter. *Urology, 1*:252, 1973.

70. Scott, F.B., Bradley, W.E. and Timm, G.W.: Treatment of urinary incontinence by an implantable prosthetic urinary sphincter. *J. Urol.*, *112*:75, 1974.

71. Shapiro, S.R., Lebowitz, R. and Colodny, A.H.: Fate of 90 children with ileal conduit urinary diversion a decade later: Analysis of complications, pyelography, renal function and bacteriology. *J. Urol.*, *55*:289, 1975.

72. Shellhammer, P.F. and Texter, J.H.: An experimental uretero-ileal anastomosis to prevent reflux. *Invest. Urol.*, *11*:319, 1974.

73. Stark, G.D. and Drummond, M.: The spinal cord lesion in myelomeningocele. *Dev. Med. Child Neurol.*, *suppl. 25 1*, 1971.

74. Stark, G.D.: Correlative studies of bladder function

in myelomeningocele. *Dev. Med. Child Neurol.*, *29*:55.

75. Stockcamp, K. and Schreiter, F.: Alpha adrenolytic treatment of the congenital neuropathic bladder. *Urol.ʿ Int.*, *30*:33, 1975.

76. Stockcamp, K.: Treatment with phenoxybenzamine of upper urinary tract complications caused by intravesical obstruction. *J. Urol.*, *113*:128, 1975.

77. Stark, G.: Pudendal neurectomy in management of neurogenic bladder in myelomeningocele. *Arch. Dis. Child.*, *44*:698, 1969.

78. Straffon, R.A., Kyle, K. and Corvalan, J.: Techniques of cutaneous ureterostomy and results in 51 patients. *J. Urol.*, *103*:138, 1970.

79. Tanagho, E.: Personal communication.

80. Tanagho, E., Jonas, U. and Heine, J.P.: Studies on the feasibility of urinary bladder evacuation by direct spinal cord stimulation. I. Parameters of most effective stimulation. *Investigative Urol.*, *13*:142.

81. Tanagho, E. and Jonas, U.: Studies on the feasibility of urinary bladder evacuation by direct spinal cord stimulation. II. Poststimulus voiding: A way to overcome outflow resistance. *Investigative Urol.*, *13*:151.

82. Thomas, V., Shelokov, A. and Forland, M.: Antibody-coated bacteria in urine and the site of urinary tract infection. *N. Eng. J. Med.*, *290*:588, 1974.

83. Timm, G.W. and Bradley, W.E.: Electromechanical restoration of the micturition reflex. *IEEE Transactions of Biomedical Engineering*, *18*:274, 1971.

84. Tsuchida, Y., Sato, T. and Ishida, M.: Radiographic anorectal function study in myelomeningocele. *J. Ped. Surg.*, *7*:50, 1972.

85. Williams, D.I. and Rabinovitch, H.H.: Cutaneous ureterostomy for the grossly dilated ureter of childhood. *Brit. J. Urol.*, *39*:696, 1967.

86. Zachary, R.B. and Lister, J.: Conservative management of the neurogenic bladder. IN Problems in Paediatric Urology, J.H. Johnston (ed.), Amsterdam, Excerpta Medica, 1972.

CARE OF THE BOWEL

Joseph A. Cox, M.D.

Patients with myelomeningoceles, in some instances, after having care for their meningomyelocele, hydrocephalus, genito-urinary tract, and skeletal problems, are left with a lingering problem of fecal incontinence. Some of these patients, as a result of their fecal incontinence, have developed excoriation of the perineal region and subsequent severe infections in the peri-anal region. In other instances, the problem has been so severe that as a last resort, the patient has been left with a permanent colostomy. Also, as the result of inadequate care of the colon and rectum, combined with the neurologic deficit, rectal prolapse has been a problem. However, over the past few years, with many of these patients having been followed and treated, plus information obtained from other groups of patients which have neurogenic ano-rectal, and spinal malformations, a body of knowledge has emerged which has led to better care for these patients. Armed with the understanding of the anatomy and physiology of the ano-rectal region, one is better equipped to cope with the problems related to neurogenic incontinence.

ANATOMY

    The ano-rectal region which we are concerned with in the

present discussion is the distal six to eight centimeters of
colon in the full-sized adult, or the distal three to four
centimeters in the infant. The ano-rectal region is essentially controlled by a dual sphincter mechanism. These
sphincters are under both voluntary and involuntary control.
The internal anal sphincter (smooth muscle) is a condensation
of the inner circular muscle of the colon and is under
involuntary control. This sphincter is innervated by
sympathetic fibers via the inferior mesenteric ganglion.
Afferent fibers from the region mediate the sensation of
rectal distention via the parasympathetic fibers of the
pelvic nerves (nervous erigens). That portion of the anal
sphincter under voluntary control (skeletal muscle) is
usually divided into two segments. The superficial segment
encircles the distal anal canal and produces a constricting
action. This constricting action is responsible for fine
control. The deep segment of the external sphincter is
closely applied to the posterior aspect of the rectum and
fans out as a broad band of attachment to the coccyx, pelvis,
and pubis. It is referred to as the pubo-rectalis sling and
is responsible for gross control via a pinch-cock mechanism.
The superficial sphincter is innervated by the perineal
branch of the fourth sacral nerve and the pudendal nerve.

NEUROPHYSIOLOGY

Much of the understanding of the neurophysiology of the
ano-rectal region is attributed to Dr. Schuster and colleagues
at the Johns Hopkins University School of Medicine. By the
appropriate placement of balloons in the ano-rectal region,
they have been able to study and record the effects of distension of various portions of the ano-rectal canal. This
has lead to an increasing understanding of the physiologic

control of continence and defecation. As the rectum fills
with stool which is propelled by the parastaltic waves, the
afferent nerves of the rectal wall and pubo-rectalis sling,
initiate a reflex relaxation of the internal sphincter.
Simultaneously, the external sphincter is contracted. In
order to maintain fine control, the external sphincter can be
voluntarily contracted.

PATHOLOGIC NEUROPHYSIOLOGY

In congenital malformations of the lumbo-sacral spine,
such as caudal regression syndrome associated with imperforate anus, myelomeningocele, or secondary traumatic lesions
of the lower spine, there is a deficiency of somatic intervention of the voluntary sphincters. The detailed study of
many patients with neurogenic incontinence with the use of
ano-rectal manometry has confirmed that the autonomic innervation of the smooth muscle is not interrupted but, the
striated external anal sphincter is weak or absent. The
result is that as the rectum begins to be filled and distended with stool, the internal involuntary sphincter relaxes,
however, there is a lack of contraction of the external anal
sphincter. This results in involuntary defecation (fecal
soilage or accidents). Clinically, digital rectal examination of these patients reveal a patulous anus with inability
to voluntarily pucker the anus.

THERAPY

Therapy to compensate for the neurogenic deficit of the
ano-rectal region is directed toward taking advantage of the
intact internal sphincter mechanism. Since it has been
established that as the rectum fills with stool, the internal
sphincter reflexly relaxes, a program of regular evacuation

of the rectum before involuntary stooling must be established.
It has been found that following a meal, one can take advantage of the gastro-colic reflex to assist in evacuating the
rectum. A suppository can be administered following a meal,
or a Saline, soap suds, or phosphate enemas can be given.
The suppository or enema is given with the child on his or
her side. This is allowed to remain in place for approximately twenty minutes. Following this, the child is placed
upon the toilet. This regimen will produce clean bottoms in
approximately fifty percent of the children. A smaller
percentage will attain regular bowel habits. In the followup
of these patients, it has been found that best results are
obtained if the bowel training is begun around three years of
age.

REFERENCES

1. Freeman, J.M.: Practical Management of Meningomyelocele.
   Baltimore, University Park Press, 1974.

2. Gross, R.E.: The Surgery of Infancy and Childhood.
   Philadelphia, W.B. Saunders Company, 1953.

3. Netter, F.H.: Nervous System, the Ciba Collection of
   Medical Illustrations, 1957.

4. Schnaufer, L., Talbert, J.L., Haller, J.A., Reid, N.C.R.W.
   Tobon, F., Schuster, M.M.: Differential sphincteric
   studies in the diagnosis of ano-rectal disorders of
   childhood. *Ped. Surg.*, *2*:538, 1967.

5. Schnaufer, L., Kumar, A.P. and White, J.J.: Differentiation and anagement of incontinence and constipation
   problems in children. *Surg. Clin. N. Amer.*, *50*:895, 1970.

6. Schuster, M.M.: Diagnostic Value of Anal Sphincter
   Pressure Measurement. Hospital Practice, pp. 115-122,
   1973.

INTERMITTENT SELF-CATHETERIZATION

Ananias C. Diokno, M.D.

In 1972 we reported a series of 12 patients with various types of bladder dysfunctions who were successfully treated by unsterile intermittent self-catheterization.[7] In 1975 we reported further observations on 218 patients with voiding dysfunctions treated by the same technique.[5] We concluded that the extremely low incidence of complications and its therapeutic efficacy clearly make clean, intermittent self-catheterization an outstanding weapon in the urological armamentarium.

The basis for intermittent self-catheterization was our belief that infection is the result of invading micro-organisms and host resistance, and that host resistance is the most important as a determinant. We postulated that most cases of urinary infection are due to some underlying structural or functional abnormality of the urogenital tract which leads to decreased tissue resistance and to bacterial invasion. Although obvious causes such as inlying catheters, urinary calculi and traumatic instrumentation can damage the structural integrity of the urothelium, we feel the most common cause of increased susceptibility to bacterial invasion is decreased blood flow to the tissue. Reduction of blood flow to the bladder can occur by increased intravesical pressures or by overdistention. The resulting ischemic

bladder is then an easy prey to invading organisms. With
these ideas, we feel that maintenance of a good blood supply
to the urinary tract by avoiding high intraluminal pressures
and over-distention is the key to prevention of urinary tract
infection and that bacterial contamination is of secondary
importance.

These ideas have led us to treat recurrent urinary tract
infections in girls[4] and women[3] with poor voiding habits by
frequent voiding to avoid bladder over-distention. The girls
with infantile bladders but good control of their sphincters
are treated by frequent voiding and anticholinergic agents
to avoid or suppress the uninhibited contraction that
abnormally increases the intravesical pressure.

METHODS AND MATERIALS

Since 1971 we have initiated intermittent catheterization in 51 patients with myelodysplasia. There were 33
females and 18 males. The youngest in the series was 7
months old and the oldest was 52 years old. Table 1 shows
the breakdown of their ages.

The majority of patients had obvious voiding difficulty
when seen. Forty-three patients were voiding by crede or
Valsalva maneuver while only eight patients were voiding
without any obvious mechanical help.

Forty-two patients had cystometric evaluation prior to
the initiation of the intermittent catheterization technique.
There were 28 patients with mixed upper and lower motor
bladders and 14 individuals with paralytic bladders. Twenty-
three patients underwent combined studies utilizing cystometry and perineal electromyography. Partial denervation of
the periurethral striated muscle was observed in twenty
patients while absent electrical activity or complete

denervation was noted in three cases.

Reasons for catheterization varied. This included recurrent urinary tract infection, deterioration of upper tracts and urinary incontinence. Patients with urinary incontinence but with normal urine and upper tracts were treated only when incontinence became a social problem. This occurred when the patient reached school age.

Follow-up period. Ten patients have been followed for more than 3 years, 11 from 2-3 years, 13 from 1-2 years, 14 from 4-12 months and 3 from 1-3 months.

CATHETERIZATION TECHNIQUE

The technique of catheterization was taught by our clinic nurse or physician assistant to the mother and the child at the same time. Initially the basic principles and goals of frequent emptying of the bladder by catheterization are discussed with the patient or parent and include: 1. decreased blood flow of any tissue weakens resistance to bacterial infection, 2. an overdistended bladder slows circulation through its wall and thus makes it susceptible to infection and, therefore, 3. to prevent or cure infection, one must empty the bladder often by frequent catheterization. Emphasis is placed upon importance of frequency of catheterization rather than sterility.

The patients are requested to report for their catheterization lesson with a full bladder, if possible. The female subject sits on the examining table with feet on the table, lower limbs flexed and knees held apart so as to help expose the introitus and urethral meatus. In the sitting position the patient is able to visualize the perineum in a mirror at the foot of the table. The labia are separated and the clitoris, urethral meatus and vaginal outlet are pointed out to the pupil. The subject is then given a 14F

plastic or rubber Robinson catheter and is instructed to
insert the catheter through the urethral meatus into the
bladder. She is directed to hold the catheter about 1-1½
inch from the tip with the dominant hand, and with the
fingers of the other hand to hold the labia apart with the
index and fourth finger while pressing on the meatus with
the third finger. The third finger is then raised from the
meatus and the catheter passed into the urethral lumen. Then
the patient is advised to partially empty the bladder, withdraw the catheter completely and recatheterize herself.
Thereafter, she is taken to the bathroom where she either
sits on the toilet seat or stands facing the toilet with one
foot on the toilet seat. She catheterizes herself several
times again until she feels confident about the procedure.

The teaching of self-catheterization to the male subject
is simple and is accomplished with the patient in the sitting
position initially and then standing. It is necessary to
apply water soluble surgical lubricant in generous fashion
to the outer terminal portion of the catheter in male
subjects in order to avoid traumatic urethritis.

Upon completion of the catheterization lesson, the pupil
is given an instruction sheet reiterating the principles and
methods involved and a list of necessary materials. The
catheter can be carried in a dry state in a plastic bag,
compact, paper towel or something comparable. No sterilizing
solution is used and no lubricant is needed for the female
subject. For the sake of cleanliness and prevention of
malodorousness, the patient, when possible washes his or her
hands with soap and water and the outer surface of the catheter with the same soapy lather and rinses the inside and
outside of the catheter with clear water. The patient is
warned never to forego catheterization when soap and water

are not available but to catheterize at the prescribed time
regardless of circumstances.

MEDICATION

Antibacterial preparations including Gantanol, Macro-
dantin and Polycillin were used during the first two to four
weeks of intermittent catheterization program. Anticholinergic agents such as Ditropan[*1] and Tincture of Belladonna
were prescribed for many of the patients with uncontrolled
bladder contractions and urinary incontinence. Alpha
adrenergic in the form of Ephedrine Sulfate[2] tablets or
elixir in a dose varying from 10-50 mg every 6 hours, was
employed to increase urethral resistance and control the
stress type of urinary incontinence seen in our patients with
significant lower motor neuron lesion.

RESULTS

Urinary Infection. Prior to being placed on the self-
catheterization regimen, only 15 percent (8/51) of the
patients had a sterile urine. Following institution of
clean, intermittent self-catheterization, the incidence of
people with sterile urines increased to 70 percent (36/51).
Seventeen percent had a negative urine without the aid of
any antimicrobial medication while 53 percent required antibiotics or chemotherapy for a varying number of times and
duration. No patient in the entire series has developed
pyelonephritis or sepsis.

Urethral False Passage and Urethritis. One patient
developed false passage at the region of the bulbous urethra

*Obtained from Marion Laboratories, Inc., 10236 Bunker Ridge
Road, Kansas City, Missouri 64137

after using an excessively large catheter. This case was
previously reported.[6] No urethritis occurred in our
patients.

Epididymitis. An 18 year-old patient developed acute
epididymitis within two weeks after starting on intermittent
catheterization. It was postulated that the inciting stimulus was probably the indwelling catheter present prior to
the self-catheterization program.

Renal Status. There were forty-two patients who had
normal pyelograms pre-catheterization and the 31 of these who
have gone long enough to have checkup urograms, continue to
show normal pyeloureterograms.

Three patients with hydroureteronephrosis in the group
of 8 with abnormal upper tracts demonstrated considerable
improvement over a period of time on self-catheterization.
The individuals with evidences of pyelonephritis remained
unchanged. As mentioned previously, no patient worsened
radiographically.

The blood urea nitrogen and serum creatinine levels
correlated well with the findings on excretory urography.

Incontinence: Only five of 51 patients in our series
persisted to have significant urinary incontinence. The
incontinence was controlled either by intermittent catheterization alone or with the addition of anticholinergic and/or
alpha adrenergic therapy. Involuntary wetting in these
people is caused by reflex bladder contractions and stress
or overflow incontinence, dissipated the chronic dermatitis
of the perineum and genitalia and, probably most important
of all, gave the patient and frequently the parents a new
outlook on life from a social point of view.

The catheterization program was abandoned in seven of
51 patients. Five patients persisted to have significant

urinary incontinence and in two patients their mothers were
unable to continue the frequent catheterization regimen.

SUMMARY AND CONCLUSIONS

Fifty-one patients with bladder and sphincter dysfunction secondary to congenital spinal cord abnormality were
treated with non-sterile technique to intermittent self-
catheterization. Marked improvement was noted in urinary
incontinence, urinary infection, renal function, bladder
emptying and, perhaps most important, the mental and
emotional status of the patient and/or parents. The extremely low incidence of complications and its therapeutic
efficacy clearly make clean, intermittent self-catheterization
an outstanding weapon in the therapy of bladder dysfunction
of myelomeningocele. It reinforces our belief regarding the
importance of host resistance in the physiopathology of
urinary infections.

REFERENCES

1. Diokno, A.C. and Lapides, J.: Oxybutynin: A new drug
    with analgesic and anticholinergic properties. *J. of
    Urol., 108*:307, 1972.
2. Diokno, A.C. and Taub, M.: Ephedrine in treatment of
    urinary incontinence. *Urology, 5*:624, 1975.
3. Lapides, J., Costello, R.T.,Jr., Zierdt, K.D. and Stone,
    T.E.: Primary cause and treatment of recurrent urinary
    infection in women: Preliminary report. *J. Urol., 100*:
    552, 1968.
4. Lapides, J. and Diokno, A.C.: Persistence of the infant

bladder as a cause for urinary infection in girls.
J. Urol., 103:243, 1970.

5. Lapides, J., Diokno, A.C., Gould, F.R. and Lowe, B.S.:
    Further observations on self-catheterizations. Accepted
    for publication to *Trans. Am. Assoc. Genito-Urinary
    Surgeons.*

6. Lapides, J., Diokno, A.C., Lowe, B.S. and Kalish, M.D.:
    Follow-up on unsterile, intermittent self-catheterization.
    Trans. Am. Assoc. Genito-Urinary Surg., 65:44, 1973.

7. Lapides, J., Diokno, A.C., Silber,S.J. and Lowe, B.S.:
    Clean, intermittent self-catheterization in the treatment
    of urinary tract disease. *J. Urol., 107*:458, 1972.

TABLE 1.

Age Distribution

7 mos. - 4 years	3
5 years - 10 years	20
11 years - 15 years	12
16 years - 20 years	10
over 20 years	6
TOTAL	51

ELECTRICAL STIMULATION OF THE
BLADDER*

Daniel C. Merrill, M.D.

The first Mentor bladder stimulator** was implanted on March 19, 1971.[2-4] During the subsequent 4 years, 32 clinical investigators from the United States and Europe have implanted over 100 of these devices in patients with a variety of different types of bladder dysfunction. A recent survey showed that bladder stimulation has been entirely successful in 55% of these patients.[5] In an additional 3% the patient's urinary dysfunction has been improved; thus, nearly 60% of these patients have benefited from bladder stimulation. This success rate is surprisingly high considering the fact that the bladders of these patients often had been subjected to years of chronic infection and over-distension, detrusor dysfunction having been present for an average of 7 years prior to implantation. It also is important to note that prior to implantation this group of patients had failed to respond to an average of 3.7 different forms of conventional therapy (intermittent catheterization, sphincterotomy, pharmacological agents, etc.). In fact, bladder stimulation often represented a last desperate

*VA Project MRIS #5674-01

**Mentor Corporation, Minneapolis, Minnesota

attempt by physician and patient to avoid supravesical diversion.

   Although it is impossible to predict the ultimate role of bladder stimulation, the clinical data accumulated to date suggest that electrical stimulation should be considered earlier in the course of the patient's disease than it has been in the past. This is so because chronic cystitis and chronic overdistension decrease and ultimately eliminate entirely the detrusor response to stimulation. The fact that implantation of a bladder stimulator is a relatively simple, safe, and noninvasive (with respect to the urinary tract) procedure is also an important consideration. In this respect, with the exception of one patient who developed grade I unilateral reflux, there has not been a single report of bladder or upper tract deterioration attributed to the implantation of a Mentor bladder stimulator. Thus, if bladder stimulation fails, all other treatment options are still open to patient and physician.

IMPLANTATION

   To implant the Mentor bladder stimulator (Fig. 1), a lower abdominal midline suprapubic incision is made and the anterior and posterior surfaces of the bladder are separated from surrounding tissue.[2] The helical electrodes are placed around the base of the bladder and the bladder wall is imbricated over the electrodes (Fig. 2). The receiver/ stimulator is placed in a subcutaneous pocket in the left or right lower quadrant of the abdomen and the electrode leads are positioned between the rectus muscles. The fascia, sub- cutaneous tissue, and skin are closed in routine fashion.

   At surgery the bladder should develop between 10 and 60 cm of water pressure during stimulation. Although the

pressure generated at surgery is not related to the ultimate
success of the procedure, the stimulator should not be
implanted if the bladder is completely unresponsive to
stimulation. The stimulator induced increase in intravesical
pressure routinely decreases during the first and second
postoperative months and, in fact, the bladder may be
entirely unresponsive to stimulation during this period.
The detrusor's responsiveness to stimulation characteristically increases thereafter and maximum excitability is
achieved at 4-6 months after surgery.[2] For this reason,
routine bladder stimulation is not recommended during the
first 3-4 postoperative months.

The following discussion on specific types of voiding
disorders is based on an analysis of the data submitted by
25 clinical investigators.[5] The conclusions drawn however,
other than the determination of success or failure in
individual patients, are my own and do not necessarily
reflect those of the independent investigators.

VESICAL HYPOTONIA OF UNKNOWN ETIOLOGY

Almost 1/3 of all implants have been made in females
with idiopathic vesical hypotonia. The primary indication
for implantation was urinary retention in each of these
patients, and 65% voided with low residuum postoperatively.
Thus, as Halverstadt has shown, vesical hypotonia is a
primary indication for bladder stimulation.[1] This is an
important observation because patients with this form of
urinary retention usually are normal except for their voiding
dysfunction and they characteristically do not tolerate
chronic inlying or prolonged intermittent catheterization.
For example, 78% of the patients in this group had failed
chronic intermittent catheterization, primarily because of

catheter induced urethral discomfort. It is important to
realize that all patients with idiopathic vesical hypotonia
will experience pain during stimulation; in 20-25% the pain
will be intolerable and result in failure of the procedure.
Unfortunately, at present the severity of stimulus induced
postoperative pain cannot be predicted accurately preoperatively.

LOWER MOTONEURON LESIONS

To date the highest success rate for bladder stimulation
(82%) has been achieved in patients with traumatic lower
motoneuron lesions. The success of the procedure in this
instance results from the fact that patients with lower
motoneuron lesions do not develop either pain or detrusor-
sphincter dyssynergia during stimulation. Thus, the stimulus
applied is not limited by pain and the urinary stream
generated by the resultant bladder contraction is not cur-
tailed by a reflex induced increase in urethral resistance.
Success in these patients is also associated with a 40%
decrease in the number and severity of bladder infections.

MULTIPLE SCLEROSIS

Bladder stimulation has been attempted in only 6
patients with multiple sclerosis to date; however, 4 of the
6 have been successful. Although multiple sclerotic patients
often develop small capacity bladders and severe urgency
incontinence, the multiple sclerotic patients in this series
all had large hypotonic bladders and retention or high
urinary residua preoperatively. In most instances the
stimulus induced reduction in residuum also was associated
with a decrease in the number and severity of bladder
infections. The results in this group of patients were

similar to the results achieved in patients with lower motoneuron lesions except that all patients with multiple
sclerosis experienced tolerable pain during bladder stimulation while pain is not a factor in patients with complete
lower motoneuron lesions.

MENINGOMYELOCELE

Twenty percent of all implants have been performed in
patients with meningomyelocele.[3] Urinary residuum was
reduced (usually to less than 5 cc's) in 75% and the severity
and number of urinary infections were reduced in 45% of these
patients. Urinary incontinence, however, was improved in
only 20% and total continence was not achieved in any patient.
This is an important observation since incontinence was the
primary reason for surgery in many of these patients. Thus,
the 35% success rate reported by individual investigators
must be tempered by the realization that most of these
patients were, for practical purposes, incontinent postoperatively. In the future a dual implant to control
continence and detrusor contractility may provide a solution
to this problem; at present, however, bladder stimulation
seems to be at best a temporizing procedure rather than a
long-term solution to the urinary problems encountered in
meningomyelocele patients. Approximately 60% of meningomyelocele patients developed tolerable pain during stimulation; however, experience to date suggests that pain will be
an infrequent cause of failure in this group of patients.

UPPER MOTONEURON LESIONS

With 2 exceptions bladder stimulation was unsuccessful
in patients with traumatic upper motoneuron lesions. Failure
primarily results from the fact that all upper motoneuron

lesion patients developed severe detrusor-sphincter
dyssynergia during electrical stimulation. Detrusor-
sphincter dyssynergia can be eliminated by phenolization of
the sacral spinal cord or pudendal neurectomy;[2] however,
these procedures most often are rejected by patient and
physician. In any case, bladder stimulation is seldom
indicated in these patients since most void satisfactorily
after sphincterotomy.

OTHER INDICATIONS

Electrical stimulation also has been successful in
patients with mixed upper and lower motoneuron lesions,
diabetes mellitus and tertiary syphilis; however, the number
of implants in each of these categories is as yet too small
to draw meaningful conclusions.

COMPLICATIONS AND SIDE EFFECTS

Erosion of the device or electrical leads through the
skin has necessitated removal of the implanted stimulator
in approximately 10% of all implantations. The incidence of
this complication, which contributed significantly to the
overall 45% failure rate, should decrease in direct relationship to the experience of the surgeon. The painful response
to stimulation described above is the primary side effect to
electrical stimulation. Stimulus induced pain occurs in all
patients with incomplete neurological injuries; fortunately,
the painful response to stimulation is tolerable in most
instances. Autonomic dysreflexia has not been a problem in
bladder stimulation.

SUMMARY

To date the Mentor stimulator has been successful in approximately 50% of all implantations, a surprisingly good result considering the fact that bladder stimulation most often has been reserved for patients with the severest type of bladder dysfunction. This treatment modality is most successful in patients who develop urinary retention as a result of traumatic lower motoneuron lesions, multiple sclerosis, or idiopathic vesical hypotonia. Bladder stimulation may also be beneficial in meningomyelocele patients; however, electrical stimulation seldom provides a permanent solution to the urinary problems of these patients since urinary incontinence is not improved by stimulation. Because of electrically induced detrusor-sphincter dyssynergia, bladder stimulation is uniformly unsuccessful in patients with upper motoneuron lesions.

REFERENCES

1. Halverstadt, D.B. and Parry, W.L.: Electronic stimulation of the human bladder: 9 years later. *J. Urol.*, *113*:341, 1975.
2. Merrill, D.C. and Conway, C.J.: Clinical experience with the Mentor bladder stimulator. I. Patients with upper motor neuron lesions. *J. Urol.*, *112*:52, 1974.
3. Merrill, D.C.: Clinical experience with the Mentor bladder stimulator. II. Meningomyelocele patients. *J. Urol.*, *112*:823, 1974.

4. Merrill, D.C.: Clinical experience with the Mentor
    bladder stimulator. III. Patients with urinary vesical
    hypotonia. *J. Urol., 113*:335, 1975.

5. Merrill, D.C.: Results of electrical vesical stimulation
    with the Mentor bladder stimulator. A survey of 25
    clinical investigators. In preparation.

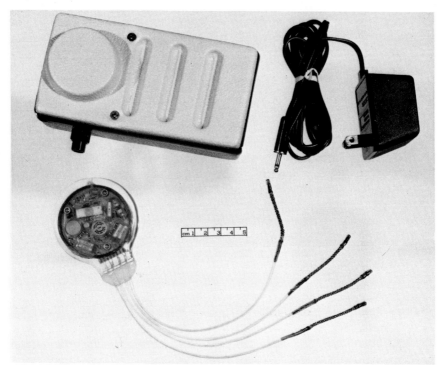

Fig. 1. Implantable Mentor adult 4-channel bladder stimulator with rechargeable external stimulator.

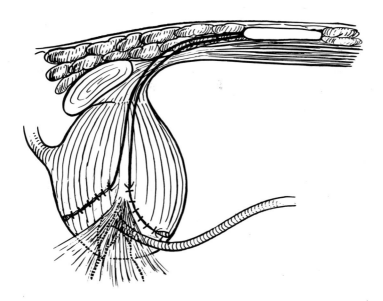

Fig. 2. Placement of the bladder stimulator's bipolar helical electrodes on either side of the left neurovascular pedical of the bladder.

EXTERNAL DEVICES FOR INCONTINENCE IN CHILDREN

George T. Klauber, M.D.

INTRODUCTION

This paper concerns external incontinence devices excluding stomal appliances described elsewhere.

The achievement of urinary control is the greatest problem and challenge in the urologic management of the myelomeningocele child and second in importance only to the preservation of renal function.

The need for suitable incontinence devices is, therefore, self-evident, apart from rendering the need for major surgical intervention unnecessary.

Temporary use of an indwelling catheter for bladder or kidney drainage is frequently useful for acute problems; long-term use of indwelling catheters is to be deprecated.

DIAPERS

The simplest device for collecting urine is the diaper, which merits more than cursory reference. Up to the age of four years, diapers are entirely age-appropriate; in addition they are suitable for application over a ureterostomy or a vesicostomy, in the infant.

Beyond four years of age, diapers become age *in*-appropriate. They also have numerous inherent disadvantages:
1. Disposable diapers are not available in a size

large enough for the older child.

2. They appear bulky because numerous diapers, at least three, must be worn to give sufficient absorbent capacity.

3. Malodor, directly or indirectly, from reusable rubber of plastic pants, is a persistent problem.

4. Changing diapers without assistance is difficult and, without adequate space, well-nigh impossible.

Bladder outflow resistance increases with age in many children with spina bifida, so that bladder expression or intermittent catheterization with or without adjunctive pharmacologic agents may become effective as the child matures. The use of diapers, or incontinence pads, is invaluable in anticipation of future continence or as a stop-gap measure for the child destined to have reconstructive surgery or prosthetic sphincter implants in the future.

URINAL

The male phallus, besides being a symbol of sexual dominance, is also a useful spout for incorporation into a urinal. Functional urinals for the incontinent female do not exist.

The ideal male urinal should be:

1. Leakproof

2. Inexpensive

3. Lightweight

4. Strong

5. Comfortable

6. Easy to wash

7. Non-traumatic

8. Odorfree

Two basic types of urinals are suitable for the male child:

1.   Condom type, which is applied to the penis like a glove.

2.   Pubic pressure type, which forms a seal around the base of the penis.

CONDOM DEVICE

Such devices are best suited for the older child with a reasonable size phallus. For the postpubertal male with a fully developed penis, a device can simply and cheaply be constructed by attaching a length of latex tubing to a prophylactic. Smaller ones can be constructed by using finger cots.

Condom type catheters named Connecticut Catheters have been designed in six sizes from 5/8" to 1¼" in diameter. To insure a proper fit, one measures the diameter of the penis and establishes the correct size.

A satisfactory method of application is to coat the shaft of the penis with tincture of benzoin, followed by a light coat of skin cement. The catheter is then rolled over the skin cement which holds it in position. The condom may be attached to a leg bag, or other type of drainage pouch.

The condom device may be removed by unrolling the catheter; the cement is usually removed during this maneuver. Some patients are able to wear a condom catheter for 2 or 3 days before replacement is necessary. A condom can be reused if carefully handled, properly cleaned and well dusted with powder before reapplication.

Condom catheters have the inherent disadvantage of twisting upon themselves, preventing urine from entering the drainage tube. This problem has been mostly avoided by the larger Connecticut, Texas and Rusch catheters, in which the apex of the condom is thickened to prevent twisting.

Reusable condoms are also available in siliconized rubber.

Since penile tourniquets are potentially dangerous, care must be taken to prevent skin breakdown.

Condom catheters by themselves are, unfortunately, not suitable for most ambulant boys.

PUBIC PRESSURE AND COMBINATION PUBIC PRESSURE CONDOM URINALS

Many such appliances are available, but most of them are designed for the adult male. Two appliances which we have found consistently acceptable are the Hill-Davol Pediatric Male Urinal[2,4] and the Down's or Byram Pubic Pressure Urinal.[1,3]

HILL-DAVOL PEDIATRIC MALE URINAL[2]

This consists of a detachable mesh suspensory of stretch fabric with an elastic waistband with Velcro fastener. A soft latex condom, or top, contains a small cone-shaped inner penile sheath which may be cut to individual size to prevent backflow. The condom passes through the pediatric suspensory and is fitted to a leg bag. Effectiveness of the Hill-Davol urinal can be improved considerably by interposing a karaya gum "collyseal" between the diaphragm or flange of the condom and the skin. This produces a urineproof seal.

Suitable patients are pre-measured with a guide known in our establishment as the "peter meter". The diaphragm and "collyseal" are custom precut to order by the supplier.

The unit is assembled by inserting the condom section of the urinal into the suspensory. The "collyseal" is moistened, placed around the base of the penis, and pressed into position. The assembled urinal and suspensory are positioned with the penis in the condom, so that the diaphragm is seated against the collyseal. The suspensory can be adjusted to give a snug fit. The leg bag is attached to

an adapter on the condom and straps are fitted around the
thigh.

An optional adapter can be attached to the lower end of
the bag and tucked into a sock. The child can then drain his
bag without undressing. He lifts his foot to the rim of the
toilet and drains the bag into the bowl.

Removal of the urinal at night and the use of diapers
is preferred by some. The same "collyseal" can be used for
up to four days.

DOWN'S AND BYRAM PUBIC PRESSURE URINALS

The Down's Pubic Pressure Urinal has been available in
the United Kingdom for approximately sixteen years.[3] Mr.
Albert Evans of Byram Surgical has recently modified and
improved this pubic pressure urinal, which may now be the most
practical appliance for many incontinent boys.[1] The pubic
pressure urinal consists of four interchangeable parts:

1. Flange with an inner sheath
2. Shaped cone
3. Belt
4. Leg bag

All are available in a variety of shapes and sizes.

The pubic pressure flange is especially useful for the
small or receding penis. The flange is firm and when the
belt is tightened, peri-penile pubic pressure pushes the
penis forward into the sheath. The flange is available in
numerous diameters from 13 to 38 mm, in 3 mm increments. A
perfect fit is, therefore, easy to accomplish. The inner
parallel-sided sheath gently grips the penis and allows for
expansion without trauma to the skin or obstruction of blood
flow. The base of the penis is again measured to select the
correct size of flange.

The pubic pressure flange is fitted with rolled rubber

understraps, which pass around both thighs and are attached
to the waistbelt.

A range of cones is available, allowing for anatomic
variations. Cones have two different bases for attachment
to the flange, either vertical or angled. Vertical cones
are suitable for the ambulant boy, whereas the cone with a
45 degree angle to the vertical allows for more protrusion
of the penis and is thus suitable for the sedentary or
wheelchair patient.

A leg bag is attached directly by a female mount to a
male threaded connector on the cone. Bags are available in
different sizes with capacities from 300 to 750 cc's. A
transverse bag has been designed for small boys to be worn
under short pants without being conspicuous.

A night drainage adaptor, or a piece of tubing, can be
fitted either to the bag or to the male threaded connector on
the cone.

The pubic pressure flange can also be used with a condom
instead of a cone. The advantages of using the condom are:

1. The ready availability of condoms does away with the
necessity of maintaining a large inventory of cones in
numerous shapes and sizes.

2. They can be fitted very easily and attached to any
leg bag, temporary or permanent.

3. They are especially lightweight.

4. They may be less traumatic to the penis.

5. They are exceedingly cheap.

The pubic pressure flange has added versatility for use
with intermittent self-catheterization, via the penile
urethra. The cone or condom may be removed, leaving the
flange in place. Intermittent catheterization may be
required for the boy with a significant residual urine,

necessitating drainage on a regular basis. Such intermittent catheterization can be performed without the patient having to undress. The patient can unzip his fly, detach the cone or condom from the flange, carry out his self-catheterization in the usual way, and reconnect the condom or cone.

The external urinal is especially suited for males with a small bladder capacity and urinary incontinence who are not candidates for the artificial sphincter or bladder augmentation procedures. The morbidity is certainly much lower than with intestinal conduit surgery. In the presence of a bladder outflow obstruction and a small bladder capacity, transurethral resection of the bladder neck and/or external sphincter prior to installation of an external collecting device should be considered rather than urinary diversion.

SUMMARY

External urinary collecting devices are by no means perfect as yet, although considerable advances have been made in the past few years. The Newington modification of the Hill-Davol condom urinal and the Byram Pubic Pressure Urinal are two examples. We hope that this presentation will encourage suitable patients to try these devices on a temporary or long term basis to achieve instant urinary control. Every myelomeningocele team of physicians and allied health professionals should have someone who is experienced in the use of these devices to give much needed help, support, advice, and encouragement to their patients.

The "Newington Urinal" and the "Byram Pubic Pressure Urinal" may be obtained from Byram Surgical, Inc., 2 Armonk Street, Byram, Connecticut 10573.

REFERENCES

1. Hall, M.H.: Appliances for the incontinent patient.
    Brit. J. Urol., *37*:4, 1965.

2. Hill, M.L. and Shurtleff, D.B.: A device for collecting
    urine in incontinent male children. *Amer. J. Dis. Child*,
    116:158, 1968.

3. Klauber, G.T. and Evans, A.: Pubic pressure urinal.
    In press, *Urology*.

4. Klauber, G.T. and Lund, S.T.: New pediatric male urinal.
    Pediatrics, *55*:134, 1975.

THE TREATMENT OF URINARY
INCONTINENCE BY ELECTRICAL PELVIC
FLOOR STIMULATION*

Daniel C. Merrill, M.D.

Electrical stimulation has now been employed to treat incontinence for over 15 years. Although Caldwell initially designed the pelvic floor stimulator to treat females with stress incontinence,[6] he and others soon extended its application to patients with postprostatectomy and neurogenic incontinence.[1,2,4,5,7,15] While this novel treatment modality has gained general acceptance in Europe, it has not been employed extensively in the United States for several reasons. First, the Marshall-Marchetti-Krantz[13] operation, or a modification of their procedure, is so successful that there seldom is an indication for electrical stimulation in females with stress incontinence. Second, the initial encouraging reports of pelvic floor stimulation in meningo-myelocele children have not been reproduced. Indeed we now know that electrical stimulation has no significant effect in denervated skeletal muscle.[15,18] Finally, Kaufman's static and Scott's volitional incontinence devices have been so popular in the United States that few American surgeons have considered alternate forms of treatment for postoperative incontinence.[10,14,16]

Recently, however, interest in pelvic floor stimulation has been increasing primarily due to laboratory studies and

*VA Project MRIS 5674-01

preliminary clinical reports which suggest that electrical
stimulation may have application in patients with urgency
incontinence, a condition which has been particularly
resistant to conventional modes of treatment.[8,18] This
exciting new application for pelvic floor stimulation is
presently being evaluated at several clinical centers.

MECHANISM OF ACTION

Passive Urinary Incontinence. In patients with passive
or outlet urinary incontinence, laboratory and clinical
studies suggest that the initial beneficial effect of stimulation results from an increase in urethral resistance. The
increase in urethral resistance recorded during stimulation
is secondary to direct and reflex activation of the pudendal
nerve innervating the external urethral sphincter and the
pelvic floor.[18] The increase in urethral resistance is
produced primarily by electrically induced skeletal muscle
contraction, the smooth muscle of the urethra and bladder
making little or no contribution in this respect.[3,18]
Contrary to what one might expect based on the rapid fatiga-
bility of most skeletal muscles, the rate of fatigue in the
external sphincter and pelvic floor skeletal muscles is
slow.[18,19] Thus, the initial increase in urethral pressure
produced by stimulation slowly decreases during the first
30-90 minutes and thereafter stabilizes at pressures 10-40 cm
of water higher than the resting (prestimulus) urethral
pressure. These pre and postfatigue increases in pressure
most likely are responsible for the initial beneficial
effects of electrical stimulation in patients with passive
incontinence.

As would be expected, in the early phase of treatment
the beneficial effects usually are lost when the patient

stops the stimulus. Many patients, however, have reported
that after 6 to 8 weeks of stimulation they remain dry for
increasing periods between stimulation.[1,7] In fact,
occasionally total urinary continence has been restored after
several months of treatment, making it possible to discontinue
the electrical stimulus entirely.[6] The mechanism of action
for this form of rehabilitation is unknown; however, it has
been postulated that such patients benefit from rehabilitation of the pelvic floor muscles in the same manner as females
with stress incontinence benefit from Kegel exercises.[11] It
has also been reported that patients occasionally are cured
after only a few days of stimulation. The mechanism of
action in the latter patients is unclear and such responses
suggest a functional rather than an organic disorder.

Active Urinary Incontinence. Cutaneous, rectal digital,
and electrical stimulation all have a depressive effect on
detrusor contractility.[8,9,12,17,18] Reflex activation of the
pelvic floor muscles via a pudendal to pelvic nerve reflex
is responsible for 20-60% of the maximal response achieved
by the implanted pelvic floor stimulator and the transrectal
stimulator.[18] The detrusor depressive effects of these
stimulus modalities may be demonstrated in normal humans and
in animals; however, the effect seems to be more pronounced
in subjects with lesions of the corticoregulatory tracts. In
either instance the electrical stimulus activates the inhibitory component of the pudendal to pelvic nerve reflex. In
decerebrate dogs and cats who developed rhythmic detrusor
contractions similar to the uninhibited contractions recorded
in patients with upper motoneuron lesions, the depressive
effect of electrical stimulation is variable and thus one can
predict that this treatment modality will not be effective in
all patients.[18] My preliminary clinical studies suggest that

detrusor inhibition may be demonstrated cystometrically in
nearly all patients; however, the clinical beneficial effects
of stimulation are achieved in less than 30% of potential
candidates. Godec and Cass[8] have had a more extensive
clinical experience with this treatment modality and have
achieved a higher cure rate. In any case, even low cure
rates are significant in patients with urgency incontinence
since they routinely fail all other forms of treatment.

Laboratory and clinical studies also show that the
depressive effect of stimulation often persists after dis-
continuation of the electrical stimulus.[8,18] The mechanism
for "reflex memory" of this type is not known; however, this
observation suggests that continual transrectal stimulation
may not be necessary to eliminate the abnormal detrusor
response to bladder distension.

METHODS OF STIMULATION

Pudendal Nerve Stimulation. Laboratory studies suggest
that the maximal increase in urethral resistance is achieved
by direct stimulation of the pudendal nerves.[18,19] This mode
of stimulation, which to date has not been employed clinically,
is superior to either transrectal stimulation or to pelvic
floor stimulation because all motor units of the pudendal
nerve are activated by the electrical stimulus.

Pelvic Floor Stimulation. Present day pelvic floor
stimulators are similar to the devices described by Caldwell
in 1963[6] (Fig. 1). The two unipolar electrodes are implanted
at the "trigger points" in the pelvic floor, one on either
side of the urethra.[15] The "trigger points" refer to the
stimulus point on the pelvic floor muscles where the maximal
visual response to stimulation is achieved with minimal
current spread to the obturator nerve. The degree of visual

muscular contraction is not necessarily related to the
success of the procedure. The receiver/stimulator is
implanted in a subcutaneous pocket in the right or left lower
quadrant of the abdomen. The implanted device has no
batteries and it is activated transcutaneously by magnetic
induction from an antenna which is taped to the abdominal
skin overlying the implanted receiver. Rechargeable batteries
provide the power supply to the pelvic floor stimulator and
the voltage delivered may be varied by the patient.

Laboratory studies suggest that the implanted pelvic
floor stimulator is more effective than the transrectal
stimulator in increasing urethral resistance,[18] thus
theoretically pelvic floor stimulation should be more effective than transrectal stimulation in patients with passive or
outlet incontinence. The pelvic floor stimulator is as
effective as the transrectal stimulator in depressing the
rhythmic contractions recorded in decerebrate animals.[18]
Similar comparisons, other than general impressions of
clinical effectiveness, have not been made in humans.

As stated above, neither pelvic floor nor transrectal
stimulation is as effective as direct pudendal nerve
stimulation in increasing urethral resistance, probably
because reflex activation of the pelvic floor skeletal
muscles is a less efficient method of activating the skeletal
muscles than is direct nerve stimulation.

Transrectal Stimulation. Transrectal stimulation is the
most popular initial mode of pelvic floor stimulation because
it is simple to apply (Fig. 2). Transrectal stimulation is
a less desirable long-term treatment modality because of the
inconvenience associated with repetitive rectal insertion and
extraction. Transrectal stimulation also induces diarrhea in
some patients, which is not a problem with the implanted

device. Thus, most patients who require continuous
stimulation for urinary control ultimately discontinue treatment or elect to have a pelvic floor stimulator implanted.

As discussed above, laboratory studies suggest that
transrectal stimulation is less effective than pelvic floor
stimulation in increasing urethral resistance; however, transrectal stimulation is as effective as pelvic floor stimulation in depressing detrusor contractions. Thus, transrectal
stimulation has particular application in patients with
urgency incontinence.

Transvaginal Stimulation. To date, transvaginal
stimulation has not proven to be a practical treatment
modality since an electrode has not been designed which will
maintain a fixed position within the vagina.[7]

PRESENT INDICATIONS FOR ELECTRICAL PELVIC FLOOR STIMULATION

Stress Incontinence. The indication for pelvic floor
stimulation in females with stress incontinence is limited
because permanent cures may be achieved in most patients with
a Marshall-Marchetti-Krantz type of surgical procedure.[13]
Thus, the patients who are primary   candidates for pelvic
floor stimulation in England are most often not considered
for electrical stimulation in the United States. There are,
however, stress incontinent patients who either refuse
surgery or are not candidates for surgery who may benefit
from transrectal stimulation. Transrectal or pelvic floor
stimulation will achieve a 50-60% incidence of significant
improvement or cure in these patients.

Postprostatectomy Incontinence. Electrical stimulation
has had limited success in postprostatectomy incontinence,
possibly because the muscular structures which must respond
to the electrical stimulation are often damaged either by the

original operative procedure or by postoperative fibrosis.
In any case, more impressive cure rates have been reported by
other surgical procedures and thus at present, electrical
stimulation is most often reserved, as it has been in stress
incontinence, either for patients who have failed more
conventional treatment modalities or for those who are not
candidates for surgery. In the latter instance, transrectal
stimulation again is attractive because it is a noninvasive
method of treatment. Electrical stimulation will achieve
significant improvement or cure in 30-40% of these patients.

Meningomyelocele & Lower Motoneuron Lesion Incontinence.
Laboratory and clinical studies show that electrical
stimulation via whatever treatment method will fail in
patients with complete lower motoneuron lesions.[3,15,18] In
my experience, electrical stimulation also has been uniformly
unsuccessful in meningomyelocele children who have been
thought to have only partial denervation of their bladders.
Similarly, in my series patients with partial lower motoneuron lesions have routinely failed to benefit from pelvic
floor stimulation.

Upper Motoneuron Lesion Incontinence. The clinical
studies presently underway suggest that patients with bladder
spasticity secondary to lesions of the corticoregulatory
tracts may be the most suitable candidates for electrical
pelvic floor stimulation. Insufficient clinical data has
been accumulated, however, to predict the ultimate cure rate
which will be achieved with electrical stimulation in
patients who suffer from active urinary incontinence. At
present, patients with bladder spasticity secondary to
multiple sclerosis, stroke, paraplegia, and quadriplegia are
all considered to be candidates for a trial of transrectal
stimulation.

SUMMARY

　　Electrical pelvic floor stimulation acts in passive or outlet incontinence by increasing urethral resistance.　The electrical stimulus, which activates the pudendal nerve directly or reflexively, may be applied by either the pelvic floor or transrectal stimulators.　Direct pudendal nerve stimulation, the most effective method of inducing pelvic floor contraction, is not employed clinically at present. Electrical pelvic floor stimulation also may have application in patients with active or detrusor incontinence because it activates the vesical inhibitory component of the pudendal to pelvic nerve reflex.

REFERENCES

1.　Alexander, S. and Rowan, D.:　Electrical control of urinary incontinence:　a clinical appraisal.　*Brit. J. Surg.*, *57*:766, 1970.

2.　Alexander, S. and Rowan, D.:　Electrical control of urinary incontinence by radio implant:　a report of 14 patients.　*Brit. J. Surg.*, *55*:358, 1968.

3.　Alexander, S. and Rowan, D.:　Closure of the urinary sphincter mechanism in anaesthetized dogs by means of electrical stimulation of the perineal muscles.　*Brit. J. Surg.*, *53*:1053, 1966.

4.　Caldwell, K.P., Martin, M.R., Flack, F.C. and James, E.D.: An alternate method of dealing with incontinence in children with neurogenic bladders.　*Arch. Dis. Child.*, *44*:625, 1969.

5. Caldwell, K.P., Cook, P.J., Flack, F.C. and James, E.D.: Treatment of post-prostatectomy incontinence by electronic implant. *Br. J. Urol.*, *40*:183, 1968.

6. Caldwell, K.P.: The electrical control of sphincter incompetence. *Lancet,* *2*:174, 1963.

7. Glen, E.: Control of incontinence by electrical devices. IN Urinary Incontinence, K.P.S. Caldwell (ed.), London, Sector, 1975.

8. Godec, C., Cass, A.S. and Ayala, G.F.: Bladder inhibition with functional electrical stimulation. *Urology,* *6*:663, 1975.

9. Groat, W.C. de, and Ryall, R.W.: Reflexes to sacral parasympathetic neurones concerned with micturition in the cat. *J. Physiol.*, *200*:87, 1969.

10. Kaufman, J.J. and Raz, S.: Use of implantable prostheses for the treatment of urinary incontinence and impotence. *Am. J. Surg.*, *130*:244, 1975.

11. Kegel, A.H. and Powell, T.O.: Physiologic treatment of urinary stress incontinence. *J. Urol.*, *63*:808, 1950.

12. Kock, N.G. and Pompeius, R.: Inhibition of vesical motor activity induced by anal stimulation. *Acta Chir. Scand.*, *126*:244, 1963.

13. Marshall, V.F., Marchetti, A.A. and Krantz, K.E.: Correction of stress incontinence by simple vesico-urethral suspension. *Surg. Gynecol. Obstet.*, *88*:509, 1949.

14. Merrill, D.C.: Surgical treatment of urinary incontinence. IN Urinary Incontinence, K.P.S. Caldwell (ed.), London, Sector, 1975.

15. Merrill, D.C., Conway, C. and DeWolf, W.: Urinary incontinence: Treatment with electrical stimulation of the pelvic floor. *Urology,* *5*:67, 1975.

16. Scott, F.B., Bradley, W.E. and Timm, G.W.: Treatment of urinary incontinence by implantable prosthetic sphincter. *Urology, 1*:252, 1973.

17. Sundin, T., Carlsson, C.A. and Kock, N.G.: Detrusor inhibition induced from mechanical stimulation of the anal region and from electrical stimulation of pudendal nerve afferents: An experimental study in cats. *Invest. Urol., 11*:374, 1974.

18. Teague, C.T. and Merrill, D.C.: Electrical pelvic floor stimulation: Mechanism of action. Submitted for publication to *J. Urol.*, 1976.

19. Teague, C.T. and Merrill, D.C.: A means of improving the effectiveness of electrical stimulation in urinary incontinence. *Proc. San Diego Biomed. Symp., 14*:465, 1975.

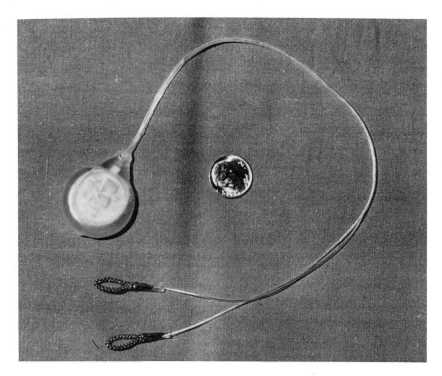

Fig. 1. Implantable Mentor pelvic floor stimulator.

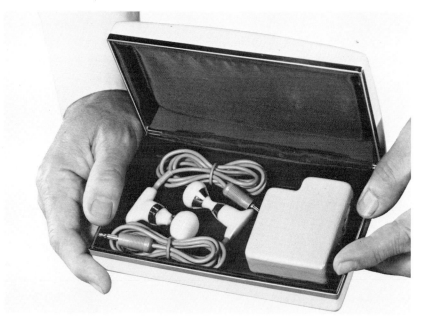

Fig. 2. Mentor transrectal stimulator, medium and large sizes.

743

TOTAL URINARY INCONTINENCE IN BOYS:
MANAGEMENT BY URETHRAL COMPRESSION

Casimir F. Firlit, M.D., Ph.D.

Urinary incontinence in children is an involved problem
to evaluate and frustrating at times to adequately manage.
Once the diagnosis of urinary incontinence is made and
characterized the most appropriate mode of therapy is at best
inadequate. Frequently, timed voiding, valsalva and crede
maneuvers, pharmacological agents, intermittent catheterization, external urethral sheaths or devices and indwelling
catheterization are modalities applied to patients with
urinary incontinence. These modalities have their short
comings. Some achieve dryness at the expense of extensive
surgery with the possibility of long-term ureteral obstruction
and renal deterioration. Others encourage urinary tract
infection, perineal and genital exchoriation, ulceration and
infection. And finally, indwelling catheterization in
addition contributes to urethral strictures and fistulae
disease.

Intermittent catheterization has become a reasonably
effective method to achieve dryness in girls with some types
of neurogenic bladders. However, boys are extremely poor
candidates because of the probability of urethral trauma.
Consequently, boys with incontinence and more so, those with
total urinary incontinence are a special management problem.

Because of our inadequacy in achieving "dryness" in boys, a
modification of the Kaufman II urethral compression technique
was made and applied in two pediatric male patients.

METHOD

Urethral compression achieved by plication of the
corpora cavernosa was performed in two boys with total
urinary incontinence. These patients were aged 5 and 9 years
and were evaluated by extensive urologic, roentgenographic
and urodynamic procedures. Both were determined to have
adequate bladder capacity, viscero ceptive sense and an
absence of internal and external urethral sphincter
mechanisms. Both were found to have flaccid bladders with
reasonable capacities. Consequently, urethral compression
was employed because of failure of all conventional
modalities and prior to performing the conduit urinary
diversion.

With the patient positioned in lithotomy, a "T" shaped
perineal incision was made over the bulbous urethra. A #10F
Robinson, straight catheter was inserted and left indwelling
so as to facilitate dissection. The bulbous urethra was
identified and freed circumferentially (Fig. A). Next the
crura of the penis was found and dissected free from its
origin along the ischial tuberosity and pubis ramus. Care
was exercised to leave the proximal most portion and neurovascular bundle of the crura intact (Fig. B). Once assured
that both crura were adequately mobilized, compression of the
bulbous urethra was achieved by plicating the crura over the
urethral bulb with interrupted 4-0 Ethiflex suture (Fig. C).
Approximately 6-8 sutures were placed and then compression
gauged by withdrawing and reinserting the 10F straight
catheter. As long as the catheter could be passed,

additional sutures were placed. Finally, when the 10F
catheter could not pass, suturing ceased. At this time it
was found that an 8F straight catheter could calibrate and
pass through the compressed urethra. This was accepted as
adequate compression. The wound was closed in layered
fashion without drains. A silastic 8F cystocath was then
placed suprapubically for post operative drainage. Convales-
cence was approximately 3-4 days. At this time the suprapubic tube was clamped and timed valsalva voiding was
instructed and initiated. Residual urine volumes were
determined intermittently. Instruction of the patient and
parents in the operation of his "new" continence mechanism
demands a considerable personal investment in time. The
patient is discharged when a good understanding of valsalva
voiding is demonstrated. Follow-up care is weekly for 2
weeks at which time the suprapubic tube is removed.

CASE REPORTS

Case I. E.R., a 6 year old white male, who shortly
after birth had excision of a presacral teratoma. Since he
has had bowel and total urinary incontinence. At 4½ years of
age urologic evaluation was sought and performed. Excretory
urography was normal. A cystogram demonstrated a bladder of
a capacity of 200cc, without evidence of vesicoureteral
reflux. A trial period with ephedrine, amphetamine, phenyl-
propanolamine and tofranil were without effect. Repeat
evaluation at age 5½ years with anal sphincter studies and
intravesical pressure studies disclosed markedly diminished
to absent external sphincter and pelvic floor EMG activity.
A bladder capacity of 225cc, absent detrusor contraction and
an excellent valsalva pressure of 85mm H_2O were determined.
Further evaluation demonstrated that he would begin dripping

per urethra when 35cc of fluid were placed in the bladder.
He could not consciously stop the dripping of urine. A trial
with an external urethral collecting device was attempted
without success. His penis was too short and small to accept
any external device. Finally, after 1½ years of ineffective
conventional therapy, urethral plication was performed in
January 1975. He retained his suprapubic catheter for two
weeks postoperatively at which time he demonstrated
proficiency in valsalva voiding.

Presently, he voids by valsalva on a timed basis every
2½-3 hours. He does experience some "vague" vesical sense of
pressure which he related to his voiding time. Residual
urine determinations have been 5-10cc on multiple determinations. Stress incontinence and overflow incontinence do
occur when his bladder volume exceeds his outflow resistance,
or if stressful activity accompanies a full bladder. However,
by planning "voiding" prior to stressful activity and by
voiding q3 hours the incidence and magnitude of "wetting" has
been remarkably reduced. Patient and family gratitude
reflect the particular success of this procedure in this
situation. Excretory urography and cystogram remained normal
at 7 months following surgery. No episodes of urinary tract
infection have occurred and no antibacterials are employed.

Case II. R.H., a 12 year old white male presented at
age 9½ years with paraplegia with bladder and bowel incontinence. Subsequent evaluation and surgery resulted in
excision of a lipomeningioma involving the lower spinal cord
and cauda equina. Following excision and decompression,
voluntary muscle control returned; however, bladder and
bowel incontinence persisted. Urologic management for the
subsequent year included attempts at crede and valsalva
voiding without success. Urine dripped continuously from an

empty bladder. Urodynamic evaluations were conducted which disclosed a bladder capacity of 400cc, good viscero ceptive pressure sense, generated valsalva pressure of 60cm H_2O and an absent detrusor response. A short trial of adrenergic agents failed to produce any improvement in bladder control. External urine collecting devices were difficult to apply because of a small penis. In May 1975 urethral plication was performed. Postoperative course was uneventful. Within two weeks valsalva voiding was mastered. He now has only rare stress incontinence while on 4 hour timed voidings. No enuresis has occurred. This patient and family are highly satisfied.

DISCUSSION

Urinary incontinence in these two patients was effectively improved by urethral plication for 10-14 months. At the present time each patient remains "dry" for 2½-4 hours with occasional episodes of minimal wetting associated with stress. Neither patient has experienced urinary tract infections or changes in excretory urography.

We are fully aware that urethral plication may in the long haul pose some problems, heretofore unforeseen. We do not know what effect continued growth and development will have on plication and compression mechanisms. However, since we feel that urinary conduit diversion in pediatric patients should be delayed as long as possible, we feel indeed justified to offer this procedure to patients with total urinary incontinence before recommending a supravesical diversion procedure.

REFERENCES

1. Kaufman, J.J.: A new operation for male incontinence.
    Surg., Gyne. & Obst., 131:295, 1970.
2. Kaufman, J.J.: Surgical treatment of post-prostatectomy
    incontinence: Use of the penile crura to compress the
    bulbous urethra. *J. Urol., 107*:293, 1972.

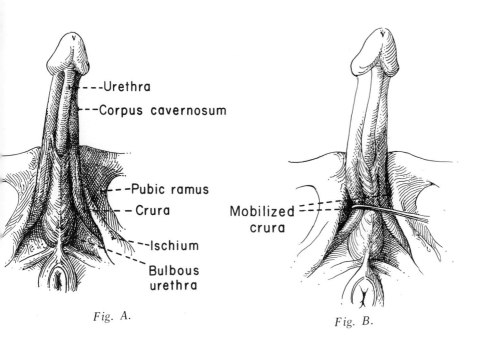

Fig. A.

Fig. B.

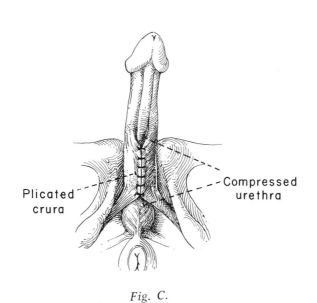

Fig. C.

THE MANAGEMENT OF NEUROGENIC BLADDER
IN PATIENTS WITH MYELOMENINGOCELE:
SPHINCTEROTOMY, BLADDER FLAP
URETHROPLASTY, AND THE ARTIFICIAL
SPHINCTER

F. Brantley Scott, M.D.

Fourteen years of urodynamic observations on patients
with neurogenic bladder dysfunction have convinced me that
the most difficult obstacle to successful management of
neurogenic bladder dysfunction is dysfunction of the urethral
sphincter. This dysfunction is manifested in two ways:
1) Contraction of the sphincter when it ought to be relaxing,
and/or 2) relaxation of the sphincter when it ought to be
contracting. Inappropriate contraction of the sphincter when
it ought to relax leads to unphysiologic bladder pressures;
this can progress to bladder trabeculation, residual urine,
reflux, bilateral hydronephrosis, and recurrent infections.
When the sphincter relaxes when it ought to contract, this of
course results in urinary incontinence. These two manifestations are usually seen in the same patient. Also, even in
those patients in whom there is no striated sphincter muscle,
because of denervation, the detrusor muscle usually lacks the
capability of contracting sufficiently to overcome that
urethral resistance caused by its inherent elasticity. I
reasoned that by removal of the influence of the sphincter,
either by transurethral sphincterotomy in the male or by
bladder flap urethroplasty in the female, voiding could be

improved. Deterrent to this approach was that incontinence
would either be worsened or brought about. However, to solve
the incontinence problem, a man-made artificial sphincter
seemed possible with current technology. Initial work began
in collaboration with William Bradley, Gerald Timm and Dipak
Kothari. Later, John Burton, Samuel Attia and others have
added to this development.[2-4]

An artificial sphincter should meet the following
standards: 1) It should be entirely implantable and accepted
by the body. 2) It must *automatically* occlude the urethra
by a force sufficient to give continence but not so as to
cause impairment of blood circulation. 3) It must
automatically increase its occlusive force on the urethra in
response to stress to prevent stress incontinence. 4) It
must open sufficiently that it offers little or no resistance
to flow during voiding. 5) It must be externally control-
lable. 6) It must open *automatically* in response to detrusor
contractions. 7) If it does not work, the patient should be
no worse off, that is, it should not be an irreversible
procedure.

These standards are met by the artificial sphincter
which has been described in previous publications. This
device will be described again sufficiently to illustrate how
the above standards were met.

THE ARTIFICIAL SPHINCTER (Fig. 1)

1. The hydraulic prosthesis is constructed of medical
grade silicone rubber and is, therefore, implantable and
acceptable by the body.

2. It is externally controlled by two subcutaneous
pumps palpably squeezed by the patient - one to open and one
to close the occlusive cuff encircling the urethra.

3. Regardless of the number of pumps rendered by the patient, valves inside the prosthesis *automatically* control the pressure inside the occlusive cuff at a level lower than diastolic arterial blood pressure. Thus, there is no impairment to the circulation to tissues gathered by the cuff.

4. In the open position, a cuff of sufficient size allows no resistance to flow. Thus, the prosthesis does not create obstruction to urinary flow during voiding.

5. As the pressures of stress increase against the bladder and toward the cuff, an equal pressure against the intra-abdominal reservoir opposes a pressure change across the valve which, therefore, does not open. Thus, the pressures inside the cuff increase only as necessary to prevent stress incontinence and without impairment of circulation.

6. Detrusor contractions which cause the bladder pressure to rise greater than diastolic blood pressure will open the artificial sphincter. This safety feature is possible since detrusor contraction increases pressure selectively against the cuff, changes pressure across the valve (no opposing pressures are transmitted via the reservoir as with stress), and opens and releases unphysiologic bladder pressures.

7. Since the prosthesis is arranged around the urethra and does not require incision into the urinary tract, there is no irreversibility to implanting this prosthesis, as for example in comparison to the ileal loop form of treatment.

PROSTHESIS RELIABILITY

Since the first human implant in 1972, the prosthesis has undergone evolutionary improvement. Increased safety, effectiveness, reliability, and percentage of clinical

success were the result of solving both surgical and
engineering problems. Some problems were better solved by
surgical methods whereas others by engineering methods; in
either case, close collaboration between the surgeon and the
biomedical engineer brought results impossible to have
achieved otherwise. Increased reliability of the device
required improvements in 1) design, 2) materials, 3) workmanship, and 4) quality control testing procedures. Though
there has been no change in the basic design concept of the
prosthesis, there have been many design changes of its
various components, all leading to improved reliability.
With each design change, the device underwent cycling for
44,000 times, equivalent to over 20 years of use. Although
constructed of medical grade silicone rubber, there are many
variations of the silicone polymer, each offering potentially
more reliability. Thus, a materials engineer maintains
constant vigilance in looking to improve the prosthesis.
Workmanship by assembly line method and by humans taking
pride in his particular assembly increased reliability.
Quality control testing procedures required special innovative engineering since a prosthesis of this sort had no
precedent with no prior established test procedures.

SELECTION OF PATIENTS

A complete urologic urodynamic evaluation of the patient
provides information for appropriate planning and staging of
procedures necessary before the artificial sphincter is
implanted. In addition to the usual history and physical
examination, this evaluation includes: 1) careful urine
cultures and antibiotic sensitivity for intense treatment of
urinary infections, 2) voiding flow rates to determine
adequacy of voiding and for evaluating, by comparison, post-

operative results, 3) cystometry to detect areflexia or
hyperreflexia (if hyperreflexic, the effect of Banthine is
assessed by repeat cystometry), 4) pressure-flow study to
determine urethral resistance, 5) urethral pressure profilo-
metry and/or sphincterometry, 6) cystoscopy, 7) voiding
cineradiography, and 8) excretory urography.

    With the results of these studies, decisions are made as
to the need for ureteral implantation, transurethral
sphincterotomy, bladder flap urethroplasty, and so forth.

TRANSURETHRAL SPHINCTEROTOMY

    Transurethral sphincterotomy relieves the male of
sphincteric dysfunction and thus improves bladder emptying.
The sphincterotomy, performed at the 12 o'clock position,
results in good urinary flow, is accompanied by little
bleeding, and does not cause impotence. This method is,
therefore, preferable to cutting the sphincter in its lateral
or posterior positions.

BLADDER FLAP URETHROPLASTY

    Although procedures such as transurethral resection,
radical urethral dilation, Collin's knife triple sphincterotomy, or a "radical" bladder neck plasty may make a patient
incontinent, these procedures do not adequately relieve the
female of urethral resistance for good voiding. The bladder
flap urethroplasty is preferable. This procedure involves:
1) splitting the entire urethra, including the meatus and
bladder neck, 2) developing a pedicle flap on the anterior
bladder surface, 3) advancing the flap to the meatus, and
thus 4) creating a large caliber urethra devoid of occlusive
circular striated sphincteric muscle. This procedure is safe
and simple in the hands of a skilled surgeon, though special

techniques are required for bladder closure.[1] A good result
leaves the patient so totally incontinent that the bladder
empties merely by assuming the erect position.

ANTIREFLUX PROCEDURE

Reflux can be cured surgically provided urethral
sphincter outlet resistance is removed by the above procedures. The technique employed in this series is basically
the Ledbetter-Politano method, except that none of the ureter
is discarded and the ureteral orifice is returned to its
original position after the ureter is re-routed and placed in
a submucosal position. A watertight bladder closure achieved
by a running horizontal extramucosal catgut suture is mandatory if the prosthesis is implanted coincidentally.[1]

RESULTS

A steady improvement in results become apparent as
surgical technique improved and surgical experience increased.
Results improved also because of better staging and better
patient selection. Improved reliability of the prosthesis
has led naturally to increased success. Of all these factors,
the reliability of the prosthesis and the experience of the
surgeon appeared to be of paramount importance. For the
latter, workshops conducted several times each year at St.
Luke's Episcopal Hospital in Houston have provided other
urologists an opportunity to learn these methods.

Only those patients who have received the artificial
sphincter are included in this series. There were 23 females
and 26 males; their ages ranged from 3 to 36 years. Of the
23 females, 19 underwent bladder flap urethroplasty. Three
of these 19 patients had had the artificial sphincter

implanted, then subsequently underwent the bladder flap
urethroplasty to improve their bladder emptying. Seven of
the 19 patients underwent simultaneous bladder flap urethroplasty, ureteral reimplantation, and the artificial sphincter
implantation. Of these seven, five had bilateral ureteral
reimplantations, whereas two had unilateral ureteral reimplantations. Two of the males underwent unilateral ureteral
reimplantation.

Those patients who voided well, had no problems of
urinary tract infections and were continent to the point
that they did not require a perineal pad (any patient who
used a pad was automatically considered a failure) were
considered successful. By these criteria, 49 patients were
evaluated. One of these was lost to follow-up, thus leaving
48. There were 30 successful patients out of the total of
48. The success rate then calculates to be 63%. Using these
same criteria and analyzing all patients who underwent the
artificial sphincter implant from June of 1972 until March of
1976, the success rate in 167 cases was 69%. Thus, the
success rate for the artificial sphincter in the myelomeningocele patients is somewhat less, probably due to multiple
surgery in more complicated cases.

MENINGOMYELOCELE ARTIFICIAL SPHINCTER '72-'76 FAILURES

Cause	Number	Candidates for Repeat
Infected prosthesis	6	6
Surgical errors	6	6
Mechanical problems	5	5
Patient selection	1	0 (mentally
	18	17 retarded)

Significantly, of the eighteen failures, seventeen of
these patients were still considered candidates for repeat

implantation of the artificial sphincter. That is, the patients were not irreversibly damaged by the failed procedure. Analysis of the failure revealed that infection of the prosthesis constituted 1/3 of the failure problems. Of the surgical errors, several were due to mistakes that would not now be made because of information learned in the early part of this series. Mechanical problems have also been improved by increased quality control in the manufacturing of the prosthesis. Thus, one would anticipate that there is improved success during current day procedures. This is borne out by the analysis of those patients done before and those done after April of 1974. April of '74 was chosen for two reasons: 1) This equally divided the 48 patients, and 2) April of '74 marked a turning point in the manufacturing of the prosthesis since most of the major changes in the design and construction of the prosthesis were made between June of '72 and April of '74, there having been very minor modifications since April of '74. Of those patients done before April of '74, there were 11/24 (45%) successes. After April of '74, there were 19/24 (79%) successes. Thus, it is apparent that there has been an improvement in the success rate. This can be attributed to increased reliability of the device, better surgical asepsis, and improved skill in rendering the surgical technique. In plotting the success rate in the 167 patients who have received the artificial sphincter (inclusive of the myelomeningocele patients), the success rate calculated according to year is as follows: 1972 - 44%, 1973 - 65%, 1974 - 82%, 1975 - 85%.

Of course, longer term follow-up will be required to further assess the long-term success of this device. However, analysis of the time intervals at which a failure was identified discloses the fact that 58% of the patients were

obvious failures within two months and 85% were failures
within 10 months. By contrast, the majority of the successful
patients have been followed for over one year. Thus, it
would appear that if there is going to be failure, it is
likely to make itself manifest within an early time interval.

Two case reports will serve to illustrate the benefit
of this prosthesis. In each instance, the patient was under
consideration for ileal loop urinary diversion.

Case #1: L.F., an eight year old girl, had experienced
recurrent infections most of her life. In spite of intermittent catheterization and antibiotics, her upper urinary
tracts displayed progressive hydronephrosis on periodic
excretory urography. Cystogram revealed bilateral reflux and
a heavily trabeculated bladder. Though her urologist was
prepared to do an ileal loop, he felt that the approach
outlined in this article was worth considering first. Therefore, the patient underwent bilateral ureteral reimplantation,
bladder flap urethroplasty, and the implantation of the
artificial sphincter. Now this patient has perfect urinary
control, her urine is free of infection, and she no longer
requires suppressive antibiotics. Her upper urinary tracts
appear to be normal (Fig. 2), and she no longer has reflux.
Although she carries a moderate residual as seen on the post-
voiding film of her excretory urogram, she has not been
plagued with further infections. Periodic urethral pressure
profiles are performed to check on the function of the
artificial sphincter to be sure that it is functioning
properly.

Case #2: G.B. is a 26 year old male with myelomeningocele. This patient had undergone two transurethral resections for the prostate and bladder neck in an effort to aid
him to urinate. In spite of this, the patient urinated very

poorly, and because of progressive bilateral hydronephrosis
and severe infections, he was advised to have an ileal loop.
Because of the patient's marked obesity (he weighed 450 lbs.),
the patient was advised to reduce his weight prior to an
ileal loop urinary diversion. After reducing to 309 lbs.,
several authorities were still reluctant to do an ileal loop
on such an obese person. He was then given a permanent
suprapubic cystostomy tube which resulted in aggravation of
his urinary tract infections with recurrent bouts of sepsis,
recurrent obstruction of the suprapubic tube, progressive
hydronephrosis, and unrelenting infection. In spite of these
indications for urinary diversion, the patient's marked
obesity was still considered a contraindication to an ileal
loop, and the patient was referred to Houston for consideration of the approach outlined in this article. Simultaneous
pressure flow and sphincter electromyographic studies
(micturition study) disclosed extremely high pressures with
poor flow, indicating high resistance due to a persistently
contracting urethral sphincter (Fig. 3).

Transurethral sphincterotomy and removal of the suprapubic tube accomplished good bladder emptying and enabled us
to free the patient of his infection and relieve him of his
hydronephrosis. In March of 1973 the artificial sphincter
was implanted. Postoperatively, the patient empties the
bladder well (Fig. 4), the hydronephrosis has disappeared,
his urinary infection has disappeared, he no longer requires
any antibiotics, and he urinates with an excellent urinary
stream (Fig. 5). Since this patient's implant in March of
1973, he has not required any revisions of the prosthesis,
and he has not leaked urine under any circumstance, either at
night or during sleep. He has been followed since March of
1973 until October 1, 1976 (43 months), and during that time

has had only one urinary tract infection in September of 1974, which cleared on ten days of Mandelamine.

DISCUSSION

A follow-up study of ten years on patients with the artificial sphincter will be required before a suitable comparison can be made between this approach and the ileal loop urinary diversion. The statistics of Shapiro, Liebowitz, and Colodny of children who had had an ileal loop for ten years do not present a very optimistic result for the ileal loop urinary diversion. Fifteen of their 90 patients were dead and five had hopeless uremia. Of the 144 living renal units, 24% had deteriorated. In fact, during this period of ten years, only 13% of their patients had remained free of all complications. Hopefully, the long-term results of the artificial sphincter will give a better outlook.

The statistics presented in this article indicate progressive improvement, consistent with improvement in surgical technique and the design of the prosthesis. Quality control procedures improving the reliability of the device have materially added to the improved success rate. Coincident with evaluating the artificial sphincter was the evaluation of the bladder flap urethroplasty. This procedure has so improved the female in voiding with a poor myelomeningocele bladder that this procedure has now become almost routine. Four patients in this series had an artificial sphincter only, and then three of four subsequently were returned to the operating room for the bladder flap urethroplasty because of persistently infected residual urines. The subsequent postoperative course of all three of these patients was dramatically reversed, thus causing us to administer this procedure in a more routine manner. The

bladder flap urethroplasty and the transurethral sphincterotomy thus represent irreversible procedures in these patients.
This is not undesirable, however, from a medical standpoint
when it is recognized that it is the neurogenic sphincter
dysfunction that causes the pathology in these patients in
the first place. Nevertheless, an artificial sphincter which
could be designed to open the urethra actively could eliminate
the need for these procedures, and for this reason, research
work is currently underway in an effort to develop such a
prosthesis.

At the time of this writing, a new modification of the
artificial sphincter is under clinical evaluation. This
modification includes the attachment of a silicone rubber
balloon which controls the pressure in the prosthesis rather
than depending upon the function of a valve. This modification offers increased reliability and safety and will permit
the design of simpler prostheses. Time will be required, of
course, to determine any adverse side effects of using this
means of controlling pressure in the artificial sphincter.

The mere fact that a number of patients are now
approaching four years since their implantation would indicate that the concept of using an internal, implantable,
hydraulically operated device to produce sufficient occlusive
pressure to the urethra for continence is sound.

The question comes to mind as to whether or not the
artificial sphincter will, in any way, inhibit growth of the
young patient. Some critics have maintained that the cuff
encircling the urethra would produce periurethral fibrosis
and constrict and inhibit the growth of the urethra. Thus
far we have seen no indication of this. The artificial
sphincter cuff size that is put in is comparable to the size
that is used in the adult. The size of the bulbs, the

reservoir, and the valves also are of the adult comparable
size. The size of the urethra following bladder flap
urethroplasty is certainly as large as one encounters in the
adult female. On several occasions we've had opportunity to
make observations with the bladder open and to look down
inside the urethra several years after the artificial
sphincter had been implanted. We find that the tissues are
soft and pliable and that there is no indication of restriction due to periurethral fibrosis nor is there any indication
of inhibition of the urethral growth. Because of these
observations, we do not feel that the age is a contraindication to the artificial sphincter.

The length of the tubing between the various components
obviously will be shorter in the very young patient versus
the adult. Because of this small length, we anticipate that
as the child grows the pumps may migrate superiorly out of
the scrotum or labia. For this reason, we place the pumps
well down into the scrotum or labia in order to allow extra
slack of silicone rubbing tubing. Hopefully, the pumps
would still be accessible for manipulation as the child
reaches his maturity years. On the other hand, if such
proves not to be the case, a simple inguinal incision with
dissection down to the tubing in the subcutaneous position
would allow reintroduction of new pumps with new valves and
new length of tubing to make the pumps again accessible to
the patient. Technically, the ideal time to do the surgery
is before the patient reaches his teenage years at about 8
to 11 years of age. At this time the bladder and bladder
neck structures are more easily accessible yet venous vessels
are less developed, making bleeding less troublesome.

Psychologically, the two critical times in the life of
the patient for continence are before he starts to school at

about age six or before he enters his teenage years, at which
time the patient grows hair on the genitalia thus trapping
bacteria and leading to offensive odors as well as wetness.
The patient's social-psychological problems coupled with the
patient's urological findings determine the timing in
considering the need for this artificial sphincter implant.
Obviously, if the patient is doing well socially and
medically, it is best not to do the artificial sphincter
implant. However, the significant change in the psychological
sense of well being on the part of the patient cannot be
underestimated. By combining transurethral sphincterotomy or
bladder flap urethroplasty with the artificial sphincter, we
are now able to offer a new outlook for this most unfortunate
group of patients.

SUMMARY

     By combining transurethral sphincterotomy in the male or
bladder flap urethroplasty in the female with the implantation of the artificial sphincter, an overall success rate of
63% has been achieved in 48 patients whose neurogenic bladder
is secondary to myelomeningocele. During the time of this
prosthesis development, there has been an improvement in the
success rate from 45% to currently 79% in this same group of
patients. This improvement in success has been attributed
to improvement in surgical skill and knowledge, more careful
selection of patients, and greater reliability of the
prosthesis.

REFERENCES

1. Baum, N., Scott, F.B. and Isaza, O.: Experimental evaluation of bladder closure technique. *Urology, 6*: 195, 1975.

2. Scott, F.B., Bradley, W.E. and Timm, G.W.: Treatment of urinary incontinence by implantable prosthetic sphincter. *Urology, 1*:252, 1973.

3. Scott, F.B., Bradley, W.E. and Timm, G.W.: Treatment of urinary incontinence by an implantable prosthetic urinary sphincter. *J. Urol., 112*:75, 1974.

4. Scott, F.G., Bradley, W.E., Timm, G.W. and Kothari, D.: Treatment of incontinence secondary to myelodysplasia by an implantable prosthetic urinary sphincter. *Southern Medical Journal, 66*:987, 1973.

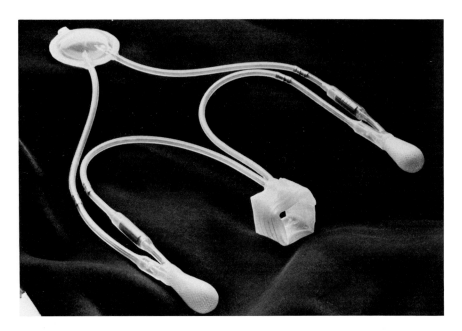

Fig. 1. The implantable artificial sphincter includes the occlusive cuff which encircles the urethra, an inflating pump, a deflating pump, and a reservoir which contains hydraulic fluid used to operate the device. Valves in the pumping mechanisms control the direction of flow of fluid, prevent over-inflation, and control the pressure in the occlusive device such that continence is obtained without interfering with blood supply to the tissues. The placement of the reservoir serves to prevent stress incontinence.

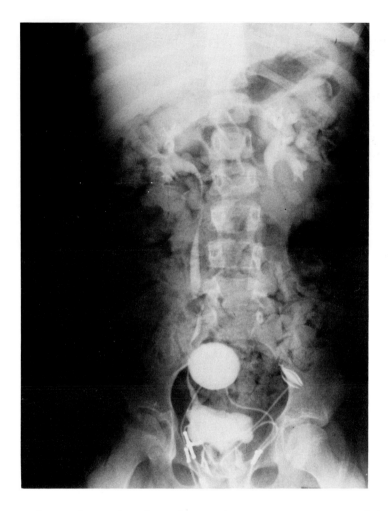

Fig. 2.   Radiographic studies showed normal upper urinary tracts and the presence of the patient's artificial sphincter reservoir. There is some post-voiding residual which is of no clinical significance since the patient maintains a sterile urinary tract without the need for antibiotics. A cystogram proved the successful treatment of bilateral reflux.

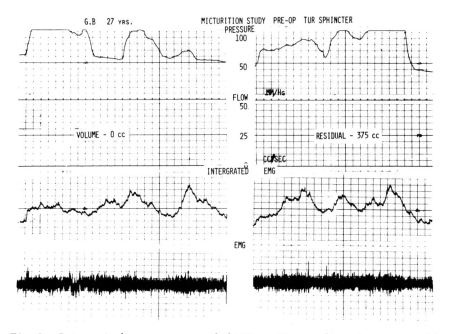

Fig. 3. Intravesical pressures exceeded 100 mmHg, yet the patient was unable to urinate; thus the resistance was infinity. The two lowermost tracings are those of sphincter activity showing that at no time did the sphincter relax, allowing voiding to occur.

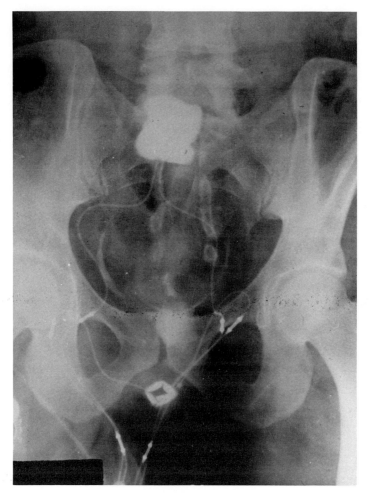

Fig. 4.   The post-voiding film shows almost complete bladder emptying, delicate normal-appearing ureters, the presence of the reservoir of the artificial sphincter, as well as the occlusive cuff which in this instance encircles the bulbous urethra.

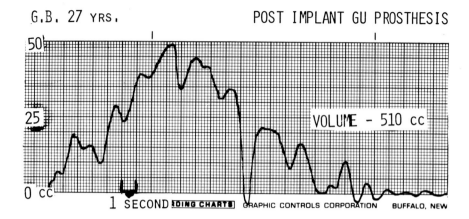

G.B. 27 YRS.   POST IMPLANT GU PROSTHESIS

50
25
0 cc
1 SECOND **IDING CHARTS** GRAPHIC CONTROLS CORPORATION   BUFFALO, NEW

VOLUME - 510 cc

Fig. 5. The normal urinary flow rate in a 27-year old man is ordinarily about 25 cc/second. This patient voids at a peak flow of about 49 cc/second, indicating excellent urinary flow with little outlet resistance.

INFECTION OF THE URINARY TRACT
IN PATIENTS WITH MENINGOMYELOCELE

Arthur T. Evans, M.D.

Patients with neurogenic spastic or atonic bladders, such as are seen in myelodysplasia, commonly harbor bacteria. One hundred percent of all patients with bladder dyskinetics have at sometime in their lives a urinary tract infection (UTI). The major cause of death in patients with meningo-myelocele is renal failure secondary to UTI. A UTI is more difficult to correct in the patient with a neurogenic bladder. Because of the high incidence of urinary tract infection in these patients, each physician providing care for myelo-dysplastic patients is obligated to be ever conscious of this threat of UTI to these patients' lives. They are therefore obligated to utilize all possible precautions to prevent bacterial innoculation of the urinary tract. They are like-wise obligated to effect, if at all possible, eradication of a urinary tract infection in the patients under discussion.

The patient with bladder dyskinetics is more prone to urinary tract infections for a number of reasons. UTI's are established by several routes: 1) hematogenous spread, 2) ascending bacteria, 3) lymphagenous spread, and 4) direct extension, as by a fistula. For emphasis, I list a fifth cause, iatrogenic infection, in order to stress its impor-tance. In the female, no doubt, urethral ascent of bacteria is ever a threat and may even be a nearly daily occurrence.

The distended ischemic walled bladder may be more susceptible
to the hematogenous metastasis of bacteria. Lymphatic spread
of bacteria to the urinary tract may occur under some unusual
conditions. Fistulous tracts, as created by the surgeon,
between the body surface or gastrointestinal tract and the
urinary transport system serve as entrances for bacteria to
the urinary transport system. The iatrogenic introduction of
bacteria by fistula production or more importantly by instrumentation needs proper assessment. There are many dyskinetic
bladders which regain their use and/or serve their purpose as
a reservoir for urine adequately because of the intermittent
or constant placement of a transurethral catheter. The placement of instruments in the bladder for endoscopy, diagnostic
x-ray studies, or drainage of the bladder can and may introduce bacteria into this organ. These procedures may be life-
saving but again may be life-threatening. Judicious and
careful utilization of urinary tract instrumentation is
essential. The same axiom holds for upper urinary tract
diagnostic studies and drainage, as well as for surgical
procedures as they relate to the bacteria which are innoculated into various portions of the urinary transport system.

Other factors play a role in influencing the colonization of bacteria in the urinary tract. Obstruction to normal
urine flow along the nephrons and the urinary transport
system facilitates the propagation of bacteria innoculated
into the stagnant or residual urine produced by the
obstruction. Obstruction may be of multiple origins in the
myelodysplastic patient. Some of these are detrusor atonia,
external sphincter spasm, urethral strictures, vesico-
uretero-renal reflux, calculus obstruction, vesicle folds
and cellules, toxic ureterectasis, inflammatory ureteral
polyps, ileal loop fibrosis, uretero-ileal fibrosis, and

nephron obstruction by fibrosis due to bacterial pyelonephritis. These and any other obstructive factors should, if
possible, be eradicated or circumvented to relieve urine
stagnation.

Another group of factors which influence continuing or
recurring urinary tract infection is reservoirs of infection
within the urinary tract. These reservoirs of bacteria serve
as a source of reinnoculation of the urinary tract. Such
conditions as calculi containing bacteria, bacterial prosta-
titis, diverticula of the transport system, infected ureteral
stumps, and septic areas within the kidney substance are
reservoirs of bacteria which must be eliminated to protect
the urinary tract from recurrence of infection.

The organisms which infect the urinary tract of the
patients under discussion are no different than those
organisms listed in any standard text as the organisms which
commonly cause urinary tract infection. A difference,
however, does exist in the incidence of infection by the
various bacteria. E. coli, which causes 80-90% of UTI
infections, is isolated only in 30-50% of urinary tracts of
patients with "neurogenic bladders". The organisms are more
commonly what I term secondary invaders. These organisms,
such as Proteus, Pseudomonas, Serratia marsescens, Provi-
dencia, Streptococcus faecalis, are more commonly seen in the
prolonged, persistent, recurring infections of the patient
with myelodysplasia. The isolated organism often changes
from one species to another, and mixed infections may often
occur. These bacteria commonly follow instrumentation or
surgical intervention and urinary diversion. I consider
them to be saprophytes. These grow - many of them - as such
naturally. They are able to establish themselves only after
there has been previous bacterial or surgical or, upon

occasion, ischemic destruction or derangement of the normal urothelium. I believe these urothelial effects alter or destroy some of the normal host defense mechanisms of the transport system. These mechanisms include urothelial acid production, possibly a mucoid protective coating, meaningful phagocytosis, mechanical transport of urine, as well as conceivably changes in the pH and composition of urine which may make the saprophytic-like organisms' proliferation more likely. E. coli, the initial opportunistic invader of the urinary tract, must set the urothelial stage for instrument innoculation of the tissue, by altering the above and possibly other host defense mechanisms of the transport system.

Infections of the urinary tract must be properly identified. Proper collection of the urine from the myelo-dysplastic patient may not be readily accomplished. A number of techniques may be utilized for a particular patient. These techniques are 1) suprapubic tap, 2) midstream voided speci-men, 3) collection apparatus, or 4) even at times catheteri-zation is essential. Greater than 10^5 colonies of bacteria per cc indicate infection in the female when the urine is collected by a midstream voided specimen. The tap specimen and the catheter-obtained specimen need not colonize nearly as many bacteria per cc to be significant. The use of sensitivity studies and culture is imperative to efficient, effective antimicrobial therapy. Bacterial typing may help identify relapse as opposed to re-infection in recurring infection. Immunofluorescent tagging may identify upper urinary tract bacteria as opposed to bladder bacteria. Gallium-67 scanning may identify septic areas as bladder or kidney infections, at least in more severe infections. The Greiss Test is 90% accurate in identifying UTI and has its greatest application, in my opinion, in identifying for the

patient the effectiveness of antimicrobial therapy and the
presence of recurrent infection at home. The dip slide
coated with nutrient and EMB agar has a place for home
culturing of urine, as does the media square on a dip stick.
The examination of the centrifuged stained sediment of urine
by the microscope has not been displaced for the experienced.
Significant bacteria can be identified with an accuracy of
85-90%. I find the culturing of urine on blood or Hinton-
Mueller agar disks with simultaneous application of sensitivity disks - a modification of Kirby-Bauer technique - very
reliable (95%). This technique provides 4-12 hour sensitivity
determinations. It is excellent for office practice. It
eliminates empirical antimicrobial prescribing.

The problem of antibiotic prescribing for UTI revolves
around the type of infection. The severity and type of
infection must be classified or identified. The most sensible
identification seems to be 1) mild to moderate simple
infection, 2) severe infections with systemic manifestation,
3) chronic infections, and 4) recurring infections. There
are no hard and fast rules for drug selection for these
infections. There is no unanimity of opinion about drug
therapy for all cases. More importantly, there are great
variances (30-76%) in the percentage of organisms, of a
specific type, that are sensitive to a certain drug in one
community as compared to another. There are even great
differences in the susceptibility of a certain bacterium to
a certain drug in a given community. This is most apparent
when community acquired bacteriuria is compared with hospital
acquired bacteriuria. Therefore, in a given urinary tract
infection, drug susceptibility testing is the most accurate
method of arriving at proper drug therapy. There may be a
question as to whether the susceptibility test should be

carried out upon an antimicrobial drug concentration obtainable in the urine or serum; but, for now, depend upon the
given testing techniques of the Kirby-Bauer techniques.
Utilize tube dilution testing and urine or serum drug
concentrations for unusual circumstances and controlled,
specific studies.

There are many idiosyncracies of antimicrobials. There
are drugs which have no determinable tissue levels, yet are
effective for treating pyelonephritis. There are drugs which
bind more with protein than others. There may be drugs which
may be more effective when there are more RBC's or WBC's in
the urine. Urine pH influences drug effectiveness. Bacteria
may affect urinary pH. There is evidence that almost any
bacterium that infects the urinary tract can, under proper
conditions, split urea to ammonia. Certain drugs have
certain toxicities, and the antimicrobial half-life must be
utilized in dosage determination in host toxic states. The
method of detoxification of a drug requires understanding.
Each antimicrobial has a package insert. These inserts today
are as nearly accurate as they are able to be as relates to
contraindications, precautions, and adverse reactions, as
well as their chemistry mode of action and detoxification,
and their indication, dosage, and their available dosage-
size capsules or pills. Read these and be familiar with the
drugs you use. This dissertation is not able to cover all of
these facts.

Understanding that susceptibility tests are the guide to
therapy, the following outline must act only as a guide for
various classifications of infection:

I. Mild to moderate infection

    A. Sulfonamides

    B. Trimethoprim-sulfamethoxazole

C. Nitrofurantoin

D. Nalidixic acid

E. Methanamine + ascorbic, mandelic or hippuric acid

F. Tetracycline

The length of therapy is optional and may be 3-14 days. Follow-up with urinalysis and possibly culture seems logical. Greiss testing aids therapy guidance.

II. Severe infection with systemic manifestation

A. Cephalosporins

B. Ampicillin/Carbenicillin

C. Gentamicin

D. Tobramycin

E. Kanamycin (specific cases)

F. Colistin

G. Rifampin (specific cases)

H. Chloramphenicol (when only drug of choice)

III. Chronic infection (long-term therapy)

A. Nitrofurantoin

B. Sulfonamides

C. Trimethoprim-sulfamethoxazole

D. Methanamine + acidification of urine

May be given in decreasing dosage or half dose for months.

IV. Prophylactics

A. Nitrofurantoin

B. Sulfonamides

C. Trimethoprim-sulfamethoxazole

D. Methanamine + urine acidification

May be given only once a day for months. May be treated only when there is acute exacerbation with drugs as in I or II.

(The dosage utilized is given in any standard text but more specifically in the package insert of the antimicrobial.) There can be no cookbook therapy for urinary tract infection, other than the susceptibility tests. The liver and renal function must be evaluated and the drug toxicities fitted to these organs' efficiencies. The standard dosage may need modification according to hepatic and renal function.

The essentials of urinary infection are 1) identify for certain that an infection is present, 2) eradicate obstructions and reservoirs of bacteria, 3) identify the organism, 4) determine the status of the patient as to severity of the infection and the general functional status of the body systems, 5) determine the bacterial antimicrobial susceptibility, and choose an appropriate drug, and 6) continue to evaluate the response of the patient to the prescribed antimicrobial. Lastly, if the infections recur or persist, do not hesitate to re-evaluate the urodynamics and the structural anatomy of the urinary transport system, as well as continually search, by finite history-taking, for a mode of re-infection.

INDICATIONS FOR CUTANEOUS
VESICOSTOMY, TECHNIQUE AND LONG TERM
RESULTS

Ananias C. Diokno, M.D.

Cutaneous vesicostomy[6] was devised in 1958 to provide
tubeless drainage of the urinary bladder for patients with
neurogenic bladder dysfunctions. Experience with this
technique has been conflicting. Numerous urologists from
different centers were unsatisfied with the results and have
abandoned this procedure.[1,5] However, at the University of
Michigan where one of the techniques for this procedure
originated, we feel that there is still a place for cutaneous
vesicostomy as a form of urinary diversion. Several precautions must be observed to obtain a successful result. The
procedure is contraindicated in the presence of obesity,
severe stress urinary incontinence, small contracted bladder
and atonic severely dilated ureters. Adult patients should
be able to apply their own device while in infants and young
children no attempt was made to apply any collecting device
except for diapers applied over the stoma.

Our first choice in the treatment of bladder dysfunction
in myelodysplastics is intermittent catheterization.
Cutaneous vesicostomy is our choice in infants and young
children with chronic urinary retention and overflow
incontinence, recurrent urinary tract infection or
deterioration of upper tracts if intermittent catheterization

fails or it cannot be performed by the parents or patient. This procedure has produced satisfactory urinary drainage, control of infection and prevention of upper tract deterioration.[4] One of the advantages of cutaneous vesicostomy is its reversibility.[8] This procedure is undertaken with the idea that as they mature, these patients can participate actively in the management of their bladder dysfunction and other forms of treatment can be instituted. This includes intermittent self-catheterization,[7] artificial urinary sphincter,[3] various forms of voiding manipulation (crede and Valsalva maneuver), drug therapy or other forms of urinary diversion.

The technique of vesicostomy varies. Blocksom[2] uses the dome of the bladder and anastomoses it to the skin. Lapides[8] uses a skin flap and incorporates it with the bladder flap in forming a vesicocutaneous fistula. Ross[9] has modified the Lapides technique and reverses the orientation of the bladder and skin flap. The purpose of using a flap of skin is to prevent stomal stenosis. We have always used the Lapides technique at our institution.

In 1971 we reported the result of 52 patients with cutaneous vesicostomy followed for five to ten years.[8] The bladder dysfunctions were secondary to spinal cord trauma, neoplasm, congenital anomalies, multiple sclerosis and bladder decompensation. There were 46 adults and six children. Seventy-seven percent (40/52 patients) were alive with good renal function. Seven patients died, two of pneumonia and five of renal failure. Of the five, four had pyelonephritis and nephrolithiasis prior to the vesicostomy. Five patients developed nephrolithiasis. Two had severe pyelonephritis prior to the vesicostomy and three were lost to follow-up.

The most up-to-date results of vesicostomy in children were reported in 1975 by Duckett, Jr. of Childrens Hospital in Philadelphia.[4] He evaluated the result of vesicostomy performed on 54 myelomeningocele children at their institution. His follow-up period was six months to ten years. Fifty-five percent of the patients were operated upon under 1½ years of age while 45 percent were between 2 and 12 years. His result showed that 54 percent (23 patients) had sterile urine with normal or improved pyelogram, 17 percent (9 patients) had infected urine with normal or improved pyelogram, 13 percent (10 patients) were failures and 4 percent (2 patients) died from non-urological complications.

Our experience as well as the recent report by Duckett, Jr. have reaffirmed our belief that vesicostomy has a place in the management of bladder dysfunctions among myelomeningocele children. This procedure has provided adequate urinary drainage and preservation of renal function. Its reversibility is an ideal feature because other more socially acceptable forms of therapy can be instituted later if found necessary. In choosing this procedure, the precautions and indications should be strictly adhered to in order to minimize failures.

CONCLUSION

Cutaneous vesicostomy is our choice in the management of bladder dysfunctions of infants and young children with recurrent urinary tract infection, chronic retention or deterioration of upper tracts provided intermittent catheterization is not feasible.

REFERENCES

1. Bell, T.E., Hoddin, A.O. and Evans, A.T.: Tubeless
    cystostomy in children. *J. Urol., 100*:459, 1968.
2. Blocksom, B.: Bladder pouch for prolonged tubeless
    cystostomy. *J. Urol., 78*:398, 1957.
3. Diokno, A.C. and Taub, M.: Experience with artificial
    urinary sphincter at Michigan. Accepted for publication
    to *J. Urol.*
4. Duckett, W. Jr.: Cutaneous vesicostomy in childhood.
    Urol. Clin. N. Amer., 1:485, 1974.
5. Ireland, G.W., Geist, R.W.: Difficulties with vesicos-
    tomies in 15 children with myelomeningocele. *J. Urol.,
    103*:341, 1970.
6. Lapides, J., Ajemian, E.P. and Lichtwardt, J.R.:
    Cutaneous vesicostomy. *J. Urol., 84*:609, 1960.
7. Lapides, J., Diokno, A.C., Lowe, B.S. and Kalish, M.D.:
    Follow-up in unsterile, intermittent self-catheterization.
    J. Urol., 111:184, 1974.
8. Lapides, J., Koyanagi, T. and Diokno, A.C.: Cutaneous
    vesicostomy: 10 year survey. *J. Urol., 105*:76, 1971.
9. Ross, G., Jr., Michener, F.R., Brady, C., Jr., et al:
    Cutaneous vesicostomy: A review of 36 cases. *J. Urol.,
    94*:402, 1965.

INDICATIONS FOR SIGMOID CONDUIT DIVERSION: TECHNIQUE AND LONG TERM RESULT

Lester Persky, M.D.

The increasing disenchantment with long term uretero-ileostomy as the prime method of urinary diversion has been engendered by a variety of difficulties. Some of these are seen early; others reflect the complications seen after years of increasing utilization of this valuable surgical tool. The early surgical problems are familiar to all of us: intestinal obstruction, prolonged ileus, eviscerations, ureteral leaks, intestinal fistulae, pyelonephritis. The later ones similarly are all too well known: stomal contracture and epithelialization, elongation of the ileal loop, stone formations, ureteral obstruction, narrowing of the intestinal anastomoses, and last but not least, deterioration of renal function with attendant loss of renal reserve. These many problems are seen especially in the myelodysplastic child in whom because of a lack of sensation or difficulty in communi-cating, fevers are often overlooked and overt obstructions not readily diagnosed.

These many challenges have made urologists, pediatri-cians, and nephrologists seek alternative routes for urinary diversion. Indwelling urethral catheters create sepsis and lead to recurrent pyelonephritis. Ureterosigmoidostomy would engender a further host of real troubles due to the

lack of a competent anal sphincter in the majority of these
infants. The cutaneous vesicostomy, although perhaps
applicable to certain situations in the neurogenic, handicapped person, has disadvantages which are almost impossible
to overcome in the minds of many workers. Cutaneous uretero-
stomies have the disadvantage of the need for separate
appliances and the threat of constriction and obstruction at
the stomal level. Utilizing nephrostomy drainage would
similarly create infection due to the presence of a foreign
body intraluminally. Therefore, other forms of diversion
have been advocated. Intermittent catheterization of the
children has been proposed and is widely used for many of
these patients. However, this does not always lead to
successful outcomes or completely obviate the need for
diversion in a certain number of these patients. An alternative to these techniques has been the use of a segment of
sigmoid in place of the ileal sleeve. The advantages,
theoretical and real, lend some weight to the argument for
the abandonment of the conventional ureteroileostomy.

The technique of the actual procedure is a relatively
direct and simple approach (Fig. 1). The large bowel is
utilized after appropriate cleansing and sterilization. The
segment to be used is separated from the remainder of the
large bowel with its blood supply intact; a two layer intestinal anastomosis restores continuity to the large intestine.
Usually an inner layer of continuous catgut and an outer
layer of interrupted silk is employed. The proximal end of
the segment is then closed similarly in two layers. The
ureters are picked up, divided close to the bladder, and the
right ureter is then brought beneath the mesentery of the
sigmoid to the left side where lateral to the sigmoid it lies
next to its mate. At this point, the ureters are spatulated

and anastomosed to the large intestinal segment. A small
muscular, extramucosal tunnel as described by Leadbetter[1] is
first made, and then the ureters are sutured to the mucosa.
The muscular layers in the region are then closed over these
ureters for a length of 2-3 centimeters. After the extraperitonealization of the anastomosis the sigmoid loop is
brought out through a stoma in the left lower quadrant.

The long term results have been good to date. Several
older studies with careful followups[2,3] have revealed a lower
incidence of stomal complications, pyelonephritis and
obstruction. Although there have been complications they
appear to be readily handled and of lesser significance.

DISCUSSION

As far as we can ascertain anti-refluxing techniques
will possibly obviate the gradual deterioration of function
seen so often in the long term followup of ureteroileostomy.
The stoma is usually of such caliber that elongation of the
loop due to obstruction is not seen and stasis is not created.
The incidence of stone disease will also probably be of less
degree and should not be a major difficulty. The success in
the prevention of pyelonephritis by the Leadbetter approach
has been demonstrated by a series of laboratory experiments
involving dogs by Richie and Skinner[4] at UCLA.

The extraperitonealization of the loop and the positioning of it lateral to the sigmoid also makes less likely the
occurrence of intestinal obstruction. It should render the
surgery easier, moreover, since there is less likelihood of
embarrassment of the lumen of the intestinal anastomosis
seen so often in small bowel surgery. One possible disadvantage is the difficulty one may anticipate in relocating
the stoma if this should be necessary. This will undoubtedly

be less of a problem than heretofore since the stoma is so uniformly adequate.

In general we must conclude that the sigmoid conduit offers an alternative means of urinary diversion when this is dictated in the myelodysplastic child. One hopes, nevertheless, that too avid an attitude will not lead to too hasty attempts at the universal application of this procedure.

REFERENCES

1. Leadbetter, W.F.: Considerations of the problems incident to the performance of uretero-ureterostomy: Report of a technique. *J. Urol.*, *73*:67, 1955.

2. Mogg, R.: Urinary diversion using the colonic conduit. *Urol. Int.*, *23*:53, 1965.

3. Hendren, Hardy: Personal communication.

4. Richie, J.P. and Skinner, D.G.: Urinary diversion: Physiologic rationale for non-refluxing colonic conduits. *Brit. J. Urol.*, *47*:269, 1975.

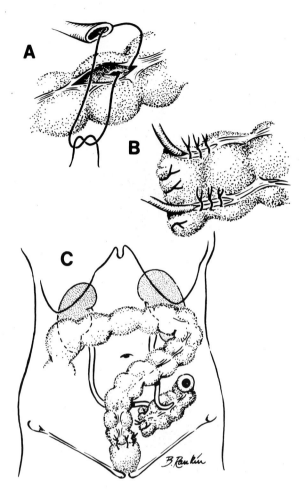

Fig. 1.

STOMAL APPLIANCES

George T. Klauber, M.D.

INTRODUCTION

A suitable urinary stomal appliance should be leakproof, comfortable, lightweight, cheap, and have adequate storage capacity. A urinary diversion can achieve maximal success only after correct selection and application of such an appliance. Various devices and equipment will be reviewed and a method of selecting appropriate equipment for the individual patient will be presented.

MEASUREMENT OF STOMAL OPENING

A urinary stoma should be measured with the patient in the recumbent and sitting positions, using a measuring guide. The stoma should first be measured with the patient lying down, using the guide aperture which permits a margin of approximately 1/16" around the stoma. The applicance aperture to be selected, therefore, has a diameter 1/8" larger than the stoma. If the stoma is oval in shape, the largest and the smallest diameters should be measured with 1/8" added to each measurement before the appliance is selected.

Intestinal stomata should be observed for peristaltic activity so that the greatest dimension is selected. The larger and more protuberant the stoma, the more important this becomes.

The patient should slowly sit up with the measuring
guide in position around the stoma, to see if any variation
in size occurs. Sitting is the most critical measuring
position, because the stoma may enlarge, indicating the need
for a larger appliance. Not infrequently, deep skin creases
may appear adjacent to the stoma when the patient is sitting.
Such creases can create lateral conduits for possible leakage
of urine under the stomal device.

Measurement for a permanent device should be made only
after post-operative edema has subsided.

If the stomal opening of the appliance is too large,
the peristomal skin becomes hyperkeratotic and scarred, and
stenosis of stoma also can result. If the opening is too
small, the stoma itself will be traumatized, ulcerated and
bleeding, and may cicatrize.

If the appliance is incorrectly centered over the stoma,
both ulceration and hyperkeratosis can occur. Hyperkeratosis
can be prevented by careful stomal fitting. Once hyperkeratosis has occurred, direct application of the appliance
over the affected area may resolve the problem.

FACEPLATES

A faceplate is designed to fit around the stoma and
against the skin. It is available in a multitude of sizes,
materials and convexities, in addition to different shaped
openings, round or oval. Such variety insures selection of
an ideal and custom faceplate for any individual. Faceplates
may be separate as part of a two piece appliance, or an
integral part of a one piece appliance.

A faceplate with a convex surface against the skin is
ideal for use over skin creases, or for a patient with
excessive subcutaneous fat. The latter fails to give

adequate resistance or support around the stoma. A convex
faceplate is hard and pushes down the peristomal skin for a
firm fit. It also requires a belt for support. A flexible
or soft faceplate cannot remain fixed on the mobile skin
overlying a thick layer of subcutaneous fat.

   Belts are not always necessary to hold a faceplate in
place, especially when the peristomal skin is firm; water-
proof adhesive tape around the edge, or skin adhesive alone
is often sufficient to hold a faceplate in position. Almost
any flat or slightly convex faceplate may be used for a
protuberant stoma emerging from a firm abdominal wall;
providing the skin does not crease in the sitting position.

SKIN ADHESIVES AND GASKETS

   Tincture of benzoin and skin cement are two of the
original adhesives in use for many years. A light coat of
benzoin or cement is applied to the faceplate with a second
coat applied to the skin around the stoma, approximating the
diameter of the faceplate. The faceplate is then placed
against the body and a good bond is usually achieved. The
disadvantage of skin cement is that it is somewhat messy to
use, and difficult to remove and clean up between changes.

   A double faced adhesive seal was the first innovative
change in the use of stomal appliances. It consists of a
disc with adhesive on both sides and is cut to the appropriate
size and shape. Protective paper is peeled from one side of
the adhesive disc and the exposed sticky surface is applied
to the faceplate. The protective paper on the other side is
then removed and the faceplate applied to the body.

   Some years ago a number of softer seals or gaskets were
introduced. The first was a karaya gum gasket consisting of
a soft mass of pure karaya gum powder in jelly form. Pure

karaya gum dissolved quickly so that the gaskets were
modified and improved by adding a number of ingredients under
the trademark of "Collyseal".

A "Collyseal" does not melt or dissolve as quickly as
the pure karaya gum seal and can be worn for five to seven
days with comfort. It is exceptionally easy both to apply
and to remove, the only requirement being to dampen the
"collyseal" with saliva or water.

Other soft seals, such as "Stomahesive" or "Reliaseals"
have been introduced; unfortunately they are expensive and
have a tendency to dissolve and coat the inside of the
urinary pouch, making it stiff and uncomfortable.

TEMPORARY APPLIANCES

Immediately after surgical construction of a urinary
stoma, a temporary appliance is recommended, because a stoma
changes in size from day to day. At first a stoma enlarges
after surgery, secondary to edema; it then shrinks as it
matures. Once matured, usually two to four weeks after
surgery, the stoma can be fitted with a more permanent
device. A temporary bag is usually transparent for easy
inspection of urine and stoma. It is affixed to the skin
by adhesive incorporated into the appliance, either with or
without a karaya gasket.

PERMANENT APPLIANCES

Permanent appliances are available in either a one or a
two piece design. A one piece appliance has the faceplate
permanently attached to the pouch. Some patients and
parents prefer the one piece appliance because it is simple
to care for and to apply. Obese children or those with
perceptual handicaps usually find a one piece appliance

easier to handle than a two piece device. One piece
appliances are available in rubber or soft vinyl plastic in
different sizes, with different convexities built into the
faceplate.

The two piece appliance is preferred by this author,
because a patient can apply a faceplate by herself and be
sure it is properly centered around the stoma. This is
particularly important with an oval or angled stoma. An
infinite variety of pouches, to fit any particular faceplate,
may be selected in all sizes, shapes and colors.

ADDITIONAL PRODUCTS

Other products are available to protect the skin from
adhesive or tape; "skin-jel" or "skin-prep" can be applied
in a thin, quick drying coat to the skin under the cement or
tape. Various deodorants and cleansing agents are available
for use with these appliances.

A night drainage bag has sufficient capacity to accommodate the urine output produced all during the night.

NEUROLOGICAL DISTURBANCES OF SEXUAL
FUNCTION AMONG PATIENTS WITH
MYELODYSPLASIA

A. Estin Comarr, M.D.

The neurophysiological principals of sexual function
have been described previously.[1] Briefly, erection is the
result of tumescence of the corpora cavernosa and the corpus
spongiosum induced by active hyperemia from arterial vaso-
dilatation.   Detumescence is caused by vasoconstriction of
the arteries.   Tumescence results from stimulation of the
cholingeric and detumescence from the adrenergic components
of the autonomic nervous system. Ejaculation consists of
seminal emission and true ejaculation.   Emission results
from contraction of the smooth muscles of the vasa deferentia,
prostate, and spermatic vesicles.   Ejaculation results from
clonic contraction of the pelvic floor muscles, including the
external urethral sphincter.   Orgasm starts with the peristalsis of the smooth muscles of the internal sexual organs and
the tonic contraction of the straited muscles of the pelvic
floor and it terminates upon completion of striated muscle
clonus.   Ejaculation and orgasm depend on autonomic and
somatic nerves.

CLASSIFICATION OF NEUROGENIC SEXUAL ACTIVITY
    Since 1946, this writer has classified myelodysplastic
patients in terms of sexual potential the same as spinal

797

cord injury patients. The diagnosis that I use can be made
at the "bedside" or in the "office". The diagnosis is based
on a somatic examination of the sacral segments of the spinal
cord; obviously, this classification has shortcomings since,
as noted in the introductory paragraph, the autonomic
nervous system plays a great role in sexual function.
However, the astute physician with experience will recognize
during this type of examination the shortcomings of making
decisions by inference and will allow for same.

   The majority of patients will fall into one of the
following classifications as a diagnosis:

I. Upper Motor Neuron Sex Complete; synonym, reflex complete
    sex
    Findings:
    (a) Positive rectal external sphincter reflex response
         by digital examination.
    (b) Absent sensation to pin prick and light touch in the
         penile skin bilaterally, scrotal skin bilaterally
         and perianal skin bilaterally.
    (c) Absent volitional contraction of the external rectal
         sphincter by digital examination.

II. Upper Motor Neuron Sex Incomplete; synonym, reflex
    incomplete sex
    Findings:
    (a) Positive rectal external sphincter response by
         digital examination.
    (b) Presence of *any* pin prick or light touch sensation
         in the penile and/or scrotal and/or perianal skin;
         and/or,
    (c) Presence of any degree of volitional contraction of
         the external rectal sphincter by digital examination.

III. Lower Motor Neuron Sex Complete; synonym, areflexic complete sex

Findings:

(a) Negative rectal external sphincter reflex response by digital examination.

(b) No sensation to pin prick or light touch in the penile skin bilaterally, scrotal skin bilaterally, and perianal skin bilaterally.

(c) No volitional contraction of the external sphincter by digital examination.

IV. Lower Motor Neuron Sex Incomplete; synonym, areflexic sex incomplete.

Findings:

(a) Negative external rectal sphincter reflex response by digital examination.

(b) Presence of any pin prick or light touch sensation in the penile, and/or scrotal and/or perianal skin; and/or,

(c) Presence of any degree of volitional contraction of the external rectal sphincter by digital examination.

From the above described classification it is self-evident that the *basic diagnosis* is dependent on the presence or absence of reflex activity of the rectal external striated sphincter.

Thus, the diagnosis that is made refers to the presence or absence of reflex activity of the external sphincter of the rectum; but by *inference*, the same diagnosis is made of the bladder and *sex*.

The term "incomplete" as used in the neurological examination is a poor term for it does not tell the reader the amount of loss of sensation or whether the loss is of pin

prick or light touch. It does not relate the degree of loss
of volitional contraction of the external sphincter. Thus,
the diagnosis if incomplete, must include for the reader, the
specific type of loss (pin prick or light touch and lateral-
ity) in the skin of the penis, scrotum and perianal sites,
and/or the degree of external sphincter volutional control.

FINDINGS OF SEXUAL FUNCTIONS AMONG SIXTEEN MYELODYSPLASTIC PATIENTS

MALES

In this study there were 11 males. The ages of the
patients studied were: 19, 20, 21, 23, 24 (two patients),
26, 30, 34, 42 and 56.

One patient had an upper motor neuron, incomplete type
of sex; six patients had lower motor neuron, complete, sex;
four patients had lower motor neuron incomplete sex.

Eight patients had balanced bladders and emptied their
bladders into an external condom collecting device, one
patient had a perianal catheter and one patient had an intraurethral catheter.

The patients were interviewed in terms of their sex
dreams. One patient did not have sex dreams of any kind.
Six patients had dry sex dreams, i.e., they dreamt of foreplay and/or intromission, but did not ejaculate or reach an
orgasm. Two patients dreamt of coitus and had ejaculation
and orgasm; however, there was no evidence of ejaculate in
the bed clothing. Two patients dreamt of coitus and did
ejaculate and have an orgasm; the ejaculate was found in the
bed clothing.

The patient with upper motor neuron, incomplete sex was
30 years of age. He had been married and was divorced after
3½ years. Dermatome testing revealed an L1 level on the

right and an L3 level on the left. Sensation was absent in
the sacral segments except for hypalgesia in the left penile
skin. He had no volitional control of the external rectal
sphincter but positive external sphincter reflex tone. He
had dry sex dreams. He had psychogenic erections which were
of short duration. He had never made an attempt at coitus.
He could not ejaculate with masturbation. He had never made
an attempt at fellatio. With cunnilingus his partner reached
an orgasm. He stated that it was "fantastic" for both of
them even though he could not ejaculate. He stated that his
partners preferred him to "normal" males because he was "so
genteel".

Six patients had lower motor neuron, complete, sex. The
ages were: 23, 24 (two), 26, 34, and 42. Three of the six
patients had dry sex dreams. Two of the six patients had
dreams of coitus with observable ejaculation (in the bed
clothing) with orgasm. One of the six patients had dreams of
coitus with ejaculation and orgasm (ejaculate not observable
in bed clothing). Four of the six patients had psychogenic
erections. Four of the six patients had occasional spontaneous erections. Two of the six patients could attain
erections via external stimulation but the erections were
only of short duration. Four of the six patients had not
made an attempt to attain erections via external stimulation.
Two of the six patients had not made attempt at coitus; four
of the six patients were able to attain intromission of which
three were able to ejaculate and reach an orgasm; the four
partners were sexually satisfied. Five of the six patients
attempted masturbation; two ejaculated and reached an orgasm.
Two of the six patients attempted fellatio; both ejaculated
and reached an orgasm. Two of the six patients attempted
cunnilingus; the two partners were sexually satisfied. One

of the six patients, 34 years of age, was married. He had
wet sex dreams wherein the ejaculate was noted in the bed
clothing. He always had psychogenic erections. He could
ejaculate and reach an orgasm during penile-vaginal coitus;
in fact, he could ejaculate up to three times during inter-
course. He could ejaculate and reach an orgasm with
masturbation and fellatio. He could always satisfy his wife
during cunnilingus. His wife was on "the pill".

Four patients had lower motor neuron, incomplete, sex.
The ages were: 19, 20, 21 and 56. One of the four patients
had wet dreams and reached an orgasm but ejaculate was not
found in the bed clothing. Psychogenic erections were attainable in the four patients. Three of the four patients had
spontaneous erections. Three of the four patients did not make
an attempt to attain erections via external stimulation; one
of the four did make an attempt but the erection was of very
short duration. Intromission was successful in the four
patients; one of the four patients had premature ejaculations
during coitus and reached an orgasm. The four patients were
able to satisfy their partners during coitus. Three of the
four patients attempted masturbation; none could ejaculate or
reach an orgasm. One of the four patients attempted fellatio;
he was unable to ejaculate; with cunnilingus he satisfied his
partner.

FEMALES

Five females were studied. The ages were: 19 (two), 28
(two) and 29. One was married.

Four females had lower motor neuron, complete, sex. One
female had lower motor neuron, incomplete, sex. Three of the
five patients had balanced bladders and used absorbent pads
and plastic panties. Two of the five patients had indwelling
intraurethral catheters. Of the four patients with lower

motor neuron, complete, bladders, two were 19 years of age
and two were 28 years of age. One of the four patients had
an indwelling intraurethral catheter; three of the four
patients wore absorbent pads and plastic panties. Two of the
four patients did not have sex dreams. Two of the four had
dry sex dreams. Two of the four patients attempted penile-
vaginal coitus of which one attained an orgasm. Only one of
the four females attempted fellatio and cunnilingus; she
stated that she performed oral sex only to please her male
partner. None of the four patients attempted masturbation.
Three of the four patients attempted foreplay of which one
reached an orgasm. Of the four patients, two had made no
attempt at coitus and therefore had no need for antipregnancy
precautions; one of the four was married and pregnant at the
time of interview and examination. The latter pregnant
patient was 28 years of age; she emptied her bladder into
absorbent pads and plastic panties. She stated that she
"could feel the penis in the vagina" and reached an orgasm.
She delivered a full term infant via caesarean section.

        One of the five female patients, age 29, had lower motor
neuron, incomplete sex. Pin prick sensation was intact in
the sacral dermatomes - clitoris, vulva and perianal sites.
She has weak volitional contraction of the external rectal
sphincter; therefore, she was incontinent of bladder and
bowel. She reached an orgasm in her dreams and stated that
she enjoyed her sex dreams better than actual coitus. She
was on the "pill" but did not enjoy coitus because it was
painful. She enjoys masturbation better via labial stimulation than clitoral stimulation. She finds fellatio distaste-
ful but performs same to please her boyfriend. Her boyfriend
performs cunnilingus but this keeps her "tense" since she has
leakage around her catheter and she is always afraid of

passing gas. She enjoys foreplay except fondling of the
nipples. She prefers her partner's digit in the vagina
rather than the penis.

DISCUSSION

It is interesting to note that of 16 patients (11 males
and 5 females) 15 patients had lower motor neuron sex; 10 had
complete and five incomplete types of sex. Only one male
patient had upper motor neuron sex. Admittedly, the majority
of myelodysplastic patients will have lower motor neuron sex;
yet, it is incumbent upon the physician to perform the
neurological examination on every one of the myelodysplastic
patients if he is to avoid missing an upper motor neuron
type. The upper motor neuron types depend on reflexogenic
erections, especially if it is complete in type. The reader
is referred to the references of this paper in order to
acquaint himself more adequately concerning upper motor
neuron, complete and incomplete, sex. Upper motor neuron sex
is found more frequently in lesions above the conus when
reflex activity is present through S_2, S_3 and S_4 segments.

Too often the physician is as guilty as non-professionals
in believing that the disabled (congenital or acquired) are
asexual. As noted from the results of our interviews, it has
been clearly shown that among the myelodysplastics the
majority of the patients are very much sexual beings.

It is this author's opinion that the physicians responsible for myelodysplasia patients' management must become
involved in their sexual future as much as any other aspect
of their care. Too many physicians appear to be uncomfortable in discussing sex. It only indicates the inadequate
training they have had in this field.

Therefore, to be a good counsellor in this field

requires knowledge in this aspect of medicine. This does not
infer that only a physician can be the counsellor. It can be
the psychologist, nurse, social worker, physical therapist,
or occupational therapist; it can be anyone of the medical
team with whom the patient has the greatest rapport. However,
there is one basic prerequisite - the counsellor must be well
trained and know what he (she) is talking about.

Once the counsellors are well trained, the parents must
be counselled; then the patient. The importance of parent
training is self-evident from the following example. One of
the five female patients in this series has a lower motor
neuron type of sex, complete. She is 28 years of age.
Interview revealed that she had no concept of her female
anatomy. She enthusiastically described how she thoroughly
enjoys her dreams of being in bed with the opposite sex. Yet,
she has never been on "a date". When asked if she would like
to go on "a date" she answered with a very emphatic "Yes, but
I am afraid that he would take advantage of me". Further
inquiry from personnel who attended her revealed that the
parents had had her always "hidden". She undoubtedly had
repeatedly been told, from a young age, about the terrible
things that boys do to girls. Yet, in spite of her teachings
from her parents, she "enjoyed" being in bed with the
opposite sex in her dreams and undoubtedly does a great deal
of fantasizing while awake. She is a sexual being who was
never guided toward sexual fulfillment.

Sexuality among these patients is just as important (if
not more so) than correction of deformities, the correct use
of braces, the prevention of pressure ulcers, bowel management and the like. Counselling should also cover the various
sexual options that are available for sexual fulfillment.

SUMMARY

    Briefly, the neurophysiology of sexual function as well
as a classification of sex among patients with neurological
disturbances has been presented. The results of sexual
interviews and examinations among 11 males and 5 females with
myelodysplasia have been presented. A plea is made that
every physician who cares for this type of patient become
involved in sexual counselling of these patients early with
the parents as well as the patients.

ADDENDUM

    Since the compilation of the statistics of the original
11 males interviewed by this writer, four additional males
have been seen that are worthy of presentation.

    One patient is a 27 year old male who has upper motor
neuron, complete, sex. His level is below T11 segmentally.
His findings are typical of this type of sex. He does not
have psychogenic erections. He has spontaneous reflexogenic
erections about once a week in the A.M. which are about two
to three minutes in duration. He has reflexogenic erections
via external stimulation which last up to five minutes.
These are available 100 percent of the time. The erections
are very firm. He has made no attempt at coitus but one can
anticipate that he will be able to satisfy his partner and
that he himself will not be able to ejaculate or have an
orgasm. He is unable to ejaculate during masturbation. He
has not had sex dreams.

    One patient is a 25 year old male with a complete lesion
below thoracic twelve segmentally. He has a perineal
urethrostomy. He states that he has dreams of coitus and
reaches an orgasm but does not ejaculate. He cannot attain
erections psychogenically but only by external stimulation

(fondling of the penis). (It is rather atypical for a lower
motor neuron complete sex patient to attain the erections
only via external stimulation; usually if erections are
attainable, it is psychogenically induced.) During coitus
he can ejaculate about four times out of 10 attempts.
Similarly, he can ejaculate about 40 percent of the time at
masturbation attempts. The duration of his firm erections
is about five minutes. He is engaged to be married.

Two patients have lower motor neuron, incomplete, sex.
One of the two patients is 16 years of age. The external
rectal sphincter is flaccid; there is volitional control of
the external rectal sphincter and pin prick sensation is
intact in the penile, scrotal and perianal dermatomes
bilaterally. The volitional control even though present
is not adequate enough to prevent a bowel movement once he
has the desire to defecate. His bladder is emptied typically
for a lower motor neuron type via strain and/or Crede. His
sex dreams are only of foreplay. He cannot ejaculate during
masturbation. He can attain firm psychogenic erections 100
percent of the time but has made no attempt at coitus. The
other patient is 18 years of age. Pin prick sensation is
lost in the sacral segments except for hypalgesia in the
scrotal dermatomes bilaterally. The external sphincter is
flaccid: there is no volitional contraction of the external
sphincter. He has psychogenic erections 95 percent of the
time; the firm erections last up to 45 minutes. He can
attain erections also via external stimulation which last up
to a half hour. His sex dreams are only of foreplay. He has
never ejaculated in a dream. One can prognosticate that he
will be able to satisfy his partner; but whether he'll be
able to ejaculate during coitus remains to be seen. He cannot ejaculate during masturbation.

REFERENCES

1. Bors, E. and Comarr, A.E.: Neurological disturbances of sexual function with special reference to 529 patients with spinal cord injury. *Urol. Survey, 10*:191, 1960.

2. Comarr, A.E.: Interesting observations among females with spinal cord injury. Proceedings of 14th Annual Spinal Cord Injury Conference of the Veterans Administration, Sunnybrook Hospital, Toronto, Ontario, Canada, October, 27-29, 1965. *Med. Serv. J. Canada, 22*:651, 1966.

3. Comarr, A.E.: Observations on menstruation and pregnancy among female spinal cord injury patients. *Paraplegia, 3*:263, 1966.

4. Comarr, A.E.: Sexual function among patients with spinal cord injury. *Urol. Int., 25*:134, 1970.

5. Comarr, A.E.: Sexual concepts in traumatic cord and cauda equina lesions. *J. Urol., 106*:375, 1971.

6. Comarr, A.E.: Sex among patients with spinal cord and/or cauda equina injuries. *Medical Aspects of Human Sexuality, 7*:222, 1973.

7. Comarr, A.E. and Gunderson, B.: Sexual function in traumatic paraplegia and quadriplegia. *Am. J. Nurs., 2*:250, 1975.

THE ADOLESCENT WITH MYELODYSPLASIA
DEVELOPMENT, ACHIEVEMENT, SEX AND
DETERIORATION*

David B. Shurtleff, M.D.
and Jan C. Sousa, M.D.

INTRODUCTION

This paper synthesizes two large groups of data. The
first describes how children born with congenital paralysis
from myelodysplasia (spina bifida aperta, myelomeningocele,
meningomyelocele, etc.) learn to become independent adults.
[11, 12] We have described our patient population in terms of
functional motor levels according to the classification of
Sharrard.[8]

We have grouped all high level lesion patients in the
first study as $L_3\uparrow$ or those with a maximum of hip flexion,
adduction and knee extension. In the second set of data we
have reported the high level lesion patients as $L_2\uparrow$ or those
with only a maximum of hip flexion and adduction and no knee
extension. The first set of data, our more recent, suggest
the overall behavior of L_3 level patients is more like L_2 and
more severely paralyzed patients. Our previous studies as
well as this current (new) study suggest that the ambulatory
learning pattern of L_3 level patients is more like that of
L_4 and L_5 level patients. Intermediately involved patients

*This study was supported in part by the National Foundation-
March of Dimes and the Shriners Hospital, Honolulu Unit.

have strong knee extension and some knee flexion from medial
hamstrings and some anterior tibialis function or L_{4-5}. The
older study, part 2, records most of these patients as L_{3-5}
including those few with knee extension only. It is apparent
that the L_{3-4} neuromotor levels are both critical for prognosis for ultimate wheelchair or brace and crutch ambulation
and difficult to determine. At this point in time we are
unsure as to whether to classify L_3 level patients with more
severely or less severely paralyzed or alone. Lack of total
numbers require they be lumped. The least paralyzed group is
relatively non-controversial; the least paralyzed group S_1↓
includes the remainder.

The second group of data describes how our adolescent
and adult patients currently function sexually, socially, at
work and in school.[9] Hopefully, these observations will
provide a basis for improving the life of these handicapped
citizens both by helping us to avoid preventable complications by treatments and by providing them with appropriate
advice.

DEVELOPMENT - THE PRE-ADOLESCENT

Four hundred and fifty one patients with myelodysplasia
have been evaluated by the University of Washington Birth
Defects Center staff over the past 19 years for an average of
three examinations each. As many as 353 observations were
recorded and stored in a Conversational Computer Statistical
Service program for later analysis.[12] From each patient's
yearly examination, a raw score measuring the level of self-
help skills, locomotion and social integration was obtained
by using a point system. The nine activities of daily living
assessed are: 1) method of locomotion, 2) type of gait or
ability to perform transfers to and from a wheelchair, 3)

transportation in the community, 4) meal management including both eating and preparation, 5) dressing, 6) hygiene, 7) urinary appliance care, 8) stool care or training, and 9) social interaction. Points were assigned for increasingly difficult steps toward independent behavior in each category. For example, a normal fully ambulatory adult drives a normal automobile for maximum points and a wheelchair bound adult must handle a wheelchair over rough terrain, accomplish all transfers and drive a hand controlled motor vehicle being given accumulative points at each step. Individuals with varying degrees of paralysis must use alternate methods to achieve the same goal.

Age ranges for achievement of each of the nine independence categories have been graphed and compared to standards for normal children as described by Alpern-Boll[1] and Gesell.[4] They are available in prepublication form from the authors. Approximately 850 evaluations of independence have been recorded for patients with different levels of paralysis and intelligence quotients above 80. As expected, paralyzed children take longer to achieve the same level of independence as their less paralyzed peers. Even minimally handicapped children take longer to master more complex procedures than non-handicapped children. Figure 1 compares hypothetical norms from data of Alpern-Boll and Gesell with children of our population who have minimal or no weakness of the lower extremities. The primary problem areas appear to be those of urine and stool hygiene training and social interaction. Developmental delay in this area has profound implications when viewed by either the classic Freudian or the more recent Erikson Developmentalist.[2]

Figure 2 demonstrates the more marked delay in development of independence for those with considerable paralysis in

the lower extremities ($L_3\uparrow$), and an intermediate group with
good knee flexion and some ankle motion (L_{4-5}), and those
with very little paralysis ($S_1\downarrow$). Marked motor impairment
has life-encompassing implications for altered development
and different life style. Independence, one of the most
important aspects of adolescent maturity is always markedly
delayed amongst the more severely paralyzed and may be
permanently beyond the reach of the congenitally paralyzed
child. Hopefully, medical-surgical therapy, as well as
special education and social programs, can improve the
learning rates and ultimate performance of such children.

In our study we found wide ranges for the earliest age
of performance for all tasks. These wide ranges stress both
the importance of appropriate age related performance and
handicap modified parental expectations. Though a few of the
children with sacral level paralysis accomplished some self-
help tasks as soon as non-paralyzed peers, most with similar
paralysis achieved performance at a delayed age. These wide
ranges of first achievement stress the importance of helping
the slower learners achieve appropriate age related activities instead of complying with expectations for the handicapped - one of the most important contributions to such
learning can be setting age-appropriate and specific
expectations. In general, our society and parents hold
expectations that are far too low. As might be expected,
their children rise to the abyss of underachievement.

Hopefully, we have arrived at the threshold of
adolescence for the myelodysplastic children with a common
understanding; i.e. children born with myelodysplasia mature
less rapidly than normal peers because their physical
impairment interferes with their ability to move about, to
socialize and to be accepted into the processes of growing up.

DETERIORATION - THE TEENAGE AND ADULT

In order to better understand the further difficulties
of passing from a delayed childhood to an imperfect adulthood, I would now like to describe the current physical and
social status of our adolescent and adult population. This
population comprises 130 individuals ranging in age from 16
to 73 years of age. The minimum age of 16 years was
arbitrarily chosen both because it fits our concept of
delayed onset of adolescence and provides a more understand-
able follow-up of data published in 1975.[9] To those original
98 cases we have added some new individuals, lost 17 to
further follow-up and will include information about 28
persons who have died (Table 1). We will restrict our
observations to those medical and surgical problems most
pertinent to sex in the teenage years.

SURVIVAL - CSF

All patients born with myelodysplasia and born prior to
1960 were ascertained by health department and hospital
records. Because a significant proportion of patients were
referred to us, or detected in chronic disease hospitals, the
sample is biased toward those with natural survival. Despite
recent prattlings, a significant number of myelodysplastic
patients survived prior to the 1950's as attested to by the
530 cases reported by Fisher et al. in 1952 (Fig. 3).[3,7,10]
Cerebrospinal fluid shunts have prolonged life for an
additional many, however. Of 23 shunted patients in our
group of patients ages 16 to 23 years, seven died from shunt
obstructions (Table 2). Two of these shunt-related deaths
occurred suddenly during adolescence. Of the 65 non-shunted
patients, only one of the 18 hydrocephalus-related deaths
occurred during adolescence. Shunts were performed on

approximately one third of the two more severely paralyzed
groups ($L_2\uparrow$ and L_{3-5}) but on only 9 percent of those with
sacral level lesions. Approximately one third of myelodysplasia patients with cerebrospinal fluid shunts develop
asymptomatic obstruction of their shunt.

SURVIVAL - RENAL

One patient died in the fourth decade of life and two
others are dying from renal failure that become evident
during adolescence (Table 3). Low grade persistent or
recurrent urinary tract infection, with or without ileal
diversion, is a preventable complication. Prevention of
upper urinary tract dilation and irreversible ureterectasis
associated with careful follow-up and maintenance of free
flow of urine are prerequisites for continued good health.
Late diversion, after onset of irreversible ureterectasis,
or lack of stomal dilation and poor follow-up of urine
infection leads to assiduous deterioration. Ileal diversion
or other urinary tract procedures are *not* definitive nor
curative. Even without operative intervention, periodic
re-evaluation is essential to maintain health and prevent
silent deterioration.

MORBIDITY - DECREASE IN FUNCTIONAL ABILITY

CNS and urinary system failures can cause both death and
increase morbidity. These two system failures, collectively,
impaired the function of only two patients amongst our older
survivors; one by quadspasticity following meningitis and
the other by the development of an incapacitating kyphosis
that could not be corrected because of renal hypertension
and impending renal failure (Table 4). The other patients
with increased morbidity suffered a complex of disorders that

could have been prevented. One group could have been helped
by early orthopedic intervention to correct or treat contractures and scoliosis. A second group could have been saved by
prevention of secondary osteomyelitis and massive tissue
destruction from pressure decubiti. A third group could have
been aided by early neurosurgical intervention to stop
progressive nerve damage from syringobulbia, lumbosacral disk
herniation or overgrowth of tissue at the site of an old
myelodysplasia repair. Figure 4 illustrates the massive disk
disease present in our septuagenarian patient who suffered
painless loss of motor function during the fifth and sixth
decades of life. Figure 5 demonstrates the mass of myelodysplastic tissue that overgrew and caused painless loss of
nerve function in a teenage college student. The fourth and
last is the group of poorly cared for, poorly motivated and
obese patients who developed urinary tract obstructions and
infections. The degree of deterioration and the relative
cause and effect of each complication vary. They have been
listed collectively in Table 4.

The interrelationship between poor care, poor compliance
and secondary complications is brought into focus further by
Table 5. The 14 patients listed represent 16 percent of
those 85 patients reviewed for this study. The majority
demonstrate dependency, low self-image and resultant poor
self-care. Of all complications reported, this group of
emotionally impaired differs most markedly from our last
report.[3] In the brief interval, nine patients have resolved
their various emotional conflicts and are doing well in
school, are now employed or have settled down to a comfortable normal life. They have been replaced by three
individuals who now appear in Table 5 because they have
developed   new   emotional   symptoms   and   are

no longer as functional as they once were.

The potential contribution of behavior disorders to
underachievement can be better appreciated when we account
for two married persons doing very poorly and three late
teenage patients who are following in that direction. All
five are mildly retarded and have been raised in foster or
group homes or institutions. All are starved for love and
affection and have been, or will be, "graduated" out into
loosely supervised group homes. The three yet to be so
graduated are all just as ill-prepared emotionally to compete
as their two predecessors who failed. They all represent a
failure of our social system.

Tables 3, 4 and 5 collectively affect only half of the
patients. Renal problems and emotional problems most afflict
those with high level paralysis $L_2\uparrow$, (33 and 24 percent
respectively). Significant loss of motor function (24 percent) and emotional problems (16 percent) afflict the intermediate group (L_{3-5}) most commonly. The three groups of
problems afflict the sacral level lesion patients approximately one in eight. (See Summary Table 3, 4 and 5).

SEXUAL ACTIVITY

Based on an abnormal child rearing and beset with the
physical and emotional problems enumerated up to this point,
it is remarkable that any of our patients have sufficient
self-confidence to enjoy any relationship with another human
being. It is pleasantly surprising to find that some of
those patients with the many problems listed are sexually
active and happily so. As Dr. Comarr has pointed out,
anesthesia of the genitalia and impotence are not preclusive
to satisfactory sex play. Just as for the traumatically
injured, the congenitally paraplegic experiences "orgasms"

by whatever description. The range of experiences related
to us (male and female interviewers with like sex patients)
are similar to those reported by Dr. Comarr. Table 6 provides the data for those sexually active in the 16 to 24 and
Table 7 for those in the 25 to 73 year old age ranges. The
passive female partner in need of no complex autonomic
nervous system function partakes far more actively - up to
89 percent of those over age 25 years - than the male - only
39 percent. Yet in that 39 percent are males who have never
had an erection. The famous French Beekeeper from Enumclaw
sired three children and satisfied two wives, both of whom
died apparently quite happy despite Julian's permanently
flail penis - a terrible secret to let out - Play Girl
editors will stoutly deny such an occurrence, I am sure! The
Beekeeper was grand. I came to know him after he read about
the recurrence risk for his defect at age 71. He came to
see about genetic counseling for himself and his third
fiancee! All of our teenage patients deserve the same
counseling: their potential for sexual enjoyment, their
potential methods of performing the sex act and, finally,
their recurrence risk factors with the potential of intrauterine diagnosis.

SUMMARY

In conclusion, it is possible to say that myelodysplasia
patients can be provided medical and surgical care that
avoids most of the complications outlined in this paper.
Table 8 summarizes the current social, economic and educational status of our 67 patients in their "delayed
adolescence" - or that transition period between childhood
and the responsibilities of adulthood. Their central nervous
systems can be closed and cerebrospinal fluid drained. Their

kyphotic spines can be corrected by a McKay Plate or
scoliotic spines held by a Dwyer Cable. Urinary tract
procedures can maintain free flow of infection free urine
with the possibility, in the near future, of a prosthetic
sphincter. Special education and training can substitute
wheelchair locomotion and hand driven appliances or automobile
for normal biped ambulation and auto. These services are not
sufficient. The myelodysplastic patient needs orientation
toward a practical and useful life goal with an appropriate
social pattern. The attainment of this total life goal
should approximate a normal sequence.

REFERENCES

1. Alpern, G.D. and Boll, T.J.: Developmental Profile.
    Indiana, Psychological Development Publications, 1972.

2. Erikson, E.H.: Childhood and Society, 2nd Ed., New York,
    Norton, 1963.

3. Fisher, R.G., Uihlein, A. and Keith, H.M.: Spina bifida
    and cranium - study of 530 cases. *Proc. of the Staff
    Meetings of the Mayo Clinic, 27*:33, 1952.

4. Gesell, A.L. and Amatruda, C.K.: Developmental Diagnosis.
    H. Knobloch, P. Pasamanick (eds.), New York, Harper and
    Row, 1974.

5. Hayden, P.W., Rudd, T., Dizmang, D., Loeser, J.D. and
    Shurtleff, D.B.: Evaluation of surgically treated hydro-
    cephalus by radionuclide clearance studies of the cerebro-
    spinal fluid shunt. *Dev. Med. Child Neurol., Suppl. 32*:
    72, 1974.

6. Kronmal, R.A., Bender, L. and Mortenson, J.: A conversa-
    tional statistical system for medical records. *J. Royal*

Stat. Soc. Series C, 19:82, 1970.

7. Laurence, K.M., Tew B.J.: Natural history of spina bifida cystica and cranium bifidum cysticum: major central nervous system malformations in South Wales, part IV. *Arch. Dis. Child., 46*:127, 1971.

8. Sharrard, W.J.W.: The segmental innervation of the lower limb muscles in man. *Ann. R. Coll. Surg. Engl., 35*:106, 1964.

9. Shurtleff, D.B., Hayden, P.W. and Chapman, W.H., et al: Myelodysplasia - Problems of long-term survival and social function. *West. J. Med., 122*:199, 1975.

10. Shurtleff, D.B., Hayden, P.W., Loeser, J.D. and Kronmal, R.A.: Myelodysplasia - Decision for death or disability. *New Eng. J. Med., 291*:1005, 1974.

11. Sousa, J.C., Gordon, L.H. and Lamers, J.Y.: An assessment of independence in myelodysplasia. Transactions of the 22nd Annual Meeting of the Orthopedic Research Society, New Orleans, ORS, Jan., 1976, pp. 164.

12. Sousa, J.C. and Shurtleff, D.B.: An assessment of independence in myelodysplasia (abstract). *Clin. Res., 24*:176A, 1976.

TABLE 1.
Total Patients

Level of Lesion	Ages 16-24 yrs.	Ages 25 yrs. plus	SUB-TOTALS	Died Infancy	Died Later	No Current Information	TOTALS
L$_2$	20	1	21	13	2	6	42
L$_{3-5}$	24	14	38	3	6	5	52
S$_1$	23	3	26	2	2	6	36
TOTALS	67	18	85	18	10	17	130

TABLE 2.

Surviving Patients 16 - 23 Years of Age

	Without Shunts				With Shunts			
	Normal I.Q. 76 &	Mental Retardation I.Q. 75 &	Dead	Total	Normal I.Q.	Mental Retardation	Dead	Total
L_2	4	6	13	23	2	7	2	11
L_{3-5}	13	6	2	21	4	1	5	10
S_1	16	2	3	21	1	1	0	2
TOTALS	33	14	18	65	7	9	7	23

TABLE 3.

Renal Failure/Problems (16%)

Level of Lesion	Age of Pt.	Urine Collection	Advanced Hydro-nephrosis	Recurrent Urinary Tract Inf.	High Blood Pressure	Other
L$_2$ ◀	20	Diaper	+	+	0	mental deficiency
	23	Late* ileal loop	+	+	+	mental deficiency kyphosis, osteoporosis
	24	Vesicotomy	+	+	+	mental deficiency
	22	Late* ileal loop	+	+	+	cephalomegaly; nephrectomy
	24	Late* ileal loop	+	+	0	nephrolithiasis
	22	Late* ileal loop	+	+	+	obesity
	21	Late* ileal loop	+	+	0	massive decubitus, loss of femur + pelvis

TABLE 3. (continued)

L$_{3-5}$	18	Sheath Collector	+	+	0	multiple musculoskeletal deformities
	30	Late* ileal loop	+	+	+	osteoporosis, kyphosis; renal failure
	36	Late* ileal loop	+	+	+	nephrolithiasis
	28	Late* ileal loop	+	+	0	nephrolithiasis
S$_1$ →	28	Late* ileal loop	+	+	+	renal transplant
	33	"natural"	+	+	+	death age 33
	20	Early* ileal loop	+	+	0	mental deficiency, poor self-care

*Late = after hydronephrosis and ureterectasis;
Early = before irreversible changes

823

TABLE 4.

Decrease in Functional Ability

Original Level of Lesion	Age of Patient At Onset	From* → To	Age Now	Cause
T_{12}	16	WC ⟶ Bed	23	obesity, kyphosis, poor hygiene, osteomyelitis of spine
L_{3-5}	8	B & C ⟶ Bed	19	CNS infection; spasticity of all four extremities
	15	B & C ⟶ WC	22	obesity, poor renal health
	19	B & C ⟶ WC	21	decubitus, osteomyelitis
	14	B & C ⟶ Bed	24	scoliosis, decubitus, osteomyelitis
	13	WC ⟶ WC	28	contractures, never ambulatory
	13	WC ⟶ WC	21	obesity, poor renal health, never ambulatory

TABLE 4. (continued)

22	Without Aides→With Aides		loss of penis from decubitus followed
	Bed	28	5 years later by progressive syringobulbia
17	B & C ——→WC	30	kyphosis, hip contractures, renal failure
20	WC ——→Bed	22	massive decubiti and osteomyelitis
S₁→			
24	B & C ——→WC	49	progressive loss of strength (disks)
49	B & C ——→WC	72(+)	progressive loss of strength (disks)
17	Without Aides→With Aides	20	progressive loss of strength (myelodysplasia)

*B & C = Braces and crutches for ambulation

WC = Wheelchair dependent

TABLE 5.

Emotional Disturbance Sufficient to Interfere With Attainment

Level of Lesion	Age of Patient	Age of Onset	Sex	Type of Problems
L_2	31	28	female	G.I. symptoms, anxiety following loss of job and fiancee
	24	15	male	"schizophrenia"
	22	childhood	female	huge head, extreme dependency; marginal I.Q.
	19	14	female	sexual fantasies, obesity; marginal I.Q.
	16	12	female	obesity; extreme dependency; school failure
L_{3-5}	21	19	male	depressed following loss of function
	28	22	male	self-abuse following loss of fiancee
	20	15	male	drug pusher, social dropout (I.Q. 150!)
	61	childhood	male	extreme dependence, non-self-care
	36	early 20's	male	extreme dependence, sexual fantasies

TABLE 5. (continued)

28	early 20's	female	poor self-image and care; acting out sexually
28	teenage	male	failure to comply with recommendations
23	teenage	female	acting out sexually
20	15	female	classic hysteria

S_1

SUMMARY TABLE

3 and 4 and 5

Level of Lesion	Number Total Patients	Number (%) With Renal Problems	Number (%) With Loss of Function	Number (%) With Emotional Problems
L_2 ←	21	7 (33%)	1 (5%)	5 (24%)
L_{3-5} →	38	4 (10%)*	9 (24%)	6 (16%)
S_1 →	26	3 (12%)	3 (11%)*	3 (12%)
TOTAL	85	14 (16%)	13 (15%)	14 (16%)

* One older patient with death due to this cause included for calculation with living.

TABLE 6.

Sexual Activity of 60 Patient - Ages 16-24 Years

		L_2 →	L_{3-5}	S_1 →
No Sex	Female	9	9	5
	Male	8	9	9
Sexually Active				
Not Married	Female	3	0	2
	Male	0	1	0
Married	Female	0	1	1
	Male	1	0	2
		4	2	5
Subtotal/Total	Female	7/30	23%	
	Male	4/30	13%	

829

TABLE 7.

Sexual Activity of 20 Patients – 25-73 Years of Age

		L_2	L_{3-5}	S_1
No Sex	Female	1	0	0
	Male	0	6	1
Sexual Activity				
Not Married	Female	0	4	0
	Male	0	1?	0
Married	Female	1	2	1
	Male	0	2	1
Subtotal/Total	Female	8/9	89%	
	Male	4/11	39%	

TABLE 8.

Current Social/Economic/Educational Status
of 67 Patients With Myelodysplasia
Ages 16-24 Years

Status	Level of Lesion	Patients With I.Q. 75 or $<$	Patients With I.Q. 76 or $>$
Home or Group Home or Institutional Care As Maximum Potential Limited Self-Care	L_2 ←	6	2
	L_{3-5} →	2	0
	S_1 →	0	0
Home or Group Home With Limited Employment Such as Sheltered Workshop	L_2 ←	6	1
	L_{3-5} →	1	1
	S_1 →	2	6

TABLE 8. (continued)

			Special Education Or Job Training		Regular School System or College
Progressing Well, Potentially Self-Sufficient	L_2 ←	0	3		1
	L_{3-5} →	0	5		14
	S_1 →	0	1		10
Employed and Self-Sufficient or Spouse	L_2 ←	0		1	
	L_{3-5} →	1		0	
	S_1 →	1		3	

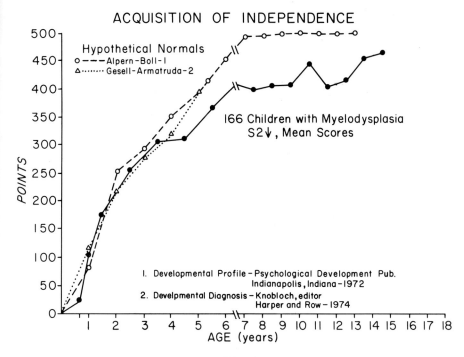

Fig. 1.

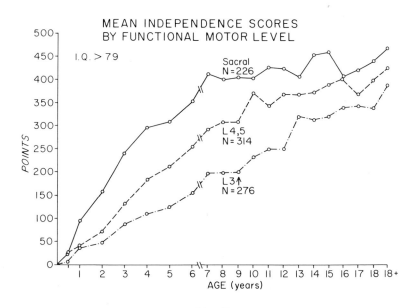

Fig. 2.

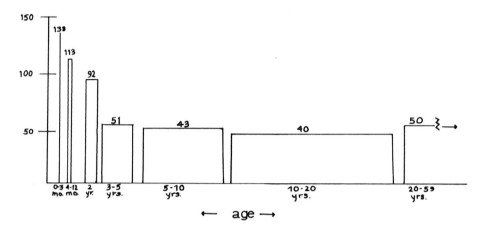

Survival
530 Myelodysplasia Patients
1952
Mayo Clinic

Fig. 3.

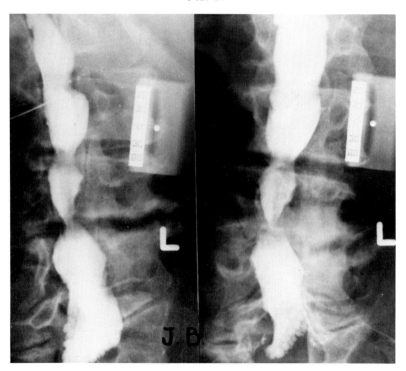

Fig. 4.

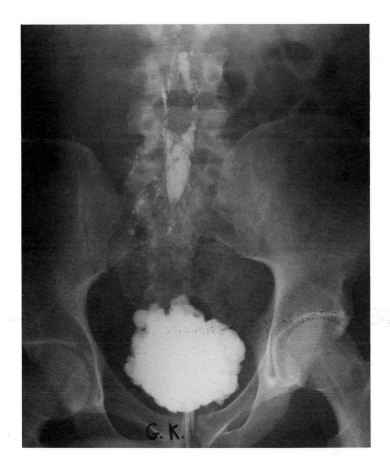

Fig. 5.

INDEX